RADIOLOGY

CASE REVIEW SERIES | Gastrointestinal Imaging

RADIOLOGY

CASE REVIEW SERIES | Gastrointestinal Imaging

Arnold C. Friedman MD, FACR, FSAR

Chief, Department of Radiology VACCHS (Fresno)
Professor of Clinical Radiology
University of California San Francisco

Stephen D. Scotti, MD

Retired Radiologist
Edina, Minnesota

Senthur Thangasamy, MD, DMRD, FRCR (UK)

Abdominal Imaging Fellow
Department of Radiology
University of Massachusetts Memorial Medical Center
Worcester, Massachusetts, USA

SERIES EDITOR

Roland Talanow, MD, PhD

Consultant Radiologist
Department of Radiology
Chrissie Tomlinson Memorial Hospital
George Town, Cayman Islands
Affiliate Professor
University of Bern
Bern, Switzerland

New York   Chicago   San Francisco   Athens   London
Madrid   Mexico City   Milan   New Delhi   Singapore
Sydney   Toronto

Radiology Case Review Series: Gastrointestinal Imaging

1 2 3 4 5 6 7 8 9 0   DSS/DSS   19 18 17 16

ISBN 978-1-259-58519-7
MHID 1-259-58519-0

This book was set in Times LT Std. by Thomson Digital.
The editors were Michael Weitz and Brian Kearns.
The production supervisor was Catherine Saggese.
Project management was provided by Sarita Yadav, Thomson Digital.
RR Donnelley was the printer and binder.

Library of Congress Cataloging-in-Publication Data

Friedman, Arnold C., author.
  Gastrointestinal imaging / Arnold C. Friedman, Stephen Scotti, Senthur Thangasamy ; series editor, Roland Talanow.
      p. ; cm. — (Radiology case review series)
  Includes bibliographical references and indexes.
  ISBN 978-1-259-58519-7 (paperback) — ISBN 1-259-58519-0
  I. Scotti, Stephen, author. II. Thangasamy, Senthur, author. III. Title. IV. Series: Radiology case review series.
  [DNLM: 1. Digestive System Diseases—diagnosis—Case Reports. 2. Digestive System Diseases—diagnosis—Problems and Exercises. 3. Diagnostic Imaging—methods—Case Reports. 4. Diagnostic Imaging—methods—Problems and Exercises. 5. Diagnostic Techniques, Digestive System—Case Reports. 6. Diagnostic Techniques, Digestive System—Problems and Exercises. WI 18.2]
  RC804.D52
  616.3'3075—dc23
                                                                    2015030987

One of my mentors told me a long time ago that academic radiologists were like stamp collectors. I find myself now near the end of my career with a very large stamp collection wondering what to do with it. The opportunity to do this book came along and it gave me the chance to share parts of my collection. I hope readers find these cases interesting, informative and useful for exam preparation. I thank my co-authors for their assistance in correcting my typos and other errors.

— Arnold C. Friedman MD, FACR, FSAR

It was a pleasure to contribute to this case review text. I owe a great deal of thanks to the other co-authors as they provided much of the case material for my contributed cases. I dedicate the work to my significant other, Valerie, who has been a great supporter through some difficult times, and to my mother, Marjorie, who sadly passed away during the period of work. She was stable as a rock, tough as nails and worked well into her 80's. She lived a good life.

— Stephen D. Scotti, MD

I gratefully acknowledge the staff radiologists in the abdominal division at University of Massachusetts Medical School for contributing interesting cases. My sincere thanks to Dr. Byron Chen for his special contributions. I also thank my co-authors Drs. Arnold C. Friedman and Stephen Scotti who took the time to edit all the cases.

Dedicated to
To my parents Thangasamy and Rajakani,
To my lovely wife Sivagamy, daughter Dheeksha and son, Nithin
To my Guru, Pinak P. Bhattacharyya

— Senthur Thangasamy, MD, DMRD, FRCR(UK)

Contents

Series Preface

Maybe I have an obsession for cases, but when I was a radiology resident I loved to learn especially from cases, not only because they are short, exciting, and fun—similar to a detective story in which the aim is to get to "the bottom" of the case—but also because, in the end, that's what radiologists are faced with during their daily work. Since medical school, I have been fascinated with learning, not only for my own benefit but also for the sake of teaching others, and I have enjoyed combining my IT skills with my growing knowledge to develop programs that help others in their learning process. Later, during my radiology residency, my passion for case-based learning grew to a level where the idea was born to create a case-based journal: integrating new concepts and technologies that aid in the traditional learning process. Only a few years later, the *Journal of Radiology Case Reports* became an internationally popular and PubMed indexed radiology journal—popular not only because of the interactive features but also because of the case-based approach. This led me to the next step: why not tackle something that I especially admired during my residency but that could be improved: creating a new interactive case-based review series. I imagined a book series that would take into account new developments in teaching and technology and changes in the examination process.

As did most other radiology residents, I loved the traditional case review books, especially for preparation for the boards. These books are quick and fun to read and focus in a condensed way on material that will be examined in the final boards. However, nothing is perfect and these traditional case review books had their own intrinsic flaws. The authors and I have tried to learn from our experience by putting the good things into this new book series but omitting the bad parts and exchanging them with innovative features.

What are the features that distinguish this series from traditional series of review books?

To save space, traditional review books provide two cases on one page. This requires the reader to turn the page to read the answer for the first case but could lead to unintentional "cheating" by seeing also the answer of the second case. Doesn't this defeat the purpose of a review book? From my own authoring experience on the *USMLE Help* book series, it was well appreciated that we avoided such accidental cheating by separating one case from the other. Taking the positive experience from that book series, we decided that each case in this series should consist of two pages: page 1 with images and questions and page 2 with the answers and explanations. This approach avoids unintentional peeking at the answers before deciding on the correct answers yourself. We keep it strict: one case per page! This way it remains up to your own knowledge to figure out the right answer.

Another example that residents (including me) did miss in traditional case review books is that these books did not highlight the pertinent findings on the images: sometimes, even looking at the images as a group of residents, we could not find the abnormality. This is not only frustrating but also time-consuming. When you prepare for the boards, you want to use your time as effectively as possible. Why not show annotated images? We tackled that challenge by providing, on the second page of each case, the same images with annotations or additional images that highlight the findings.

When you are preparing for the boards and managing your clinical duties, time is a luxury that becomes even more precious. Does the resident preparing for the boards truly need lengthy discussions as in a typical textbook? Or does the resident rather want a "rapid fire" mode in which he or she can "fly" through as many cases as possible in the shortest possible time? This is the reality when you start your work after the boards! Part of our concept with the new series is in providing short "pearls" instead of lengthy discussions. The reader can easily read and memorize these "pearls."

Another challenge in traditional books is that questions are asked on the first page and no direct answer is provided, only a lengthy block of discussion. Again, this might become time-consuming to find the right spot where the answer is located if you have doubts about one of several answer choices. Remember: time is money—and life! Therefore, we decided to provide explanations to *each* individual question, so that the reader knows exactly where to find the right answer to the right question. Questions are phrased in an intuitive way so that they fit not only the print version but also the multiple-choice questions for that particular case in our online version. This system enables you to move back and forth between the print version and the online version.

In addition, we have provided up to three references for each case. This case review is not intended to replace traditional textbooks. Instead, it is intended to reiterate and strengthen your already existing knowledge (from your training) and to fill potential gaps in your knowledge.

However, in a collaborative effort with the *Journal of Radiology Case Reports* and the international radiology community Radiolopolis, we have developed an online repository with more comprehensive information for each case, such as demographics, discussions, more image examples, interactive image stacks with scroll, a window/level feature, and other interactive features that almost resemble a workstation. In addition, we are planning ahead toward the new Radiology Boards format and are providing rapid-fire online sessions and mock examinations that use the cases in the print version.

I am particularly proud of such a symbiotic endeavor of print and interactive online education and I am grateful to McGraw-Hill for giving me and the authors the opportunity to provide such a unique and innovative method of radiology education, which, in my opinion, may be a trendsetter.

The primary audience of this book series is the radiology resident, particularly the resident in the final year who is preparing for the radiology boards. However, each book in this series is structured on difficulty levels so that the series also becomes useful to an audience with limited experience in radiology (nonradiologist physicians or medical students) up to subspecialty-trained radiologists who are preparing for their CAQs or who just want to refresh their knowledge and use this series as a reference.

I am delighted to have such an excellent team of US and international educators as authors on this innovative book series. These authors have been thoroughly evaluated and selected based on their excellent contributions to the *Journal of Radiology Case Reports*, the Radiolopolis community, and other academic and scientific accomplishments.

It brings especially personal satisfaction to me that this project has enabled each author to be involved in the overall decision-making process and improvements regarding the print and online content. This makes each participant not only an author but also part of a great radiology product that will appeal to many readers.

Finally, I hope you will experience this case review book as it is intended to be: a quick, pertinent, "come to the point" radiology case review that provides essential information for the radiology boards in the shortest time available, which in the end is crucial for preparation for the boards.

Roland Talanow, MD, PhD

Preface

I have accumulated a lot of cases during 33 years of academic radiology practice and 3 years of residency. A desire to share them and avoid their going to waste had nagged me. Therefore, I accepted when approached by Dr. Talanow to write a GI radiology case review book. I chose cases that illustrate common manifestations of common diseases, unusual manifestations of common diseases, and common manifestations of unusual diseases. I tried to pick cases that were "gettable." I think this book will be most useful to radiologists preparing for boards and recertification. I hope readers will find it challenging and entertaining as well as instructive.

Arnold C. Friedman MD, FACR, FSAR
Stephen D. Scotti, MD
Senthur Thangasamy, MD, DMRD, FRCR(UK)

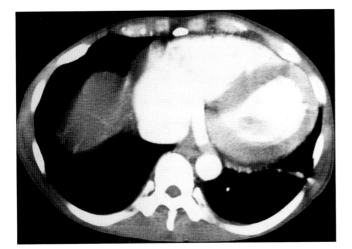 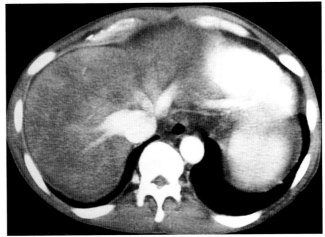

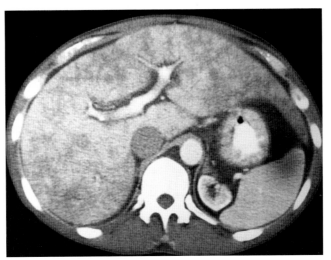

1. What is the most likely diagnosis?

2. What is the most common liver enzyme
   elevation in congestive hepatopathy?

3. What ultrasonographic appearance has been
   described in acute hepatitis and congestive
   hepatopathy due to pulmonary hypertension?

4. Apparent diffusion coefficient values have
   been described as what in acute hepatic
   hepatopathy?

5. What is the classic CT appearance of
   congestive hepatopathy?

Case ranking/difficulty:

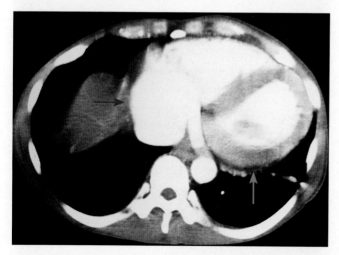

Axial contrast-enhanced CT shows cardiomegaly with right atrial enlargement (*red arrow*) and left ventricular hypertrophy (*green arrow*).

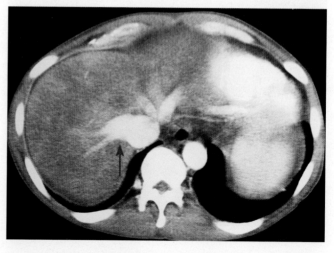

Contrast-enhanced CT shows dilated inferior vena cava and hepatic veins (*red arrow*) with reflux of contrast from the right atrium.

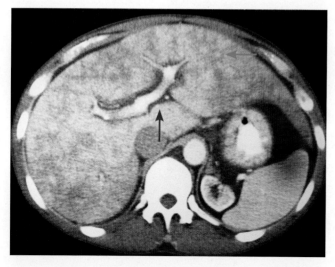

Contrast-enhanced CT shows fairly classic findings of passive hepatic congestion with periportal edema (*red arrow*) and an inhomogeneous enhancement pattern with linear and curvilinear areas of hypodensity (*green arrow*).

Answers

1. Hepatic veno-occlusive disease, Budd-Chiari syndrome, and passive hepatic congestion are all disorders in the spectrum of hepatic venous outflow obstructive disorder. In veno-occlusive disease the obstruction is at the sinusoidal level, in Budd-Chiari syndrome the obstruction is at the level of the hepatic veins and the inferior vena cava, and in passive hepatic congestion it is at the cardiac level.

In the case at hand the hepatic veins and inferior vena cava are patent, and the reflux of contrast into the inferior vena cava, dilatation of the inferior vena cava, and cardiomegaly point to passive hepatic congestion.

Wilson disease and Osler-Weber-Rendu do cause hepatic disease, but not a venous outflow obstruction problem.

2. An elevated bilirubin level (mostly unconjugated) is the most common liver enzyme abnormality related to congestive hepatopathy. Serum transaminases may be mildly elevated, but not to the degree seen in acute viral hepatitis.

3. Although classically described in acute viral hepatitis, a "starry sky" pattern on ultrasound can also be seen on congestive hepatopathy. This is related to hypoechoic parenchyma and echogenic portal venules.

4. Diffusion-weighted MRI imaging can show increased diffusion and slightly elevated apparent coefficients in congestive hepatopathy related to pulmonary hypertension.

5. There is usually a constellation of CT findings in congestive hepatopathy, including:
   • Dilated IVC and hepatic veins with reflux of contrast from the right atrium.
   • Inhomogeneous contrast enhancement giving a mosaic appearance.
   • Linear and curvilinear areas of decreased enhancement.
   In later phases, the appearance of the liver is more homogeneous.

Pearls

- Hepatic dysfunction, either acute or chronic, related to primary right-sided cardiac disorder, including cardiomyopathy, pericardial disease, valvular disorder, and cor pulmonale.
- Acutely may be reversible. Chronically evolves into "cardiac cirrhosis."
- In the spectrum of hepatic venous outflow obstruction along with veno-occlusive disease and Budd-Chiari syndrome.
- Most easily recognized by noting dilated inferior cava and hepatic veins along with reflux of contrast into the inferior vena cava and hepatic veins during early contrast enhancement phase.
- "Nutmeg liver" with mosaic inhomogeneous pattern of enhancement on CT and MRI that becomes more normal in later phases.

Suggested Readings

Abu-Judeh HH. The "starry sky" liver with right-sided heart failure. *AJR Am J Roentgenol.* 2002;178(1):78. Epub 2002/01/05. doi: 10.214/ajr.78..780078.

Alvarez AM, Mukherjee D. Liver abnormalities in cardiac diseases and heart failure. *Int J Angiol.* 2011;20(3):135-142. Epub 2012/09/04. doi: 10.055/s-0031-1284434.

Bayraktar UD, Seren S, Bayraktar Y. Hepatic venous outflow obstruction: three similar syndromes. *World J Gastroenterol.* 2007;13(13):1912-1927. Epub 2007/04/28.

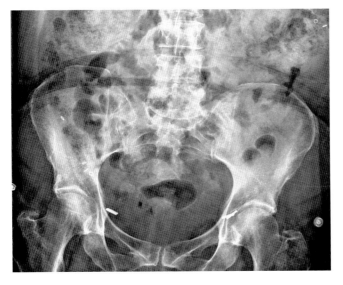
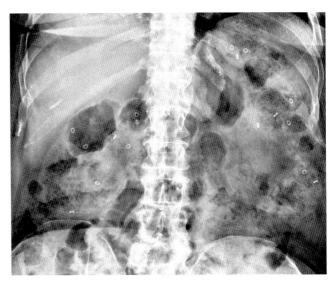
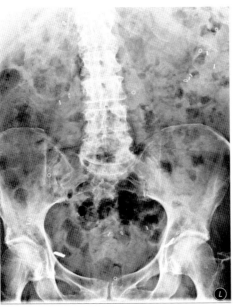
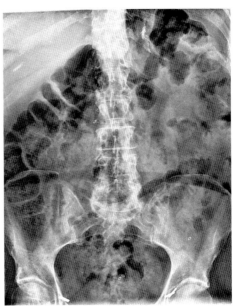

1. What is the purpose of this study?

2. What is the name of the markers?

3. What are the radiographic manifestations in colonic inertia?

4. What are the causes of outlet delay?

5. What are the secondary causes of chronic constipation?

Case ranking/difficulty: 🌰

Answers

1. The purpose of this study is to assess the colonic transit time.

2. The name of this radiopaque marker is Sitz markers.

3. In cases of colonic inertia, the markers will be scattered throughout the colon.

4. Rectal prolapse, fecal impaction, megarectum/colon, and pelvic floor dyssynergia are the causes of outlet delay.

5. Medication, diabetic, hypercalcemia, hypoparathyroidism, neurological disorder, and obstructive bowel disease are the secondary causes of chronic constipation.

Suggested Readings

Bove A, Pucciani F, Bellini M, et al. Consensus statement AIGO/SICCR: diagnosis and treatment of chronic constipation and obstructed defecation (part I: diagnosis). *World J Gastroenterol.* 2012 Apr;18(14):1555-1564.

Gore RM, Szucs RA, Wolf El, et al. Miscellaneous abnormalities of the colon. In: RM Gore, MS Levine, eds. *Textbook of Gastrointestinal Radiology.* 3rd ed. Philadelphia, PA: Saunders Elsevier; 2008:1708-1729.

Saberi H, Asefi N, Keshvari A, Agah S, Arabi M, Asefi H. Measurement of colonic transit time based on radio opaque markers in patients with chronic idiopathic constipation; a cross-sectional study. *Iran Red Crescent Med J.* 2013 Dec;15(12):e16617.

Pearls

- This test helps differentiate colonic inertia and outlet obstruction.
- If <5 to 6 markers retained on day 5, suggest normal colonic transit time.
- Subtotal colectomy may be performed in cases with isolated slow segmental colonic transit time who are resistant to medical treatment.

2 weeks history of abdominal pain and diarrhea
H/o hypertension and coronary artery disease

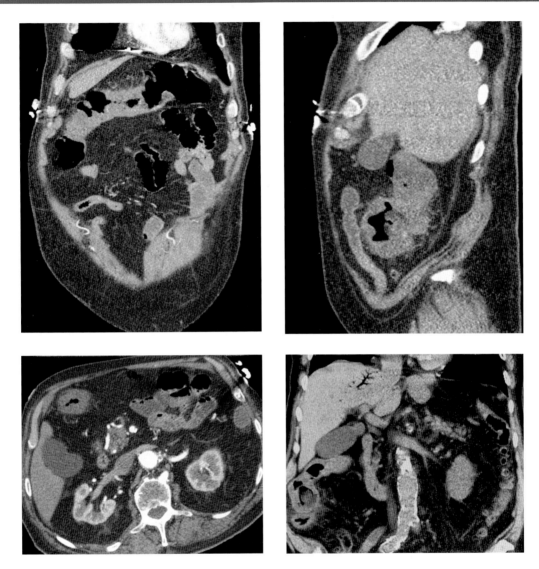

1. What are the findings?

2. What is the best diagnosis?

3. What are the two common sites of involvement of ischemic colitis?

4. What are the possible complications of ischemic colitis?

5. What is the best diagnostic test?

Case ranking/difficulty: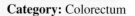

Category: Colorectum

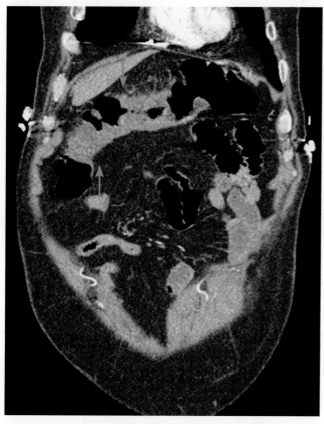

CTA abdomen shows circumferential segmental wall thickening of the proximal transverse colon (*green arrows*). The wall is relatively high density and does not show intramural gas.

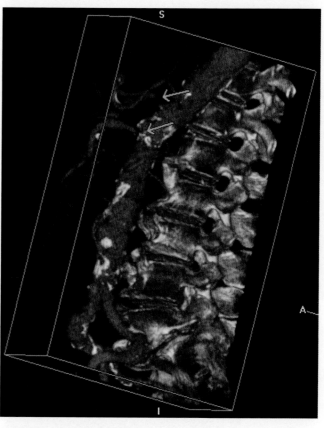

3D volume rendering image reveals complete occlusion of the celiac artery and severe short segment stenosis of the superior mesenteric artery (*green arrows*).

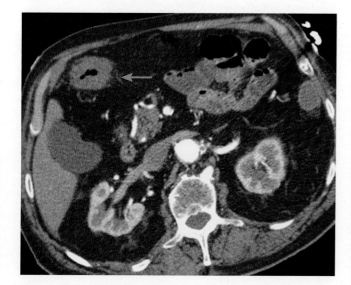

CTA abdomen axial image shows the circumferential wall thickening in the proximal transverse colon (*green arrow*).

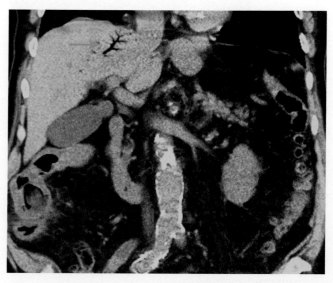

The same patient noncontrast coronal CT image (performed 5 hours earlier) shows portal venous air in the left lobe of the liver (*green arrow*). There is cecal wall thickening with fat stranding and no ascites.

Answers

1. Circumferential wall thickening in the cecum and proximal transverse colon and air within the portal vein are the radiographic findings.

2. This is ischemic colitis. It can occur on the right side in 10% to 20% of cases.

3. Splenic flexure and rectosigmoid junction are watershed areas and commonly involved in ischemic colitis.

4. Perforation, bowel necrosis, stricture, and death are the possible complications of ischemic colitis.

5. CT findings are nonspecific and can be seen in other infectious and inflammatory colitides. Colonoscopy is more sensitive and specific than barium enema.

Pearls

- Useful diagnostic features: acute abdominal pain, bloody stool, and negative stool culture.
- Segmental colonic wall thickening in an elderly patient after a hypotensive episode is highly suspicious for colonic ischemia.
- Mucosa and submucosa are most sensitive to ischemia.
- Rectal involvement is rare due to rich collaterals.
- The possibility of subsequent infarct or perforation cannot be predicted by CT findings alone.
- Most ischemic episodes resolve without any complication.

Suggested Readings

Balthazar EJ, Yen BC, Gordon RB. Ischemic colitis: CT evaluation of 54 cases. *Radiology*. 1999 May;211(2): 381-388.

Horton KM, Corl FM, Fishman EK. CT evaluation of the colon: inflammatory disease. *Radiographics*. 2000;20(2):399-418.

Thoeni RF, Cello JP. CT imaging of colitis. *Radiology*. 2006 Sep;240(3):623-638.

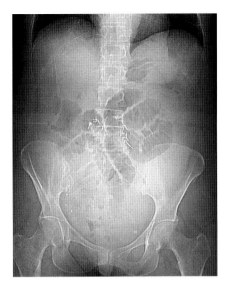
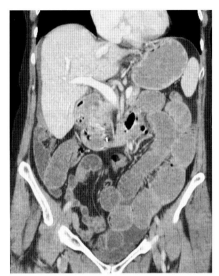
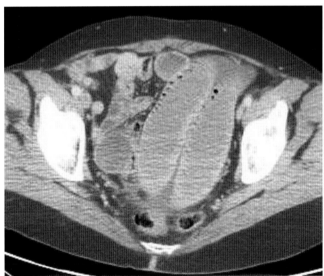
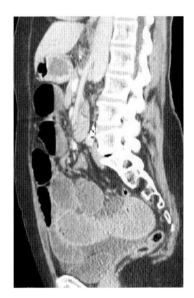

1. What is the diagnosis?

2. What is the probable level of obstruction?

3. What is the most likely etiology?

4. What are the potential complications of small bowel obstruction?

5. What are the radiological findings of closed-loop obstruction?

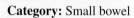
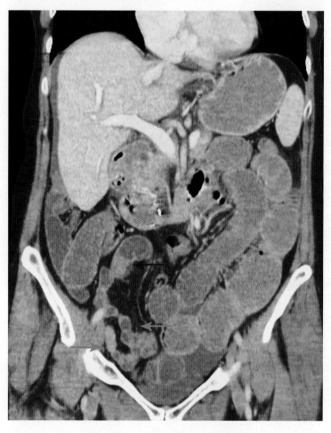

Coronal CT image demonstrates fluid-filled distended small bowel loops, transitional zone at the right lower quadrant (*red arrow*), and collapsed distal ileal loops (*green arrows*).

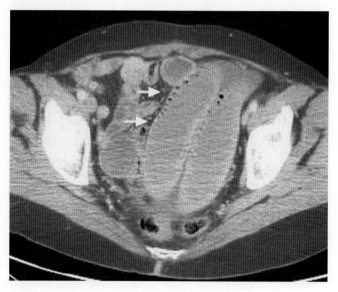

Axial CT image shows dilated fluid-filled ileal loops with string of pearls sign (*white arrows*), highly suggestive of mechanical obstruction. This sign is rarely seen in paralytic ileus and acute gastroenteritis.

Answers

1. Dilated proximal small bowel with collapsed distal bowel with right lower quadrant transition is diagnostic of small bowel obstruction.

2. Dilated jejunum and collapsed distal ileum point to the ileum as the level of obstruction.

3. The absence of etiological finding at the transition zone points to an adhesion as the cause of the obstruction. Small bowel feces sign is helpful to locate the transition point.

4. Perforation, strangulation, infarction, and sepsis are potential complications of small bowel obstruction.

5. "U"-shaped distended bowel loops, twisting of mesenteric vessels and bowel wall, and tapering ends at two points are signs of closed-loop obstruction.

Pearls

- On plain radiography, equal to or >3 air fluid levels of >3 cm raises the suspicion of mechanical obstruction.
- Use of oral contrast may help differentiate between complete and incomplete obstruction.
- Bowel ischemia is more common with adhesive band than matted adhesions.
- Strangulation is much more common in closed-loop obstruction than simple obstruction. Mortality up to 25% if untreated for >36 hours.
- In most cases of acute small bowel obstruction, CT scan helps decide whether the patient requires urgent surgery or conservative management.
- By imaging findings alone, it may not be possible to differentiate low- from high-grade obstruction.

Suggested Readings

Hong SS, Kim AY, Byun JH, et al. MDCT of small-bowel disease: value of 3D imaging. *AJR Am J Roentgenol*. 2006 Nov;187(5):1212-1221.

Nicolaou S, Kai B, Ho S, Su J, Ahamed K. Imaging of acute small-bowel obstruction. *AJR Am J Roentgenol*. 2005 Oct;185(4):1036-1044.

Stallmann HP, Borstlap J, Bollen TL. Water-soluble contrast agents in small bowel obstruction: a useful discriminator. *AJR Am J Roentgenol*. 2012 Dec;199(6):W783.

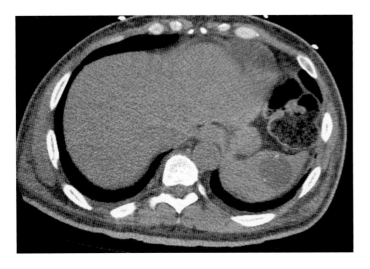 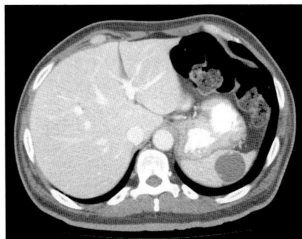

1. What is the most likely diagnosis?

2. What is the general size threshold for consideration of treatment?

3. What entities are considered primary splenic cysts?

4. Can one definitively distinguish a primary splenic cyst from a secondary cyst on CT? True or false.

5. Name possible treatments for splenic cysts.

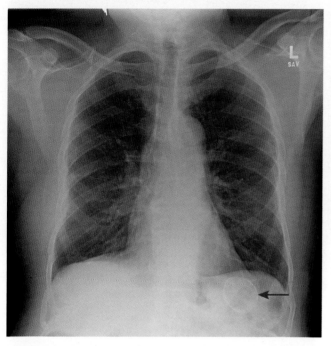

A 67-year-old male, supplemental case. PA chest image shows left upper quadrant mass (*red arrow*) with peripheral, somewhat irregular calcification.

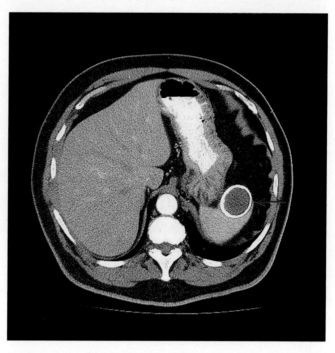

Axial contrast-enhanced CT shows a low-density nonenhancing splenic mass with peripheral calcification (*red arrow*).

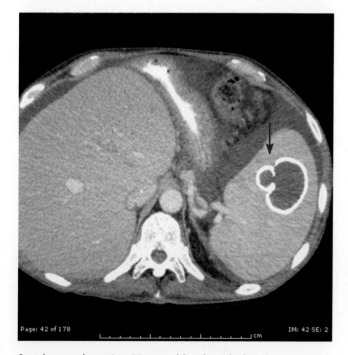

Supplemental case in a 55-year-old male with chronic hepatocellular disease. Axial CT shows water density cyst with fractured calcified wall (*arrow*).

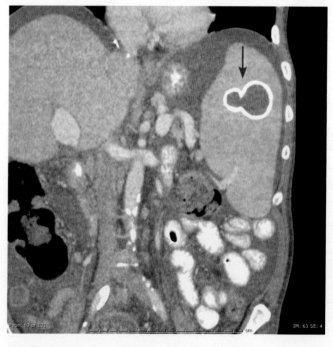

Supplemental case in a 55-year-old male with chronic hepatocellular disease. Coronal CT shows irregular water density cyst with irregular wall (*red arrow*).

Answers

1. A splenic cyst is the most likely diagnosis. Hemangiomas and lymphangiomas could be considered, but they usually have a density higher than that of water and they enhance in some fashion. Splenic hemangiomas can enhance in a manner similar to hepatic hemangiomas, although it may not be as nodular as noted in the liver. Lymphangiomas have septae that can enhance and are often more complex than a simple cyst. Lymphoma can have multiple patterns within the spleen, including simple splenomegaly, but a solitary near water density lesion would be unusual. A hydatid cyst is usually more complex with daughter cysts and there may be disease elsewhere.

2. In the surgical literature a threshold size for consideration of intervention is 5 cm, although any symptomatic cyst could also be considered.

3. There have been several classification systems for splenic cysts. These have frequently been based on whether or not the cyst has an endothelial lining, whether they a parasitic or nonparasitic and on the etiology. A useful classification is one that designates congenital cysts (sometimes called epithelial or epidermoid cysts) and benign tumors (hemangiomas, lymphangiomas, and dermoid cysts) as primary cysts and other acquired cysts (such as from trauma, infection, infarction, or pancreatitis) as secondary cysts.

4. Although there may be some clues, it is generally not possible to distinguish between primary and secondary splenic cysts on CT. A contributory clinical history may be more helpful than the imaging findings. Fortunately, the distinction is not that important from a clinical perspective.

5. Treatment is undertaken depending on size and symptoms, generally considered if size is greater than 5 cm or if there are symptoms. Splenectomy, partial splenectomy, cystectomy, marsupialization, and percutaneous drainage are options. In order to preserve splenic function, 20% to 25% of the splenic tissue needs to be preserved.

Pearls

- Primary and secondary cyst classification, with secondary cysts being "acquired" through trauma, infarct, infection, or pancreatitis, primary cysts being congenital (sometimes called epidermoid or epithelial cysts) or neoplastic (hemangiomas, lymphangiomas, dermoids).
- Cysts are also divided into parasitic and nonparasitic cysts.
- Differentiation between primary and secondary cysts is difficult by imaging alone.
- 5 cm diameter is used as threshold for consideration of resection.

Suggested Readings

Adas G, Karatepe O, Altiok M, Battal M, Bender O, Ozcan D, et al. Diagnostic problems with parasitic and non-parasitic splenic cysts. *BMC Surg*. 2009;9:9. Epub 2009/05/30. doi: 10.1186/1471-2482-9-9.

Elsayes KM, Narra VR, Mukundan G, Lewis JS, Jr., Menias CO, Heiken JP. MR imaging of the spleen: spectrum of abnormalities. *Radiographics*. 2005;25(4):967-982. Epub 2005/07/13. doi: 10.1148/rg.254045154.

Kamaya A, Weinstein S, Desser TS. Multiple lesions of the spleen: differential diagnosis of cystic and solid lesions. *Semin Ultrasound CT MR*. 2006;27(5):389-403. Epub 2006/10/20.

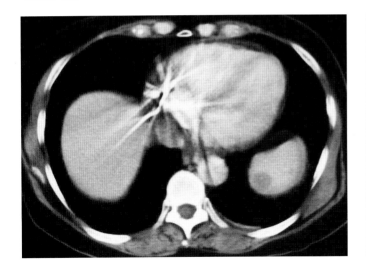 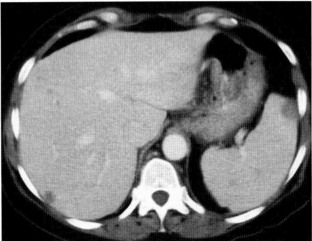

1. What is the most likely diagnosis?

2. What three criteria constitute B symptoms?

3. What are some commonly used criteria for defining splenomegaly?

4. What criteria are often used on PET/CT to define hypermetabolic splenic activity?

5. What type of lymphoma is sometimes responsive to treatment of *H pylori* infection?

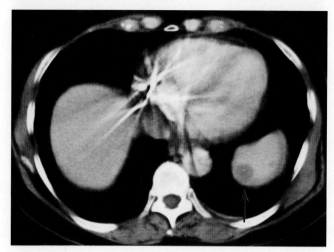

Portal venous phase CT shows round, well-marginated, hypodense mass within the spleen (*red arrow*).

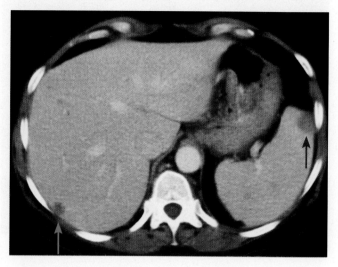

Portal venous phase CT shows round, well-marginated, hypodense mass within the spleen (*red arrow*) and in the liver (*green arrow*). There are additional less well-defined hypodense foci in the spleen.

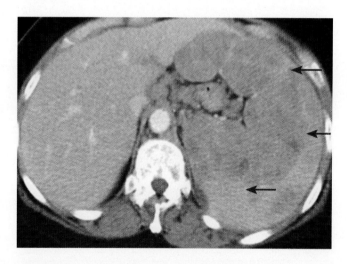

A 50-year-old female with night sweats and weight loss, supplementary case. Portal venous phase CT shows large hypodense mass occupying the majority of the spleen (*red arrows*) and other hypodense foci.

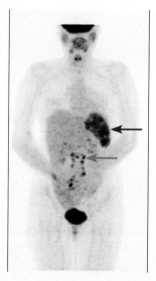

A 26-year-old female with non-Hodgkin lymphoma, supplementary case, PET. There is nodular diffuse increased uptake within the spleen (*red arrow*) along with multiple hypermetabolic retroperitoneal lymph nodes (*green arrow*).

Answers

1. The best diagnosis is lymphoma. Primary splenic lymphoma is rare and accounts for approximately 1% of cases of lymphoma, so most cases represent secondary involvement of the spleen. The spleen is secondarily involved about 1/3 of the time in Hodgkin and non-Hodgkin lymphoma.

   Disseminated infection from tuberculosis, fungus, or bacteria could be considered, and a history of immunosuppression would be contributory. The lesions from an infectious etiology would be somewhat less dense than lymphoma on CT.

2. Unexplained fever greater than 38 degrees C, night sweats, and a 10% weight loss from baseline over 6 months are "B symptoms," and serve as a marker for potentially more advanced disease. It is part of the Ann Arbor staging system for lymphoma.

3. Opinions and criteria vary. The pathologic definition is a spleen that weighs more than 250 g in an adult. A commonly used guideline is a craniocaudal length greater than 13 cm, although this entails some inherent inaccuracy as spleens have variable shapes. Other criteria include calculation of a splenic index or a splenic weight. The splenic index is the product of the length, width, and depth, with an upper range of 480 cm^3. From this value you can approximate a weight by multiplying by pi/6, the adjustment for the volume of a prolate ellipse, although this is still somewhat inaccurate.

A more accurate formula is splenic volume = $(0.36 \times W \times T \times L) + 28$, where W is the width, T is the thickness, and L is the length.

4. When assessing the spleen on PET/CT it is useful to compare splenic activity to liver activity. In general, if splenic activity is greater than that of the liver it suggests abnormal hypermetabolic activity in the spleen, not necessarily lymphoma. Some practitioners will use the actual SUV, with a cutoff of around 2.3 to 2.5.

5. A significant number of cases of gastric MALT (mucosa-associated lymphoid tissue) are related to infection with *H pylori*, and some respond to treatment of the primary *H pylori* infection without the need for chemotherapeutic agents.

Pearls

- Typically hypodense or hypointense nodules or masses on contrast-enhanced CT or contrast-enhanced MRI, although there may simply be splenomegaly or even a normal-sized spleen without evident lesion. Four patterns described.
- PET/CT is helpful in initial staging and treatment response monitoring, particularly for aggressive disease categories.
- Sarcoidosis and granulomatous disease can be a bit of a mimic on PET/CT with hypermetabolic nodes and a hypermetabolic spleen.

Suggested Readings

Benter T, Klühs L, Teichgräber U. Sonography of the spleen. *J Ultrasound Med*. 2011;30(9):1281-1293. Epub 2011/08/31.

de Jong PA, van Ufford HM, Baarslag HJ, de Haas MJ, Wittebol SH, Quekel LG, et al. CT and 18F-FDG PET for noninvasive detection of splenic involvement in patients with malignant lymphoma. *AJR Am J Roentgenol*. 2009;192(3):745-753. Epub 2009/02/24. doi: 10.2214/ajr.08.1160.

Saboo SS, Krajewski KM, O'Regan KN, Giardino A, Brown JR, Ramaiya N, et al. Spleen in haematological malignancies: spectrum of imaging findings. *Br J Radiol*. 2012;85(1009):81-92. Epub 2011/11/19. doi: 10.1259/bjr/31542964.

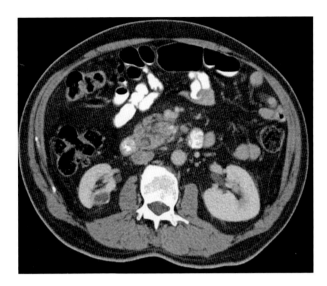 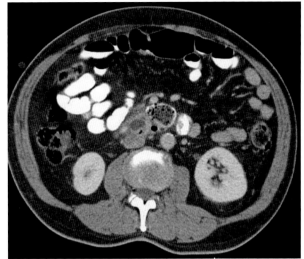

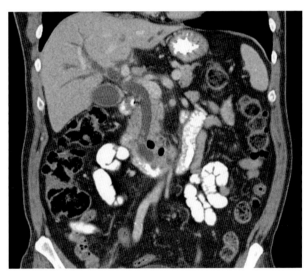

1. What is the primary finding concerning the bile ducts?

2. What is the difference between primary and secondary common duct stones?

3. What is the preferred noninvasive test in the evaluation of choledocholithiasis?

4. What is a useful adjustment that can be made with the window/level settings when looking for common duct stones?

5. Name two of the more common complications of ERCP.

Case ranking/difficulty: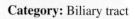

Category: Biliary tract

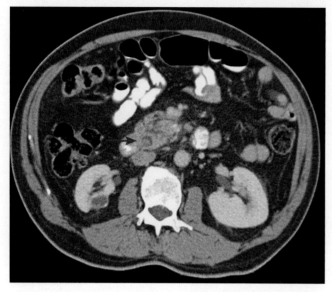

Axial CT shows round dependent soft tissue density in the distal common bile duct (*red arrow*).

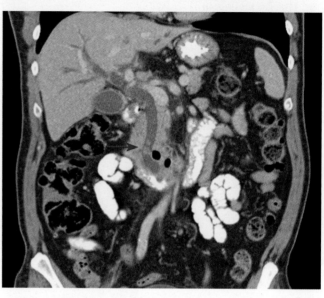

Coronal CT shows intrahepatic and extrahepatic biliary ductal dilatation and multiple filling defects within the distal common bile duct (*red arrow*).

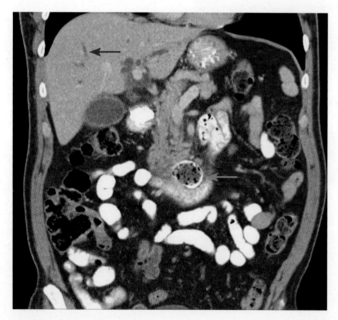

Coronal CT showing intrahepatic biliary ductal dilatation (*red arrow*) and duodenal diverticulum (*green arrow*).

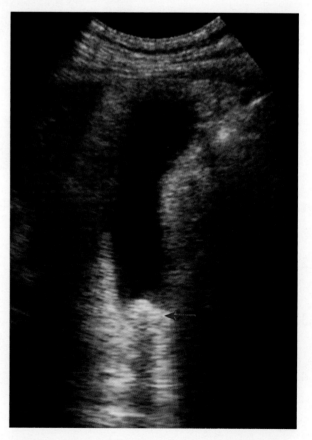

Echogenic shadowing gallstone within the gallbladder neck (*red arrow*).

Answers

1. There is intrahepatic and extrahepatic biliary ductal dilatation, but the primary finding is multiple densities within the distal common bile duct related to common duct stones, choledocholithiasis.

2. It is true that primary stones are usually pigment stones, but the main point is that primary stones form within the bile ducts whereas secondary stones migrate from the gallbladder through the cystic duct and into the bile ducts.

3. Ultrasound is very sensitive in the detection of gallstones, but the sensitivity in the detection of common duct stones is suboptimal and operator dependent. CT has a fairly high sensitivity, but it involves the use of ionizing radiation. MRCP is very sensitive in the detection of common duct stones, approaching 100% for all but small stones, and it does not involve the use of ionizing radiation. ERCP is invasive.

4. Just as certain window/level settings are useful in the detection of subdural hematoma, it is useful to set window/level settings specifically when looking for common duct stones. A level set to the HU of bile in the common bile duct with a window of 150 is helpful.

5. ERCP is relatively safe, but complications do occur. Pancreatitis is the most common complication and the exact incidence varies depending on the definition of pancreatitis, biochemical or clinical. The incidence is in the range of 3% to 5%. Cholangitis is much less frequent, but is also a potential complication.

Pearls

- Ultrasound is less sensitive in the detection of choledocholithiasis than is computed tomography or magnetic resonance cholangiopancreatography. MRCP is the preferred noninvasive modality.
- Variable density of stones on computed tomography. Only small minority can be seen on plain film.
- Look for indirect signs such as biliary ductal dilatation and clinical parameters as clues.

Suggested Readings

Freitas ML, Bell RL, Duffy AJ. Choledocholithiasis: evolving standards for diagnosis and management. *World J Gastroenterol.* 2006;12(20):3162-3167.

Kondo S, Isayama H, Akahane M, Toda N, Sasahira N, Nakai Y, et al. Detection of common bile duct stones: comparison between endoscopic ultrasonography, magnetic resonance cholangiography, and helical-computed-tomographic cholangiography. *Eur J Radiol.* 2005;54(2):271-275. Epub 2005/04/20. doi: 10.1016/j.ejrad.2004.07.007.

Wong HP, Chiu YL, Shiu BH, Ho LC. Preoperative MRCP to detect choledocholithiasis in acute calculous cholecystitis. *J Hepatobiliary Pancreat Sci.* 2012;19(4):458-464. Epub 2011/10/11. doi: 10.1007/s00534-011-0456-8.

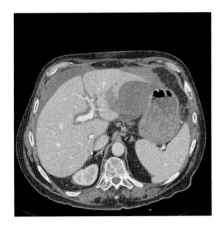 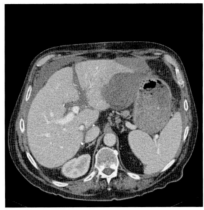 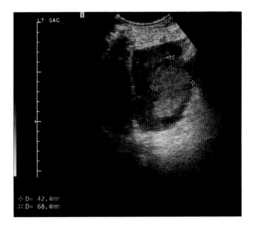

1. What happened after the patient's biopsy?

2. What is the most common serious complication related to percutaneous liver biopsy?

3. What options are there for the management of hemorrhage in this setting?

4. According to the consensus guidelines for periprocedural management of coagulation status and hemostasis risk in percutaneous image-guided interventions, what is the lower limit of platelet count for percutaneous liver biopsy?

5. According to the consensus guidelines for periprocedural management of coagulation status and hemostasis risk in percutaneous image-guided interventions, what is the recommended INR for percutaneous liver biopsy?

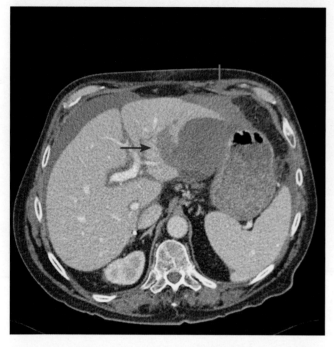

Portal venous phase CT shows acute intraparenchymal (*red arrow*) and subcapsular (*green arrow*) hemorrhage involving primarily the left hepatic lobe contiguous with the biopsy tract. There is periportal fluid and right perihepatic fluid as well.

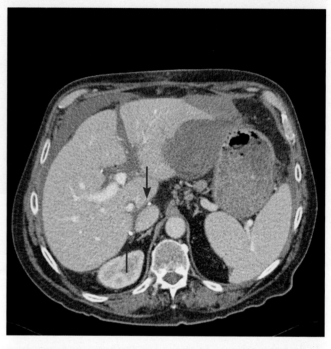

Similar image at a slightly lower level shows similar findings. Note the surgical clips around the IVC related (*red arrows*) to liver transplant. It is a transplant liver.

Answers

1. There is a large amount of intraparenchymal and subcapsular hemorrhage related to the biopsy. Some of the perihepatic fluid on the right is ascites, but some is also likely hemorrhage. The hemorrhage is well seen on the ultrasound as well as an echogenic mass with unsharp margins.

2. Gallbladder injury and pneumothorax are serious complications, but they are rare and in some series occur more commonly when ultrasound guidance is not used. The pleural space does extend quite far inferiorly and it is possible to puncture the lung during a biopsy. Hemorrhage is the most common serious complication of percutaneous liver biopsy.

3. Simple observation is unwise. A significant amount of blood has been lost internally. In most cases, this could probably be managed with IV fluids and observation. Depending on the patient's status blood transfusion is another option. If the bleeding continues or the patient is unstable interventional embolization or surgery may be necessary.

4. For percutaneous biopsy the consensus guidelines are that the platelet count should be greater than 50,000.

5. The consensus guidelines recommend an INR value less than 1.5.

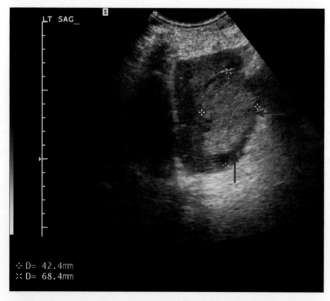

Sagittal ultrasound image through the left hepatic lobe demonstrates echogenic hemorrhage within the left hepatic lobe (*red arrows*). Other images demonstrate the subcapsular component.

Pearls

- Percutaneous liver biopsy is a relatively safe procedure with a low incidence of complications.
- Hemorrhage is the most common serious complication and can usually be managed with intravenous fluids or transfusion. Rarely, interventional embolization or surgery may be required to stop hemorrhage.
- Platelet count greater than 50,000 and INR less than 1.5 are consensus guidelines regarding coagulation parameters.

Suggested Readings

Cakmakci E, Caliskan KC, Tabakci ON, Tahtabasi M, Karpat Z. Percutaneous liver biopsies guided with ultrasonography: a case series. *Iran J Radiol.* 2013;10(3):182-184. Epub 2013/12/19. doi: 10.5812/iranjradiol.13184.

Caldwell S, Northup PG. Bleeding complication with liver biopsy: is it predictable? *Clin Gastroenterol Hepatol.* 2010;8(10):826-829. Epub 2010/07/06. doi: 10.1016/j.cgh.2010.06.010.

Patel IJ, Davidson JC, Nikolic B, Salazar GM, Schwartzberg MS, Walker TG, et al. Consensus guidelines for periprocedural management of coagulation status and hemostasis risk in percutaneous image-guided interventions. *J Vasc Interv Radiol.* 2012;23(6):727-736. Epub 2012/04/20. doi: 10.1016/j.jvir.2012.02.012.

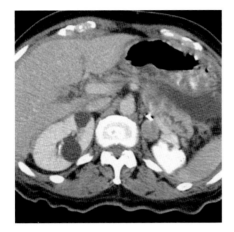
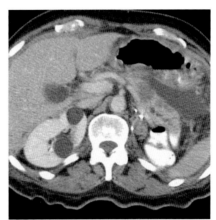

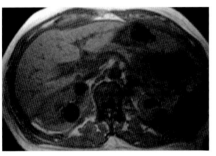
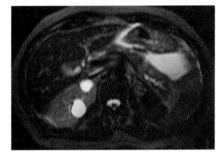
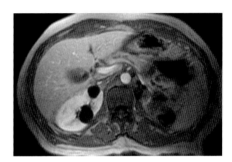

1. What is the most likely diagnosis regarding the pancreas?

2. Where does pancreatic cancer rank in terms of cancer mortality?

3. What tumor marker is used clinically in relation to pancreatic cancer?

4. Names three signs, two clinical and one radiologic, that pertain to pancreatic cancer.

5. Name two risk factors for pancreatic cancer that are common and modifiable.

Case ranking/difficulty: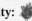

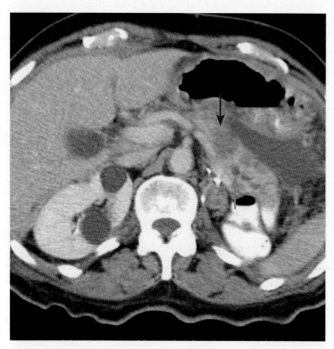

CT at slightly different level again shows a hypodense mass within the midbody of the pancreas (*red arrow*) and ductal dilatation involving the tail of the pancreas (*green arrow*). Left nephrectomy and left adrenal mass related to metastatic renal cell carcinoma are again noted.

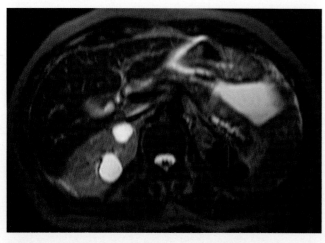

T2W fat sat image, mass is not well seen but is slightly hyperintense. The dilated duct in the tail of the pancreas is somewhat better seen on the T2W image (*red arrow*).

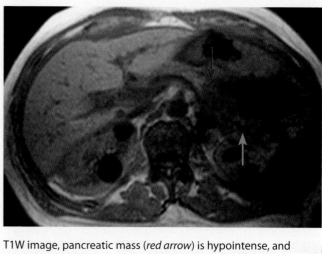

T1W image, pancreatic mass (*red arrow*) is hypointense, and ductal dilatation is faintly seen (*green arrow*).

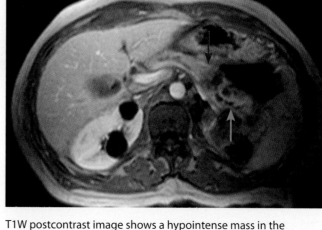

T1W postcontrast image shows a hypointense mass in the midbody of the pancreas (*red arrow*) and ductal dilatation within the tail (*green arrow*).

Answers

1. Findings are typical for duct cell adenocarcinoma of the pancreas. It is hypodense on CT and hypointense on T1W/T1W+c MRI. There is upstream ductal dilatation related to the desmoplastic character of the tumor and upstream obstruction. Islet cell tumors and carcinoid tumors often enhance more than native pancreas as they are hypervascular tumors. The other tumors are cystic neoplasms with distinguishing features.

2. In terms of incidence pancreatic cancer ranks 12 among all cancers. However, the survival statistics are very poor and it ranks fourth among all cancers in terms of overall mortality. It ranks behind lung, colorectal, and breast cancer.

3. CA 19-9 is a tumor marker that is often positive in pancreatic cancer, although it can be elevated because of other neoplasms or some benign causes. The utility is that it can be used to monitor disease activity in patients in whom it is initially elevated and who have undergone treatment.

4. There are a number of signs, both clinical and radiologic, that pertain to pancreatic cancer. Trousseau sign is migratory thrombophlebitis that sometimes occurs in patients with pancreatic cancer and other malignancies. Courvoisier sign refers to a nontender palpable gallbladder, something that can be seen when there is a pancreatic head mass obstructing the common bile duct. The double duct sign refers to a dilated common bile duct and a dilated main pancreatic duct secondary to a pancreatic head tumor.

5. There are numerous risk factors for pancreatic cancer. Many of these are hereditary and therefore not modifiable.

However, smoking and obesity are risk factors for pancreatic cancer and these are modifiable.

Pearls

- Ranks 12th in cancer incidence but fourth in cancer deaths.
- Trousseau sign, migratory thrombophlebitis.
- Courvoisier sign, nontender palpable gallbladder.
- Double duct sign, dilated biliary and pancreatic ducts secondary to pancreatic tumor.
- CA 19-9 is a tumor marker that is often positive in pancreatic cancer, although not specific.
- 5-Year survival is dismal, around 6%.

Suggested Readings

Bronstein YL, Loyer EM, Kaur H, Choi H, David C, DuBrow RA, et al. Detection of small pancreatic tumors with multiphasic helical CT. *AJR Am J Roentgenol.* 2004;182(3):619-623. Epub 2004/02/21. doi: 10.2214/ajr.182.3.1820619.

Morgan DE, Waggoner CN, Canon CL, Lockhart ME, Fineberg NS, Posey JA, 3rd, et al. Resectability of pancreatic adenocarcinoma in patients with locally advanced disease downstaged by preoperative therapy: a challenge for MDCT. *AJR Am J Roentgenol.* 2010;194(3):615-622. Epub 2010/02/23. doi: 10.2214/ajr.08.1022.

Tamm EP, Silverman PM, Charnsangavej C, Evans DB. Diagnosis, staging, and surveillance of pancreatic cancer. *AJR Am J Roentgenol.* 2003;180(5):1311-1323. Epub 2003/04/22. doi: 10.2214/ajr.180.5.1801311.

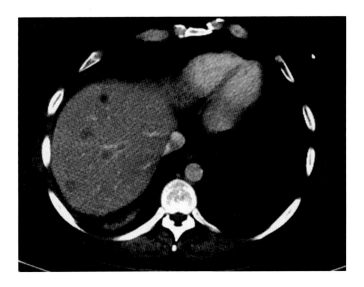 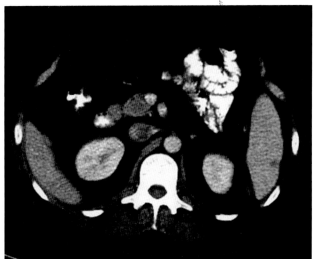

1. What is the most likely diagnosis?

2. What is the approximate incidence of hepatosplenic candidiasis in patients with leukemia?

3. Besides blood cultures and tissue specimens, what other techniques can be used to make a diagnosis?

4. Which is the best imaging modality?

5. What relatively routine blood test is often elevated in hepatosplenic candidiasis?

Case ranking/difficulty: 🦠

Category: Liver

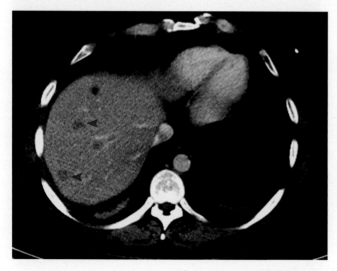

Axial portal venous phase CT shows multiple small hypodensities of nearly equal size scattered randomly throughout the liver (*red arrowheads*).

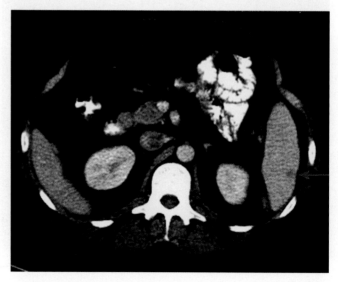

Axial portal venous phase CT shows a single hypodense lesion within the spleen that is similar in size to the hepatic lesion (*red arrow*). Other lesions were also present.

Answers

1. Given the history and the presence of multiple small hypodensities in the liver and spleen, disseminated candidiasis is the most likely diagnosis. Lymphoma is usually larger and not so round in appearance. Metastatic disease is a thought, but tends to be larger, often has some peripheral enhancement, and a splenic lesion would be unusual. Biliary hamartomas (also called von Meyenburg complexes) are a thought, but if prior imaging is available that would be helpful as they would not evolve. A comet-tail artifact has been described on US, and MRCP may be helpful as they appear as cystic lesions usually. Caroli disease manifests as fusiform and saccular dilatation of the bile ducts.

   The key is the clinical setting and the imaging appearance.

2. The historical incidence was somewhat higher with reports in the range of 3% to 29%. However, leukemia patients now receive prophylaxis for fungal infection and this has resulted in a decrease in the incidence of hepatosplenic candidiasis in patients so that the range is around 3% to 7%.

3. Historically, blood culture and biopsy were used to make a diagnosis. Blood culture is problematic because cultures may take some time to grow, and the same applies to tissue specimen. Biopsy also carries the risk of hemorrhage or other complications. PCR techniques have been used to make a more rapid diagnosis.

4. MRI is considered the preferred modality, with T1W postcontrast images being the most sensitive. In practice, multidetector CT is used more often given the availability and cheaper cost. Ultrasound is problematic, although there are reports of it being useful. Plain films and cholangiography have no role in the evaluation.

5. Not surprisingly, alkaline phosphatase levels are often abnormal in patients with hepatic disease. Other liver enzyme levels may be abnormal but often are not.

Pearls

- Typically occurs in patients with hematologic malignancies or in immunocompromised patients.
- Patients sometimes not symptomatic until neutropenia is recovering.
- Imaging appearance can vary with the neutrophil count, becoming more conspicuous as the patient recovers.
- Healed lesions can calcify.

Suggested Readings

Kirby A, Chapman C, Hassan C, Burnie J. The diagnosis of hepatosplenic candidiasis by DNA analysis of tissue biopsy and serum. *J Clin Pathol*. 2004;57(7):764-765. Epub 2004/06/29. doi: 10.1136/jcp.2003.015347.

Mortelé KJ, Segatto E, Ros PR. The infected liver: radiologic-pathologic correlation. *Radiographics*. 2004;24(4): 937-955. Epub 2004/07/17. doi: 10.1148/rg.244035719.

Semelka RC, Shoenut JP, Greenberg HM, Bow EJ. Detection of acute and treated lesions of hepatosplenic candidiasis: comparison of dynamic contrast-enhanced CT and MR imaging. *J Magn Reson Imaging*. 1992;2(3):341-345. Epub 1992/05/01.

61-year-old female status post rectopexy and sigmoid resection for rectal prolapse 1 week ago

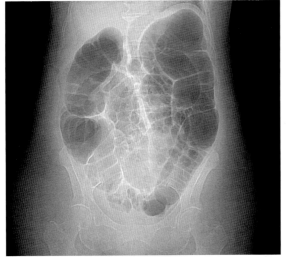
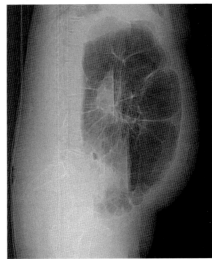
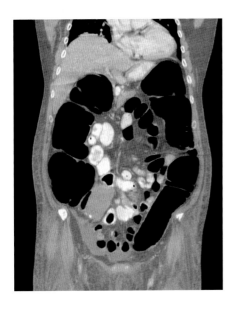
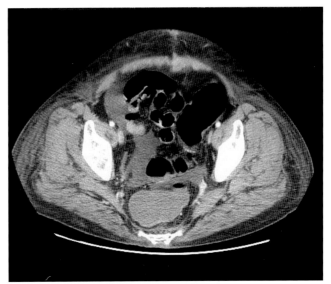

1. What is the most likely diagnosis?

2. Which part of the bowel is generally the last to recover function after abdominal surgery?

3. What is the 3-6-9 rule?

4. What should one evaluate when reading a CT for bowel obstruction?

5. How long does an ileus have to be present to be considered prolonged?

Case ranking/difficulty:

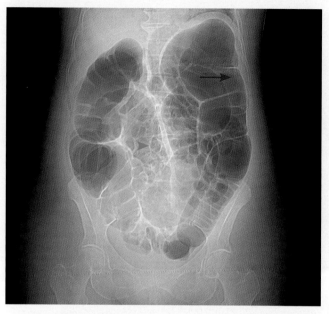

Scout image from CT examination of the abdomen to evaluate for obstruction. Dilated colon (*red arrow*) with multiple more normal appearing loops of small bowel noted centrally (*green arrowhead*).

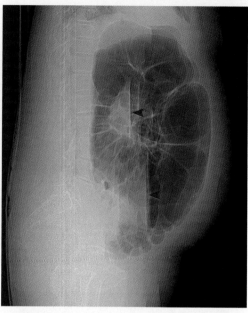

Lateral scout image from CT examination of the abdomen shows multiple dilated loops of colon along with multiple air fluid levels (*red arrowheads*).

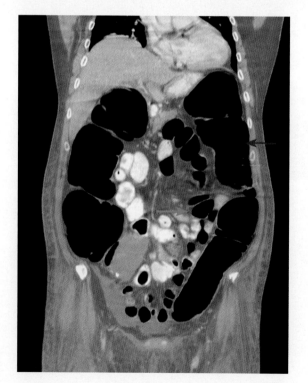

Portal venous phase CT with oral contrast shows dilated colon (*red arrow*) and normal caliber loops of small bowel (*green arrow*).

Answers

1. A dilated colon with normal appearing small bowel loops, no transition point, and no obstructing lesion identified in conjunction with a postoperative state is most consistent with postoperative ileus. There is nothing to suggest small bowel obstruction, gastric outlet obstruction, colonic obstruction, or closed-loop obstruction.

2. Within the abdomen, small bowel is the first part of bowel to recover function. This is followed by the stomach and then by the colon, so the colon is the last part of the bowel to recover function.

3. It is a convenient rule of thumb used for threshold values when evaluating for bowel obstruction on plain radiographs. 3 cm is the diameter threshold for the small bowel, 6 cm is the threshold value for the colon, and 9 cm is the threshold value used for the cecum.

4. All of the items mentioned should be evaluated when interpreting a CT obtained for bowel obstruction. The presence or absence of obstruction should be confirmed. If present, one needs to identify a transition point. In some instances this may require tedious analysis of the bowel and viewing multiplanar reconstructions of the examination. One should determine the severity of the obstruction, namely whether it is high grade or low grade. If possible, a cause should be identified,

and complications such as a closed-loop obstruction or strangulation should be looked for.

5. There is not complete agreement on the definition of prolonged ileus. Typically, unrestricted clear fluids are administered after slightly more than 2 days in patients who have undergone abdominal surgery. A useful guideline for the definition of prolonged ileus is ileus lasting more than 5 to 6 days after surgery.

Pearls

- Proportional dilatation of the small bowel and colon without a transition point seen in postoperative ileus.
- Plain radiography is not very helpful in identifying a transition point when there is bowel obstruction. Rule of 3s and 3-6-9 rules for plain radiography interpretation.
- CT to identify transition point or other etiology in cases of obstruction. Useful for further characterization in cases of bowel obstruction.

Suggested Readings

Artinyan A, Nunoo-Mensah JW, Balasubramaniam S, Gauderman J, Essani R, Gonzalez-Ruiz C, et al. Prolonged postoperative ileus-definition, risk factors, and predictors after surgery. *World J Surg.* 2008;32(7):1495-1500. Epub 2008/02/29. doi: 10.1007/s00268-008-9491-2.

Mullan CP, Siewert B, Eisenberg RL. Small bowel obstruction. *AJR Am J Roentgenol.* 2012;198(2):W105-W117. Epub 2012/01/24. doi: 10.2214/ajr.10.4998.

Silva AC, Pimenta M, Guimarães LS. Small bowel obstruction: what to look for. *Radiographics.* 2009;29(2): 423-439. Epub 2009/03/28. doi: 10.1148/rg.292085514.

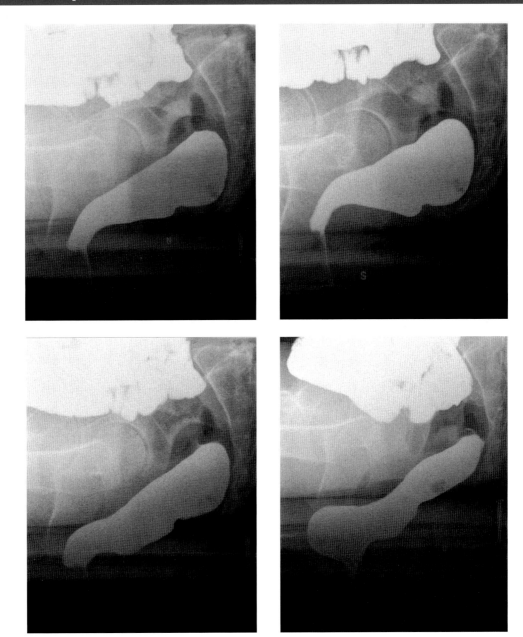

1. What is this study?

2. What are the indications for this study?

3. What are the radiographic manifestations of rectocele?

4. What is the muscle responsible for maintaining the anorectal angle?

5. What is the role of MR defecography?

Case ranking/difficulty: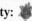

Category: Colorectum

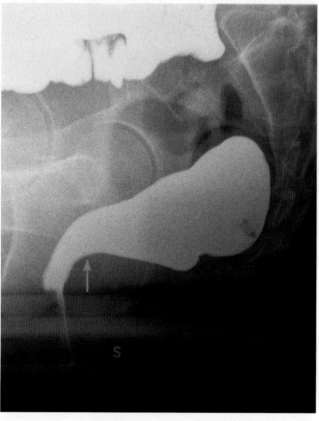

During squeeze, the ARA is lessened. Note the prominent puborectalis impression (*arrow*).

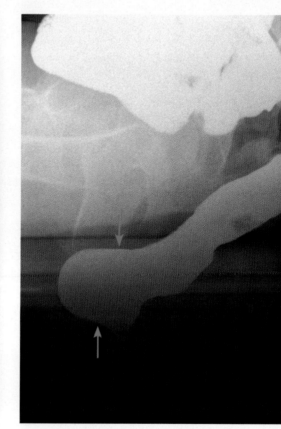

Image during defecation. Rectocele was diagnosed by measuring the anterior bulging (*green arrows*) more than 2 cm.

Answers

1. Defecography or evacuation proctography.

2. Chronic constipation, unexplained rectal or anal pain, suspected rectal prolapse, fecal incontinence, and sensation of incomplete evacuation.

3. Anterior bulging of rectum into the vagina. To be significant, the anterior bulge should be more than 2 cm from the line drawn along the anterior wall of anal canal.

4. The puborectalis maintains the anorectal angle (around 95° in resting state) and thereby rectal continence. During defecation, it relaxes and the AR angle widens to approach 180°.

5. MRI is useful for surgical planning, suspected multicompartmental defects and those patients in whom radiation is a concern.

Pearls

- Conventional defecography is the gold standard for detection of pelvic floor hernia.
- MRI can be used whenever there are multicompartmental defects and while planning for surgery.

Suggested Readings

Fielding JR. Practical MR imaging of female pelvic floor weakness. *Radiographics*. 2002;22(2):295-304.

Kim AY. How to interpret a functional or motility test—defecography. *J Neurogastroenterol Motil*. 2011;17: 416-420.

Reginelli A, Di Grezia G, Gatta G, et al. Role of conventional radiology and MRI defecography of pelvic floor hernias. *BMC Surg*. 2013;13 suppl 2:S53.

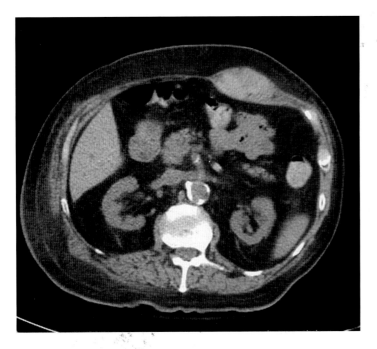 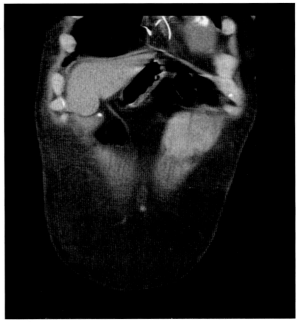

1. What is the most likely diagnosis?

2. What is Fothergill sign?

3. What is a grade III rectus hematoma?

4. Name two other rectus muscle masses that could be considered in the differential diagnosis.

5. What risk factor do most patients with rectus sheath hematoma have?

Case ranking/difficulty:

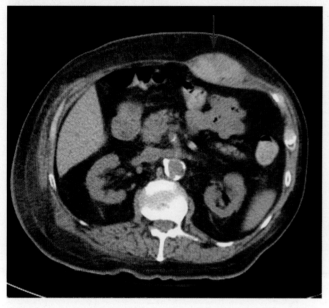

Noncontrast axial CT image shows a soft tissue density (slightly hyperdense) mass within the left rectus sheath (*arrow*).

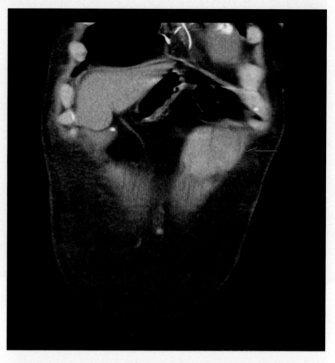

Reformatted coronal noncontrast CT image shows slightly hyperdense soft tissue density mass contained within the left rectus sheath (*red arrow*).

Answers

1. Based on the appearance alone of a hyperdense mass within the rectus sheath, a rectus sheath hematoma is the best diagnosis. The history of trauma in a patient on anticoagulation therapy makes the diagnosis even more certain. Additional imaging with US could be helpful by demonstrating no vascular flow within the mass.

   An abscess would not be so dense on CT and would be relatively hypoechoic or have heterogeneous echogenicity on US. The patient would also be more ill, likely with an elevated WBC count and fever.

   A desmoid tumor is a thought, although there may be a history of prior surgery, and the mass would not be so dense and would have some vascularity.

   An endometrioma would not occur in a male patient.

   A solitary fibrous tumor is rare, and it would not be so dense, and there would be some vascularity.

2. Fothergill sign refers to a unilateral abdominal wall mass involving the rectus muscle which does not change with flexion of the rectus muscle. It is a useful sign in diagnosing a rectus hematoma in patients presenting with acute abdominal pain.

3. There is a grading system for rectus muscle hematomas. Grade I hematomas are intramuscular, unilateral with no dissection. Grade II hematomas are bilateral with some dissection but no extension into the peritoneum

or prevesical space. In general, grade I and grade II hematomas can be treated conservatively with management of coagulation status (if the patient is anticoagulated), bedrest, and transfusion if necessary.

Grade III hematomas have some fascial dissection and extension into the prevesical space and peritoneum. Grade III hematomas more often require aggressive measures such as embolization or surgery.

4. Although rare, desmoid tumor (also called aggressive fibromatosis) can arise from the rectus muscles and manifest as a soft tissue density mass involving the muscle. Endometrial implants (endometriomas) occasionally occur within the rectus sheath, being implanted there after gynecologic or obstetrical surgery. In the right clinical setting an abscess is a possibility.

   Lymphoma and a solitary fibrous tumor in this location are rare.

5. Although trauma and a recent bout of coughing or straining are risk factors for rectus sheath hematoma, anticoagulation is more common and the majority of patients who present with a rectus sheath hematoma has that risk factor.

Pearls

- In most cases there is a history of anticoagulation.
- Typically occurs in elderly women, or as the result of coughing or physical exertion (eg, tennis players, weight lifters).
- If there is abdominal mass that stops at the midline (linea alba), this is a clue to the diagnosis, although not definitive.

Suggested Readings

Alla VM, Karnam SM, Kaushik M, Porter J. Spontaneous rectus sheath hematoma. The *West J Emerg Med*. 2010;11(1):76-79. Epub 2010/04/23.

Berna JD, Garcia-Medina V, Guirao J, Garcia-Medina J. Rectus sheath hematoma: diagnostic classification by CT. *Abdom Imaging*. 1996;21(1):62-64. Epub 1996/01/01.

Cherry WB, Mueller PS. Rectus sheath hematoma: review of 126 cases at a single institution. *Medicine*. 2006;85(2):105-110. Epub 2006/04/13. doi: 10.097/01.d.000216818.3067.a.

68-year-old male with abdominal pain and distention

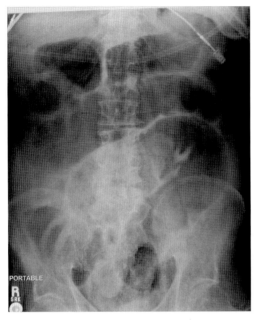
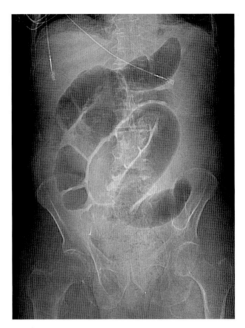
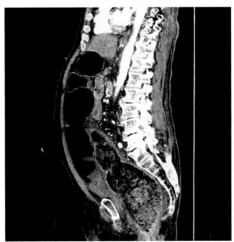

1. If the patient was unable to pass feces, what would you call this?

2. In the setting of a nursing home or extended care facility what is the prevalence of fecal impaction?

3. What is stercoral colitis?

4. What is a reported mortality rate in perforation related to stercoral colitis?

5. Where are most cases of stercoral colitis located?

Case ranking/difficulty: 🍁

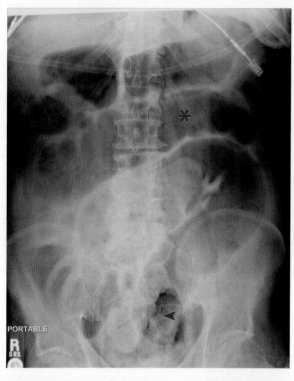

Portable AP image of the abdomen shows multiple dilated loops of large bowel (*asterisk*) with a large amount of fecal material having a mottled appearance noted within the rectum (*red arrowhead*).

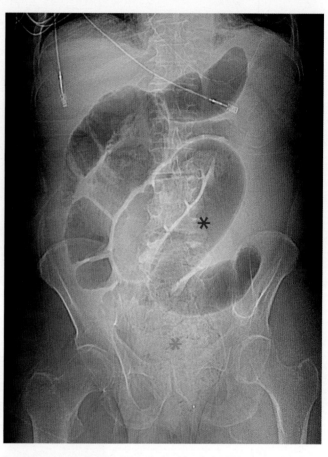

Scanogram prior to CT of the abdomen shows dilated loops of large bowel (*red asterisk*) and fecal material having a mottled appearance within the rectum (*green asterisk*).

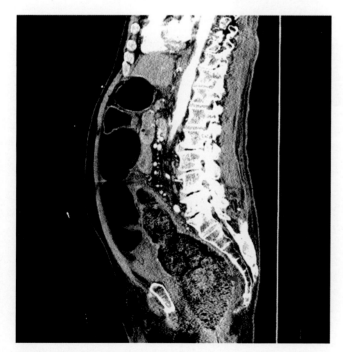

Reformatted midline sagittal CT image shows a large amount of fecal material having a mottled appearance within the rectosigmoid (*red arrowhead*). More proximal colon is also dilated.

Answers

1. From a clinical standpoint this would be called fecal impaction. In some cases patients are able to pass more liquid feces around the immobile obstructing mass, but the hardened mass remains and they still may require manual methods for disimpaction.

2. In one report, the reported value was approximately 8.8%. This was the value reported for fecal impaction and not for simple constipation. Overall, fecal impaction is much more common in the hospital setting and in extended care facilities.

3. Stercoral colitis results from pressure exerted by fecal material upon the containing bowel. It is usually focal or multifocal and is thought to essentially be an ischemic colitis resulting from the mass effect and pressure exerted by the fecal mass. It can result in focal ulceration, focal wall thickening, and frank perforation.

4. A reported mortality rate in perforation related to stercoral colitis is 35%. This emphasizes the importance of preventing the disease altogether by treating fecal impaction promptly, and the importance of detecting evolving stercoral colitis to prevent progression.

5. Not surprisingly, most cases of stercoral colitis are located within the sigmoid colon and the rectum. This makes sense since this is where the impacted fecal material is most often located.

Pearls

- Fecal impaction usually adequately managed medically.
- Stercoral colitis is a possible complication of fecal impaction and has characteristic imaging features.

Suggested Readings

Araghizadeh F. Fecal impaction. *Clin Colon Rectal Surg*. 2005;18(2):116-119. Epub 2005/05/01. doi: 10.1055/s-2005-870893.

Arce DA, Ermocilla CA, Costa H. Evaluation of constipation. *Am Fam Physician*. 2002;65(11):2283-2290.

Heffernan C, Pachter HL, Megibow AJ, Macari M. Stercoral colitis leading to fatal peritonitis: CT findings. *AJR Am J Roentgenol*. 2005;184(4):1189-1193. Epub 2005/03/25. doi: 10.2214/ajr.184.4.01841189.

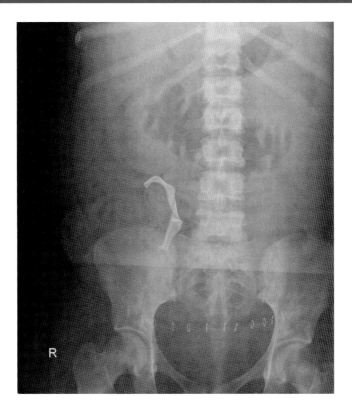

1. What is the most likely diagnosis?

2. In approximately what proportion of surgeries does a retained foreign object occur?

3. What surgical device accounts for the majority of retained foreign objects?

4. A correct count in the operating room effectively excludes a retained foreign object. True or false.

5. In the cases that prompted litigation in the *New England Journal* report what was the average settlement amount?

Case ranking/difficulty:

Category: Peritoneum

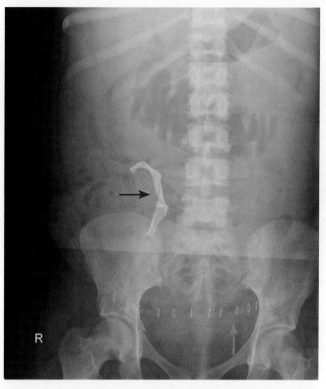

AP abdominal image showing staple line (*green arrows*) related to recent C-section and retained laparotomy sponge (*red arrow*).

Answers

1. The postoperative study shows skin staples related to recent C-section, and there is a radiopaque marker strip overlying the right lower quadrant corresponding to a laparotomy sponge. The image is otherwise consistent with postoperative state.

   If one is unfamiliar with the radiographic appearance of possible retained foreign objects it is helpful to create a reference image or two on a PACS system to serve as a reference.

2. Reports vary since reporting and documentation may vary. However, a good estimate is 1:5500 surgeries as noted in the study from the Mayo Clinic. The *New England Journal of Medicine* study reports values of 1 in 8000 to 1 in 18000 inpatient operations, but this is based on malpractice claims and likely underestimates the frequency.

   In terms of a raw number of cases, 1500 annually is one estimate, although the actual number is likely significantly greater.

3. The most commonly retained device is a surgical sponge. These come in a variety of sizes and shapes but they all have an attached radiopaque marker that allows them to be identified on a radiograph. Sponges are sometimes difficult to identify at the time of surgery as they may blend in with the surrounding tissue or be otherwise hidden from view.

4. In the Mayo Clinic study the majority of retained foreign objects occurred in the setting of a correct count of instruments, sponges, and needles, so the answer is false. Routine postoperative survey imaging in all patients undergoing some surgical procedures is an important part of a program aimed at reducing the incidence of postoperative retained foreign objects.

5. In the *New England Journal of Medicine* report there were 47 cases that prompted litigation, and the average settlement amount of these cases was $52,581. For all cases with retained foreign objects the median date of detection was the 21st day after surgery.

Pearls

- Gossypiboma refers to foreign object, such as cotton matrix object or sponge left behind postoperatively.
- Sponges have radiopaque markers.
- Absorbable material such as Surgifoam and Gelfoam may persist for months after surgery, and may resemble an abscess.

Suggested Readings

Cima RR, Kollengode A, Garnatz J, Storsveen A, Weisbrod C, Deschamps C. Incidence and characteristics of potential and actual retained foreign object events in surgical patients. *J Am Coll Surg.* 2008;207(1):80-87. Epub 2008/07/01. doi: 10.016/j.amcollsurg.007.2.47.

Gawande AA, Studdert DM, Orav EJ, Brennan TA, Zinner MJ. Risk factors for retained instruments and sponges after surgery. *N Engl J Med.* 2003;348(3):229-235. doi: 10.056/NEJMsa021721.

Joint Commission on Accreditation of Health Care Organizations. Focus on five, preventing retained foreign objects, improving safety after surgery. Joint Commission Perspectives on Patient Safety. March 2006;6(3):11

Upper abdominal fullness

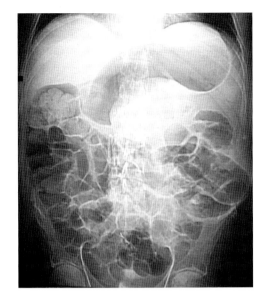

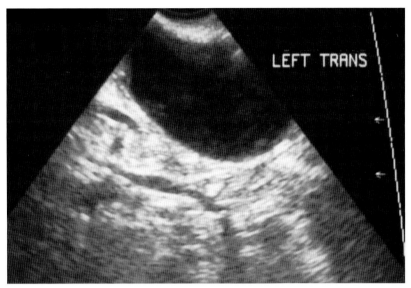

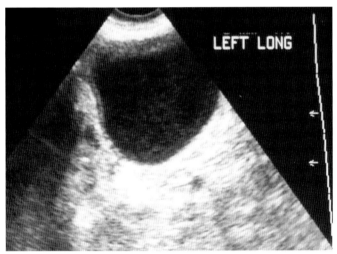

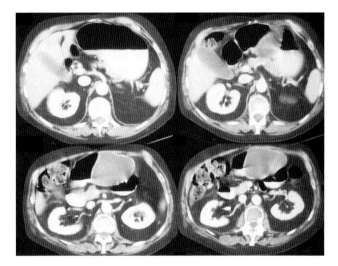

1. What is the most likely diagnosis given the history and images?

2. Approximately what percentage of all gastrointestinal duplications are gastric duplications?

3. What is the primary entity in the differential diagnosis for a gastric duplication cyst?

4. What are the three diagnostic criteria for a duplication cyst?

5. What is the most common location for gastrointestinal duplication cysts?

Case ranking/difficulty:

Category: Stomach

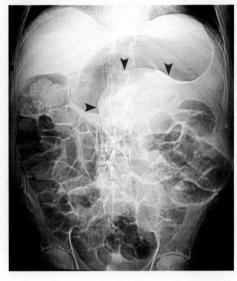

AP radiograph shows a large extraluminal mass deforming the contour of the greater curvature of the stomach (*red arrowheads*).

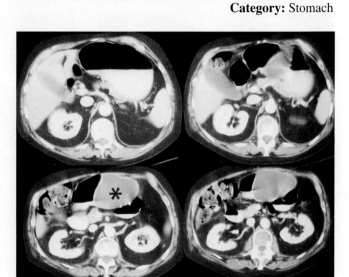

Contrast-enhanced CT demonstrates a large fluid density mass contiguous with the greater curvature of the stomach (*red asterisk*).

Answers

1. Given the cystic appearance, contiguity with the stomach, and appearance on ultrasound examination, the most likely diagnosis is a gastric duplication cyst. The patient is of relatively advanced age for diagnosis, but the findings are otherwise consistent with a duplication cyst.

2. Gastrointestinal duplications are not that uncommon. The most common location is the ileum. Gastric duplications are relatively uncommon and account for only approximately 5% to 7% of gastrointestinal duplications. The most common location is the greater curvature of the stomach.

3. Given that duplications usually have fluid contents, adenocarcinoma, GIST, leiomyosarcoma, and gastritis should not be considered. Pancreatic pseudocyst is a consideration.

   It may be difficult to distinguish between a pseudocyst and a duplication if one is not able to establish the intimate connection of the mass with the stomach (in the case of a duplication) or separate the mass from the stomach (in the case of a pseudocyst). There have been cases that were preoperatively misidentified as a pseudocyst when in fact there was a duplication cyst.

4.
   1. Intimate attachment to the GI tract (sharing muscle wall and blood supply)
   2. Layer of smooth muscle in the wall
   3. Epithelial lining resembling some part of GI tract

   Communication with the bowel lumen is not a criterion. While most do not communicate with the bowel lumen, some do.

5. The small intestine is the most common location for gastrointestinal duplication cysts. It accounts for approximately 44% of the total.

Pearls

- Bowel signature (inner echogenic layer, outer hypoechoic layer) useful ultrasound finding in suggesting the diagnosis.
- Usually simple fluid contents, although may be variable depending on the presence of hemorrhage or complications.
- Possible synchronous abnormalities.

Suggested Readings

Agha FP, Gabriele OF, Abdulla FH. Complete gastric duplication. *AJR Am J Roentgenol.* 1981;137(2):406-407. Epub 1981/08/01. doi: 10.2214/ajr.137.2.406.

Cheng G, Soboleski D, Daneman A, Poenaru D, Hurlbut D. Sonographic pitfalls in the diagnosis of enteric duplication cysts. *AJR Am J Roentgenol.* 2005;184(2):521-525. Epub 2005/01/27. doi: 10.2214/ajr.184.2.01840521.

Lee J, Park CM, Kim KA, Lee CH, Choi JW, Shin BK, et al. Cystic lesions of the gastrointestinal tract: multimodality imaging with pathologic correlations. *Korean J Radiol.* 2010;11(4):457-468. Epub 2010/07/02. doi: 10.3348/kjr.2010.11.4.457.

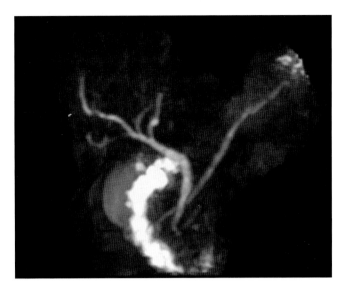

1. What is the diagnosis?

2. What is the incidence of this condition in ERCP series?

3. What is the best noninvasive test for diagnosing pancreatic divisum?

4. What are the CT findings suggestive of this condition?

5. What is the role of secretin in secretin-enhanced MRCP?

Case ranking/difficulty: 🐾

Answers

1. The lack of communication between dorsal and ventral ducts and draining of most of the pancreas by the dorsal duct are diagnostic of pancreas divisum.

2. Two percent to 8% in ERCP series, 4% to 14% in autopsy series.

3. MRCP is much more sensitive than CT and uses heavily T2-weighted (fluid-sensitive) sequences.

4. Pancreatic head enlargement, fat cleft between ventral and dorsal pancreas, no communication between ventral and dorsal pancreatic ducts, and dominant dorsal duct sign, all suggest pancreas divisum on CT.

5. Secretin transiently increases the tone of the sphincter of Oddi and stimulates pancreatic exocrine secretion.

Suggested Readings

Reinbold C, Bret PM, Guibaud L, Barkun AN, Genin G, Atri M. MR cholangiopancreatography: potential clinical applications. *Radiographics*. March 1996;16(2):309-320.

Tirkes T, Sandrasegaran K, Sanyal R, et al. Secretin-enhanced MR cholangiopancreatography: spectrum of findings. *Radiographics*. November-December 2013;33(7):1889-1906.

Vitellas KM, Keogan MT, Spritzer CE, Nelson RC. MR cholangiopancreatography of bile and pancreatic duct abnormalities with emphasis on the single-shot fast spin-echo technique. *Radiographics*. July-August 2000;20(4):939-957; quiz 1107-8, 1112.

Pearls

- Pancreas divisum (PD) is the most common congenital pancreatic duct anomaly.
- Pancreas divisum may simulate pancreatic head mass and ERCP should precede biopsy of an isodense head mass.
- Pancreatic divism as a cause of acute pancreatitis is controversial.
- MRCP is accurate in depicting pancreatic ductal abnormalities including PD and can be improved by postsecretin imaging.

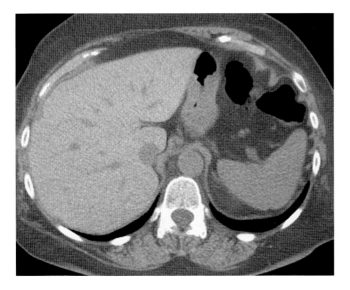 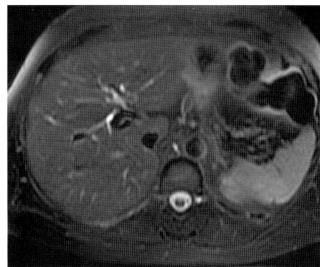

1. What is the most likely diagnosis?

2. What are the possible sequelae of amiodarone accumulation in the liver?

3. What other organs may be affected by amiodarone toxicity?

4. What are the other causes of diffuse increased liver density?

5. What is the normal liver density?

Case ranking/difficulty:

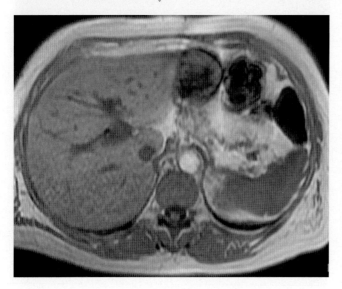

MR T1W in-phase image shows normal liver signal.

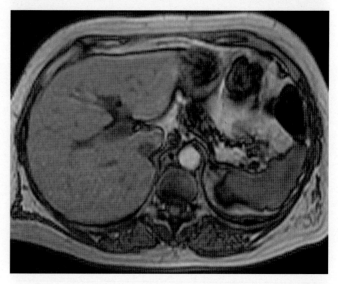

MR T1W out-of-phase image shows no liver signal increase (which would be expected if this were iron overload) compared to MR in-phase image.

Answers

1. Amiodarone deposition in the liver. It is one of the causes of generalized increase in liver density. In hemochromatosis, there will be signal loss in liver on GRE and T2W images.

2. Transient asymptomatic raise in serum aminotransferase, symptomatic hepatitis, liver cirrhosis, and liver failure are the possible sequelae of amiodarone deposits in the liver.

3. Lung, thyroid, heart, nervous system, skin, and cornea may be affected by amiodarone toxicity.

4. Hemochromatosis, glycogen storage disease, Wilson disease, hemosiderosis, gold therapy, and thorotrast are the other causes of diffuse increased liver density.

5. The normal liver density is 55 to 65 HU, about 10 HU higher than spleen. Liver density >75 HU is suspicious for hemochromatosis or other cause of increased hepatic density.

Pearls

- Generalized increased liver density +/− high-density lung opacities in a patient on amiodarone therapy should rise the possibility of its toxicity.
- No liver signal change on out-of-phase MR image compared to MR in-phase image in amiodarone deposition.

Suggested Readings

Kojima S, Kojima S, Ueno H, Takeya M, Ogawa H. Increased density of the liver and amiodarone-associated phospholipidosis. *Cardiol Res Pract.* 2009;2009:598940.

Lee W, Ryu DR, Han SS, et al. Very early onset of amiodarone-induced pulmonary toxicity. *Korean Circ J.* 2013 Oct;43(10):699-701.

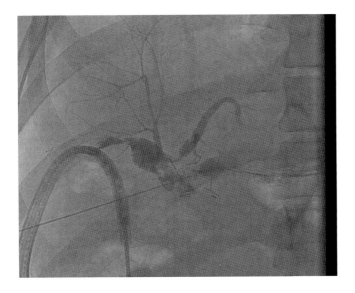
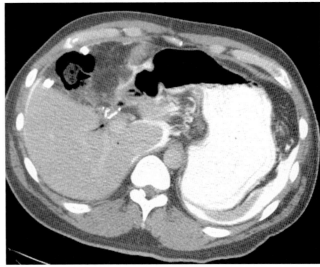
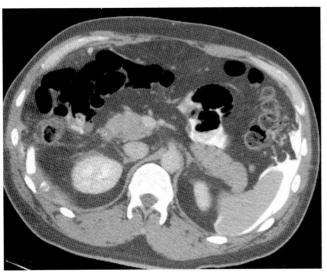
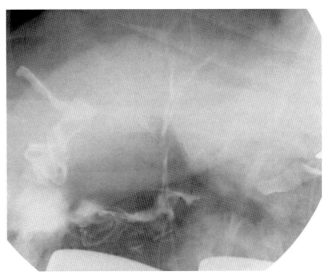

1. What are the most likely diagnoses?

2. What is the initial investigation of choice for suspected biliary leak?

3. Which is the best method of investigation for low CBD injuries?

4. What is the most common location of abscesses due to dropped gallstones?

5. What are the possible sequelae of dropped gallstones?

Case ranking/difficulty:

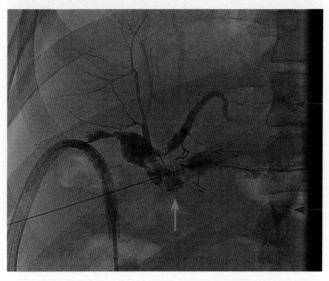

Contrast injection during PTC demonstrates opacification of nondilated intrahepatic biliary ducts and proximal common hepatic duct only up to the surgical clips (*green arrow*) and contrast leak into the subhepatic space (*red arrows*). Since the distal biliary duct is not opacified beyond the surgical site, this is most likely biliary transection.

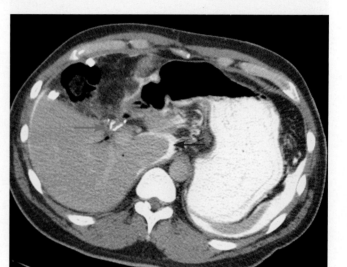

Axial CT after PTC demonstrates spillage of contrast into the peritoneal cavity (*red arrow*) due to biliary leak. Surgical clips (*green arrow*) are present in the GB fossa.

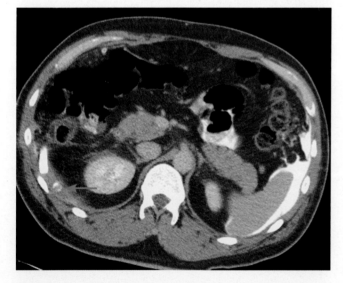

Axial CT after PTC also shows a calcification in Morrison pouch due to dropped stone (*green arrow*).

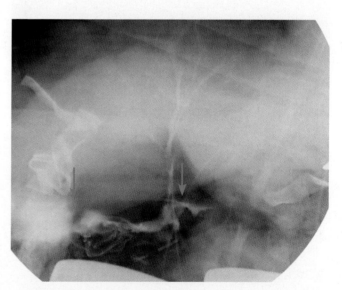

Operative cholangiogram shows flow of contrast from the proximal common hepatic duct into the subhepatic space (*green arrows*).

Answers

1. Biliary leak and dropped stone. There is spillage of contrast from PTC into the peritoneal cavity and also minimal air within the biliary tree. This is most likely from biliary leak. Intraoperative cholangiogram shows definite subhepatic contrast leak, which further confirms the diagnosis of biliary leak. A dropped stone is noted in the hepatorenal space. On CT a retained surgical sponge (gossypiboma) appears as a heterogeneous spongiform mass with wavy strips and air bubbles.

2. Both US and CT scan are useful to detect and localize a fluid collection, ascites, or biliary duct dilatation. ERCP and PTC can then be performed for a biliary leak depending on the level of injury, low or high.

3. ERCP. It can diagnose and treat most low ductal injuries.

4. The most common location of abscesses due to dropped gallstones is posterior and inferior perihepatic.

5. Dropped stones are most frequently asymptomatic. However, they can develop into intra-abdominal abscess around liver. Treatment is surgical removal rather than percutaneous drainage. Dropped stones can migrate to subdiaphragmatic space or into the pleural cavity.

Pearls

- Postsurgical complications are less common with laparoscopic (vs open) technique. However, biliary duct injuries are more common (×2) in laparoscopic surgery.
- Most of the low ductal injuries can be diagnosed and treated by ERCP.
- PTC is helpful to delineate the anatomy before surgery in high biliary duct injuries and serves as a biliary diversion.
- Most of the dropped gallstones are clinically silent, but can develop into abscess and fistula.

Suggested Readings

Bharathy KG, Negi SS. Postcholecystectomy bile duct injury and its sequelae: pathogenesis, classification, and management. *Indian J Gastroenterol*. 2014;33(3):201-215.

Jabłońska B, Lampe P. Iatrogenic bile duct injuries: etiology, diagnosis and management. *World J Gastroenterol*. 2009 Sep;15(33):4097-4104.

Nayak L, Menias CO, Gayer G. Dropped gallstones: spectrum of imaging findings, complications and diagnostic pitfalls. *Br J Radiol*. 2013 Aug;86(1028):20120588.

Intermittent dysphagia

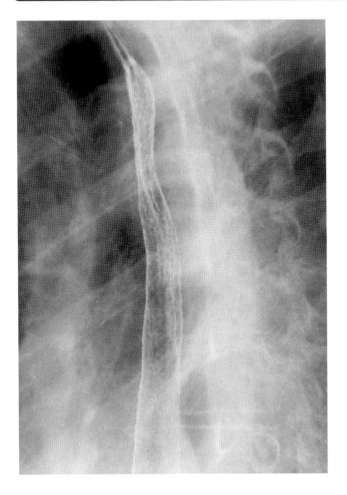 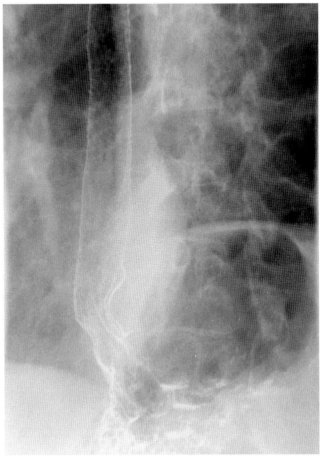

1. What is the most likely diagnosis?

2. What is the usual age demographic for patients with glycogen acanthosis?

3. Up to what percentage of elderly patients undergoing double-contrast esophagrams may have glycogenic acanthosis?

4. What size range do nodules in glycogenic acanthosis have?

5. On endoscopy, what appearance does glycogenic acanthosis have?

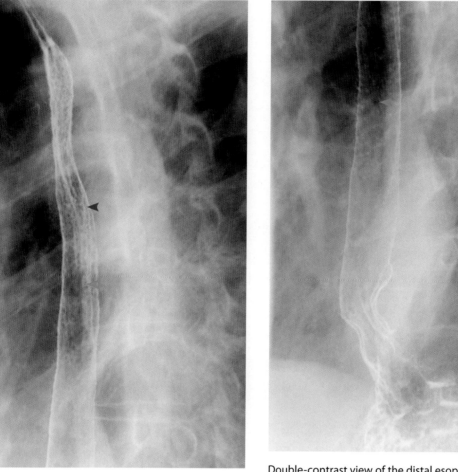

Slightly collapsed double-contrast image of the midesophagus shows longitudinal folds with scalloped margins (*red arrowhead*) as well as small nodules several millimeters in diameter (*green arrowhead*).

Double-contrast view of the distal esophagus (slightly more distended) demonstrates a nodular pattern with nodules a few millimeters in diameter (*green arrowhead*). When overdistended this may not be well visualized.

Answers

1. Glycogenic acanthosis is the most likely diagnosis. The patient's age is concordant with that, and the presence of longitudinal folds with scalloped margin and small nodules fits. Nodules are fairly randomly distributed, but may also be more evident in the midesophagus.

   Candida esophagitis is a consideration, although the nodules in glycogenic acanthosis are more round in appearance when compared to more linear plaques in *Candida* esophagitis. Patients may also be immunocompromised.

   Pill-induced esophagitis is usually more focal, there may be a history, and there may be ulceration.

   Herpes esophagitis usually manifests as multiple small, superficial ulcers in the upper or midesophagus without plaques. Patients may also be immunocompromised.

Reflux esophagitis is often distal with strictures and possibly ulceration. Barrett esophagus may occur.

2. Glycogenic acanthosis may be considered a benign degenerative condition related to the accumulation of cytoplasmic glycogen within esophageal squamous epithelium. The peak occurrence is in the fifth and six decades.

3. Reports vary, but the upper limit reported is nearly 30% of patients in an elderly population, so it is a very common condition and can be viewed almost as a part of normal aging with no malignant potential. Much lower numbers have also been reported (3.5%).

4. The nodules in glycogenic acanthosis range in size from 2 to 15 mm, although they are usually smaller than that upper limit. They tend to be of a similar size within the

same patient. Plaque-like lesions can occur, but these are less common.

5. On endoscopy, glycogenic acanthosis appears as discrete white nodules, occasionally as lumpy folds or plaques. They can be missed on endoscopy if the mucosa is not ideally distended or not carefully examined.

Pearls

- Benign condition related to accumulation of cytoplasmic glycogen within squamous epithelium.
- Might be confused with *Candida* esophagitis.

Suggested Readings

Ghahremani GG, Rushovich AM. Glycogenic acanthosis of the esophagus: radiographic and pathologic features. *Gastrointest Radiol.* 1984;9(2):93-98. Epub 1984/01/01.

Glick SN, Teplick SK, Goldstein J, Stead JA, Zitomer N. Glycogenic acanthosis of the esophagus. *AJR Am J Roentgenol.* 1982;139(4):683-688. Epub 1982/10/01. doi: 10.214/ajr.39..83.

Levine MS, Rubesin SE. Diseases of the esophagus: diagnosis with esophagography. *Radiology.* 2005;237(2):414-427. doi: 10.148/radiol.372050199.

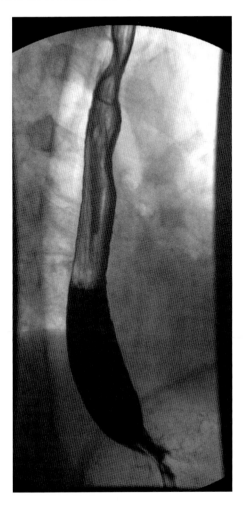 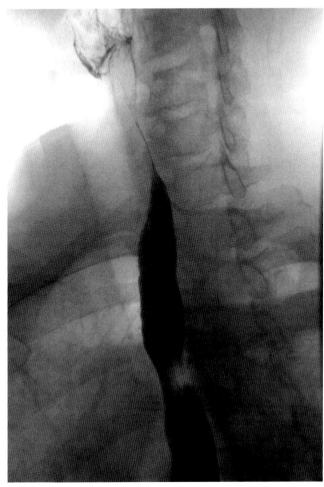

1. What is the most likely diagnosis for the first case?

2. What potentially catastrophic complications can occur?

3. At what age does dysphagia lusoria usually present?

4. An aberrant right subclavian artery can pass between the esophagus and the trachea. True or false.

5. At what level is the extrinsic impression upon the esophagus typically seen?

Case ranking/difficulty:

Category: Esophagus

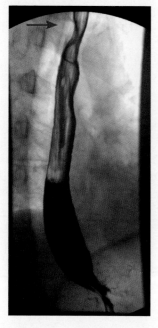

Oblique esophagram shows a mild extrinsic compression upon the posterior aspect of the esophagus at the level of the aortic arch (typically about the fourth thoracic vertebra, *red arrow*).

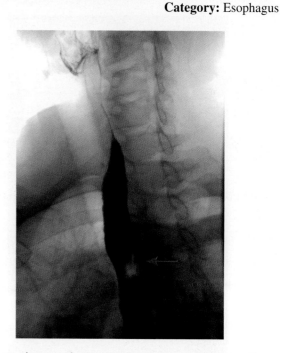

Oblique esophagram shows an extrinsic compression upon the posterior aspect of the esophagus at the level of the aortic arch (*red arrow*).

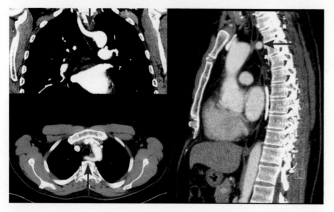

Same case, composite CT scan in coronal, axial, and sagittal planes shows the aberrant right subclavian artery crossing from the left to the right side, in this case behind the trachea and the esophagus (*red arrows*).

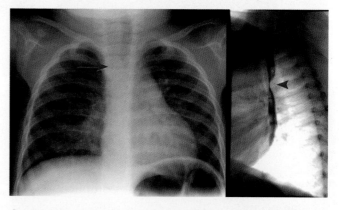

Companion case, pediatric patient, AP chest, and esophagram from a pediatric patient with difficulty swallowing and eating. Plain radiograph shows a right aortic arch (*red arrow*), and lateral esophagram shows extrinsic impression on the esophagus posteriorly (*red arrowhead*), in this case from an aberrant left subclavian artery.

Answers

1. The esophagram is highly suggestive, and the CT clearly demonstrates an aberrant right subclavian artery passing behind the esophagus and the trachea. The CT excludes a pulmonary sling, vascular ring, right arch, and normal branching.

   The reported incidence of an aberrant right subclavian artery is approximately 0.5% to 2% of the population.

It is the most common aortic arch branching anomaly, and it is usually asymptomatic. It is a relatively common finding (25%) in patients with Down syndrome.

2. Of the entities mentioned, fistula formation to the esophagus or trachea is the most serious and potentially fatal complication. Such cases are rare but there are case reports.

Esophageal and tracheal obstructions tend to be incomplete or are usually not life threatening.

3. Dysphagia lusoria tends to be present in older patients. The reason for this is not entirely clear, but it may be related to the stiffening and noncompliance of the aging aberrant right subclavian artery. Rarely, it can present in children.

4. True. Although in most cases (80%) the artery passes posterior to the esophagus, in rare cases it can pass between the esophagus and the trachea or anterior to the trachea.

5. The extrinsic impression upon the esophagus is typically at about the forth thoracic vertebral level and near the level of the aortic arch. These are both around the same level. The aberrant vessel runs inferosuperiorly from left to right as it crosses the mediastinum to the right side.

Pearls

- Most cases of aberrant right subclavian artery are asymptomatic.
- Presents in old age, patients in seventh and eighth decade.
- May manifest in children (rarely).
- Characteristic extrinsic impression upon the esophagus at about the fourth thoracic vertebral level.

Suggested Readings

Donnelly LF, Fleck RJ, Pacharn P, Ziegler MA, Fricke BL, Cotton RT. Aberrant subclavian arteries: cross-sectional imaging findings in infants and children referred for evaluation of extrinsic airway compression. *AJR Am J Roentgenol.* 2002;178(5):1269-1274. Epub 2002/04/18. doi: 10.214/ajr.78..781269.

Janssen M, Baggen MG, Veen HF, et al. Dysphagia lusoria: clinical aspects, manometric findings, diagnosis, and therapy. *Am J Gastroenterol.* 2000;95(6):1411-1416. Epub 2000/07/14. doi: 10.111/j.572-0241.000.2071.

Ka-Tak W, Lam WW, Yu SC. MDCT of an aberrant right subclavian artery and of bilateral vertebral arteries with anomalous origins. *AJR Am J Roentgenol.* 2007;188(3): W274-W275. Epub 2007/02/22. doi: 10.214/ajr.5.694.

49-year-old male with epigastric pain, jaundice, elevated liver function tests

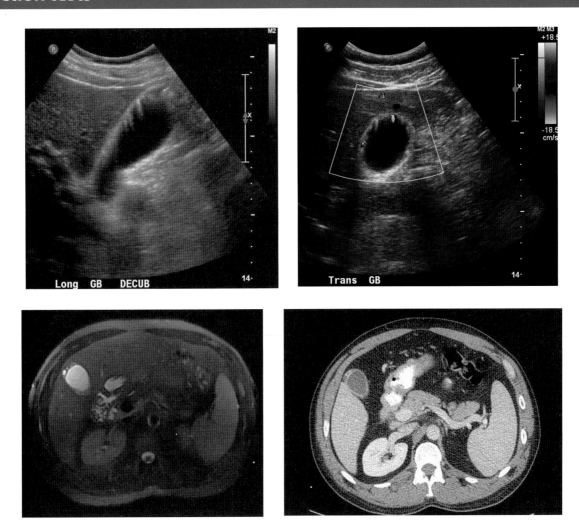

1. What is the most likely diagnosis?

2. What causes the rosary sign described on enhanced CT in adenomyomatosis?

3. What entities fall under the more general term hyperplastic cholecystosis?

4. In approximately what percentage of cholecystectomy specimens is adenomyomatosis present?

5. What features of a polypoid lesion in the gallbladder are concerning for malignancy?

Case ranking/difficulty:

Category: Gallbladder

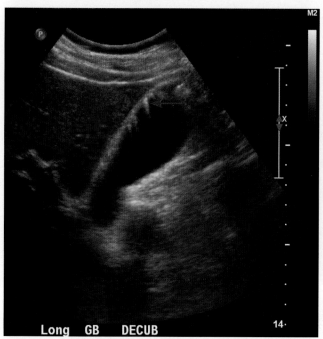

Longitudinal ultrasound image through the gallbladder shows echogenic round foci within the gallbladder wall producing multiple "comet tail artifacts" distally (*red arrow*). There is also mild apparent wall thickening.

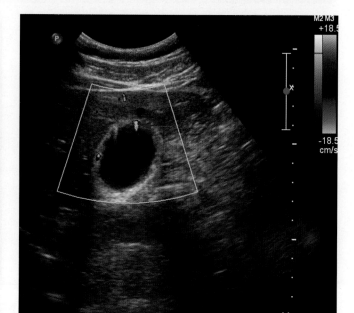

Transverse color Doppler ultrasound image through the gallbladder shows "twinkle sign" or "color comet tail artifact" arising from focus of adenomyomatosis within the gallbladder wall (*red arrow*).

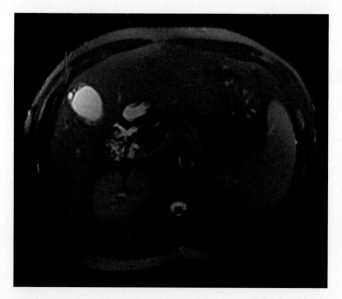

T2W MRI through the gallbladder shows focus of high signal abnormality within the gallbladder wall corresponding to intramural mucosal diverticula (Rokitansky-Aschoff sinuses) (*red arrow*). When numerous, this is the so-called "pearl necklace sign."

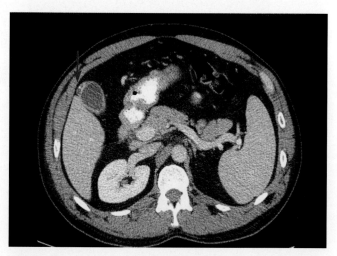

Axial CT showing intramural low density corresponding in intramural mucosal diverticula (*red arrow*).

Answers

1. There are numerous findings and signs that point to a diagnosis of adenomyomatosis, including echogenic foci in the wall demonstrating comet tail and color comet tail signs, foci of high T2W signal within the wall on MRI, and low density within the wall on CT.

    The case shown does not exhibit cholelithiasis or focal mass to suggest carcinoma, and there is no evidence of cholangitis or cholecystitis.

2. The rosary sign is caused by enhancement of the proliferative mucosal epithelium lining the Rokitansky-Aschoff spaces, so one sees a central hypodensity with a surrounding ring-like enhancing epithelium, surrounded by unenhanced hypertrophied muscle coat. It can be seen on enhanced CT of patients with adenomyomatosis.

3. Gallbladder cholesterolosis and gallbladder adenomyomatosis are forms of hyperplastic cholecystosis.

    Gallbladder cholesterolosis can be diffuse or focal. When diffuse it usually cannot be seen by imaging but pathologically corresponds to "strawberry gallbladder." When focal it usually causes cholesterol polyps, which can be multiple and large in size, although usually less than 5 mm. Gallbladder adenomyomatosis is related to hyperplastic changes involving the mucosa with prominent Rokitansky-Aschoff sinuses.

    Adenomatous polyps, inflammatory polyps, and villous adenomas are not forms of hyperplastic cholecystosis and represent other types of polyps or precancerous lesions.

4. Reports vary, but it is in the range of 5.0% to 8.7%, so it is a relatively common finding in pathologic specimens. One should note that coexistent gallstones and gallbladder disease are also very common, in some series up to 90% of cases.

5. Cholesterol polyps are usually less than 10 mm in diameter and they are more often multiple than solitary. They may have other features suggesting cholesterolosis as well. However, they do comprise approximately 50% of polypoid lesions within the gallbladder. Features that are concerning for a polypoid lesion are size greater than 10 mm, vascular flow velocity greater than 20 cm/s, and a solitary lesion.

Pearls

- "String of pearls" or "pearl necklace" on MRI corresponding to Rokitansky-Aschoff sinuses.
- Echogenic foci with gallbladder wall thickening, "comet-tail" reverberation artifact originating in the gallbladder wall.
- "Rosary sign" on CT.

Suggested Readings

Boscak AR, Al-Hawary M, Ramsburgh SR. Best cases from the AFIP: Adenomyomatosis of the gallbladder. *Radiographics*. 2006;26(3):941-946. Epub 2006/05/17. doi: 10.148/rg.63055180.

Chao C, Hsiao HC, Wu CS, Wang KC. Computed tomographic finding in adenomyomatosis of the gallbladder. *J Formos Med Assoc*. 1992;91(4):467-469. Epub 1992/04/01.

Ching BH, Yeh BM, Westphalen AC, Joe BN, Qayyum A, Coakley FV. CT differentiation of adenomyomatosis and gallbladder cancer. *AJR Am J Roentgenol*. 2007;189(1): 62-66. Epub 2007/06/21. doi: 10.214/ajr.6.866.

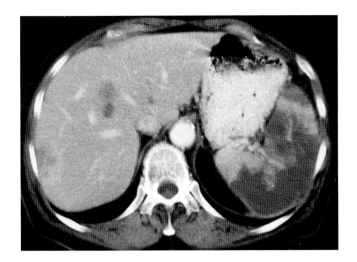 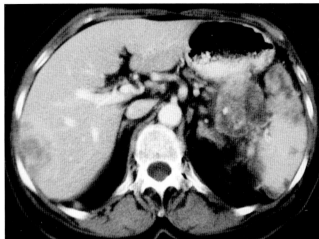

1. What is the most likely diagnosis regarding the spleen?

2. What etiology do patients older than 40 tend to have for splenic infarction?

3. What is a rim sign in the context of splenic infarction?

4. What is Kehr sign?

5. What nuclear medicine scan can be used to diagnose splenic infarction?

Case ranking/difficulty: 🦪

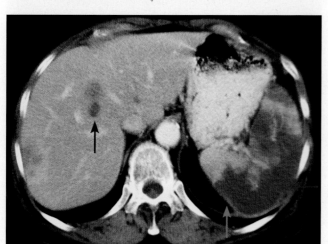

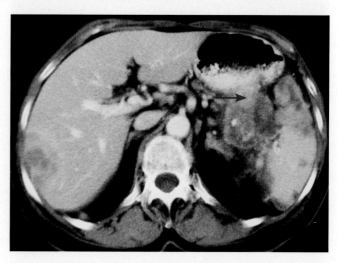

Axial portal venous phase CT demonstrates fairly well-demarcated low density regions within the spleen (*red arrow*) along with enhancing capsular margin of the spleen seen best posteriorly (*green arrow*). Also noted are multiple low-density areas within the liver related to metastatic disease (*blue arrow*).

Axial portal venous phase CT demonstrates a large mass in the tail of the pancreas (*red arrow*) encircling the splenic artery. Multiple smaller splenic infarcts and liver metastases are again noted.

Answers

1. The images and history are most consistent with splenic infarction, particularly when there is splenic capsule enhancement.

   Splenic lymphoma is usually more round or mass like, with disease outside of the spleen. Splenic cysts are usually solitary well-defined masses with density near water or slightly greater. Splenic lacerations are usually more linear with disruption of the splenic capsule and significant hemorrhage. Splenic abscesses can be solitary or multiple, but there is usually a contributory history.

2. Thromboembolic phenomena predominate in patients older than 40. One should be cognizant of the possibility that there may be emboli to other organs in such cases (eg, bowel, kidney, brain).

   In patients less than 40 underlying hematologic diseases, such as sickle cell disease or chronic myelogenous leukemia, are often underlying causes.

3. When nearly the entire spleen is infarcted there is persistent arterial supply to the capsule of the spleen, resulting in enhancement of the capsule and nonenhancement of the parenchyma. This is called a "rim sign" and is probably best seen when nearly the entire spleen is infarcted.

4. Kehr sign is a type of referred pain related to peritoneal and diaphragmatic irritation in the setting of left upper quadrant abdominal disease. The pain is referred to

the left shoulder, and it classically is related to splenic rupture, but it may occur in other conditions.

5. Although not commonly used any longer, a Tc 99m sulfur colloid scan has been used and can be used to diagnose splenic infarct. An infarct would appear as a photopenic defect in the spleen, although it might be difficult to differentiate that from an abscess or other space-occupying lesion.

Pearls

- Younger patients tend to have an underlying hematologic condition.
- Older patients tend to have an embolic source.
- The patient with embolic source may have emboli in other organs.

Suggested Readings

Balcar I, Seltzer SE, Davis S, Geller S. CT patterns of splenic infarction: a clinical and experimental study. *Radiology*. 1984;151(3):723-729. doi: 10.148/radiology.51..718733.

Goerg C, Schwerk WB. Splenic infarction: sonographic patterns, diagnosis, follow-up, and complications. *Radiology*. 1990;174(3 pt 1):803-807. Epub 1990/03/01. doi: 10.148/radiology.74..406785.

Jaroch MT, Broughan TA, Hermann RE. The natural history of splenic infarction. *Surgery*. 1986;100(4):743-750. Epub 1986/10/01.

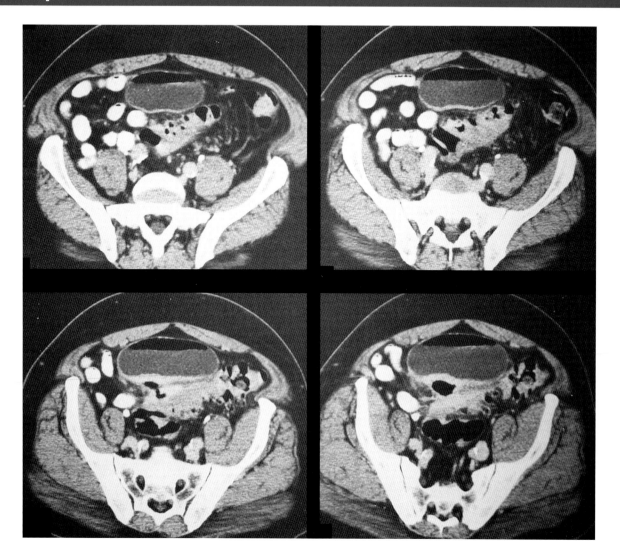

1. Based on top-left figure, what is the most likely diagnosis?

2. What are some of the causes of colovesical fistula besides diverticulitis?

3. What are the clinical features of colovesical fistula?

4. What are the CT findings of colovesical fistula other than direct demonstration of the fistula?

5. How should the CT be conducted in suspected colovesical fistula?

Case ranking/difficulty:

Category: Colorectum

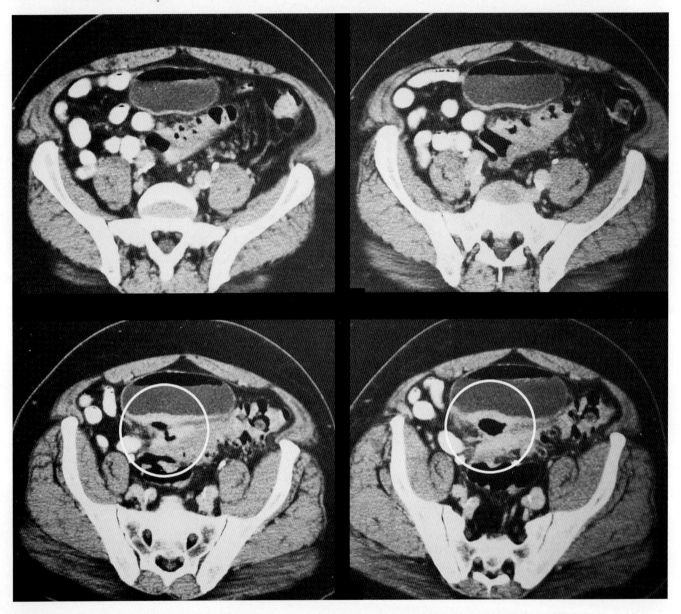

All images show a thick-walled sigmoid with diverticula and an air-fluid level in the bladder. Lower right shows a small gas-containing mass between the sigmoid and the bladder (*circle*) and lower left shows the gas-containing fistula (*circle*). Bottom two images show minimal pericolic fat infiltration.

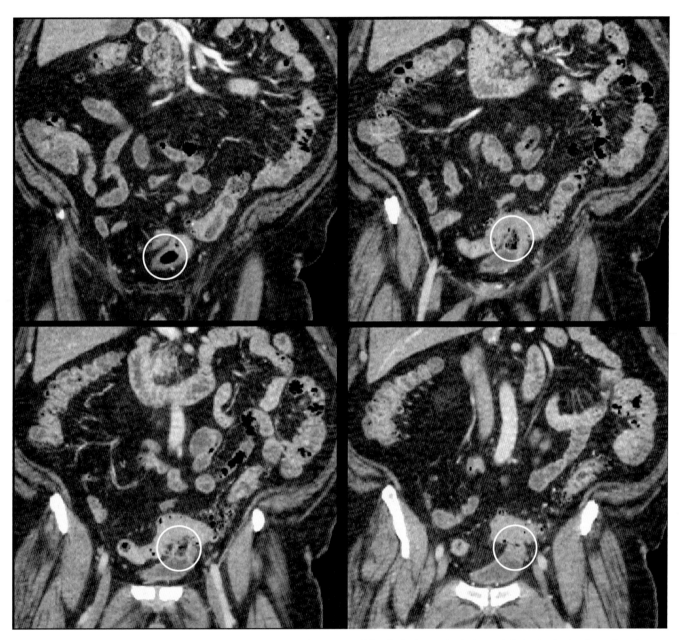

Different case illustrating value of coronal images in display of colovesical fistula findings. Cephalocaudal tile display in the order of top left, top right, bottom left, bottom right. Air in the bladder (*circle top left*), gas-containing mass between bladder and thickened diverticula containing colon (*circles top right and bottom left*), and bladder wall focal mass-like thickening (*circle lower right*).

Answers

1. Absence of intramural gas mitigates against emphysematous cystitis. A colovesical fistula is clearly shown along with gas in the bladder lumen. There is sigmoid wall thickening and diverticula pointing to diverticulitis, which is also statistically the most common cause of colovesical fistula.

2. Fistulas between the bladder and large bowel most often occur due to diverticulitis (65%), GI or GU neoplasms (usually colon carcinoma), or inflammatory bowel disease. Radiation therapy, pelvic surgery, and foreign bodies are less common causes. Infections including tuberculosis and syphilis, common in the past, are now rare causes of colovesical fistula.

3. The clinical presentation of colovesical fistula may include recurrent cystitis, pneumaturia, fecaluria, fever, and abdominal pain.

4. Although CT often fails to demonstrate the fistula itself, other suggestive findings are usually seen:

   1. Intravesicle gas in the absence of recent instrumentation

   2. Focal bladder wall thickening adjacent to a diseased segment of colon

   3. Sigmoid wall thickening and diverticula and extraluminal mass

   4. Pericolic stranding

   5. Oral or rectal contrast in the bladder

5. At least for the first phase scanning should be performed after oral (or rectal) administration of contrast but before intravenous contrast can be excreted into the bladder. Rescanning after active urination and defecation may be useful when a suspected fistula is not demonstrated on the initial scan. Urine specimens obtained after a nondiagnostic CT or barium enema can be centrifuged. Specimen radiograph(s) of the centrifuge tube(s) are performed and if barium is seen precipitating at the bottom of the tube(s), the diagnosis of a fistula is established.

Pearls

- Colovesical fistula causes gas only in the bladder lumen, not within the wall.
- Emphysematous cystitis causes gas in the bladder lumen; there will usually be intramural gas as well.
- CT often fails to demonstrate the fistula itself but other suggestive findings are usually seen: intravesical gas, focal bladder wall thickening adjacent to diseased segment of bowel (usually thickened sigmoid with diverticula), and extraluminal mass. Pericolic stranding may or may not be obvious.
- CT should be performed prior to bladder instrumentation since intravesical gas is a key finding.
- Scanning should be performed after oral (or rectal) administration of contrast but before intravenous contrast can be excreted into the bladder. That way any high-density material in the bladder proves colovesical fistula.
- Since diverticulitis usually involves the sigmoid colon, consequent colovesical fistulas tend to involve the left posterior portion of the bladder.

Suggested Readings

Horton KM, Corl FM, Fishman EK. CT evaluation of the colon: inflammatory disease. *Radiographics*. March-April 2000;20(2):399-418.

Joseph RC, Amendola MA, Artze ME, et al. Genitourinary tract gas: imaging evaluation. *Radiographics*. March 1996;16(2):295-308.

Pickhardt PJ, Bhalla S, Balfe DM. Acquired gastrointestinal fistulas: classification, etiologies, and imaging evaluation. *Radiology*. July 2002;224(1):9-23.

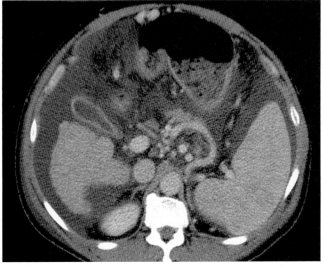
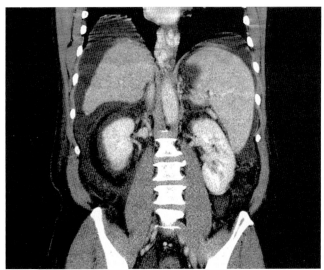
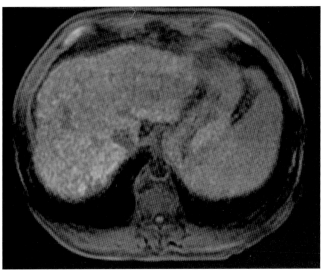
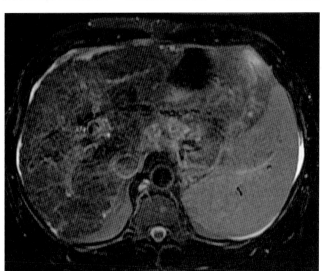

1. What is the most common cause of portal hypertension in Western countries and the correct diagnosis in this case?

2. What is the most accurate sign of liver cirrhosis on ultrasound?

3. What is the specificity of caudate/right lobe ratio >0.65 in detection of liver cirrhosis?

4. What are the signs of portal hypertension on imaging?

5. What is the normal hepatic vein pressure gradient (HVPG)?

Case ranking/difficulty: 🌰

Answers

1. Cirrhosis is the most common cause of portal hypertension in Western countries whereas schistosomiasis is the leading cause of portal hypertension in Africa and portal vein thrombosis the leading cause in India. Only 10% of cases in the West are due to a noncirrhotic etiology.

2. Surface nodularity is the most accurate sign of liver cirrhosis on ultrasound.

3. 100%. However, the sensitivity ranges from 40% to 80%. It is least sensitive in alcoholic cirrhosis and most sensitive in cirrhosis due to hepatitis B.

4. Dilated portal (>13 mm), superior mesenteric (>12 mm) and splenic veins (>11 mm), splenomegaly, ascites, and portosystemic collaterals are signs of portal hypertension.

5. Normal hepatic vein pressure gradient is 1 to 5 mm of Hg; 5 to 9 mm of Hg is subclinical portal hypertension; >10 mm of Hg is clinical portal hypertension; >12 mm of Hg has risk of variceal bleeding. For each 1 mm of Hg increase in HVPG, there is an 11% higher risk of clinical decompensation.

Pearls

- Differentiation of hepatic fat from fibrosis is difficult on sonography: both can show coarse, increased echotexture. MRI is much better at accurate depiction of fatty versus fibrotic liver.
- Notch in the right posterior liver lobe is more common in alcoholic liver cirrhosis.
- Recanalization of paraumbilical vein is only seen in portal hypertension.
- In case of hepatofugal portal flow, the liver is only supplied by the hepatic artery.
- Gamna-Gandy bodies are microhemorrhages within the splenic follicle, a feature of chronic portal hypertension which can be seen in MRI as diffusely scattered low signal foci.

Suggested Readings

Berzigotti A, Seijo S, Reverter E, Bosch J. Assessing portal hypertension in liver diseases. *Expert Rev Gastroenterol Hepatol.* 2013 Feb;7(2):141-155.

Jung KS, Kim SU. Clinical applications of transient elastography. *Clin Mol Hepatol.* 2012 Jun;18(2):163-173.

Poca M, Puente A, Graupera I, Villanueva C. Prognostic markers in patients with cirrhosis and portal hypertension who have not bled. *Dis Markers.* 2011;31(3):147-154.

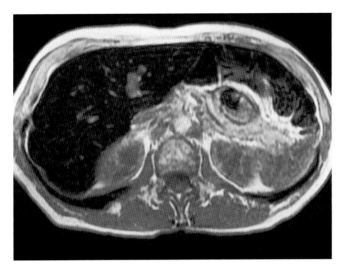 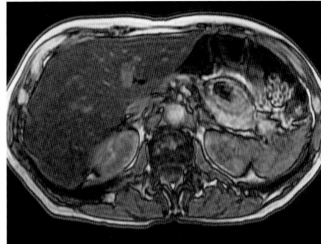

1. What is the diagnosis?

2. Which is most sensitive MRI sequence for detection of hemochromatosis?

3. What are the causes of generalized increased liver density in CT?

4. What is the role of MRI in cases of hereditary hemochromatosis?

5. What are the complications of hereditary hemochromatosis?

Case ranking/difficulty: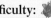

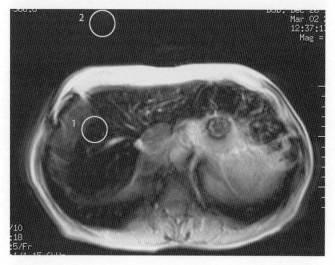

MRI GRE images: measured value of liver and air in different TEs was used to calculate the iron load (*circle*).

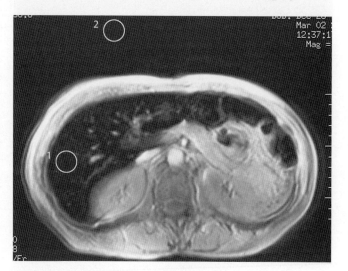

MRI GRE images: measured value of liver and air in different TEs was used to calculate the iron load (*circle*).

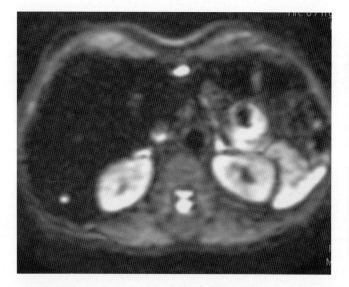

Axial DWI image shows generalized liver signal loss.

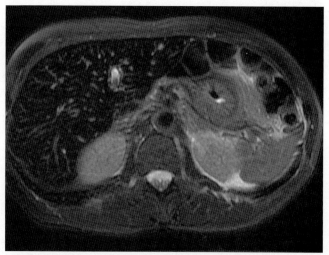

Axial MRI T2W image shows signal loss in liver.

Answers

1. Hereditary hemochromatosis is the best diagnosis to explain the generalized liver signal increase on the out-of-phase image compared to the in-phase image. In hepatic steatosis, there is diffuse signal decrease on the out-of-phase image.

   Heterogeneous signal intensity, nodular liver outline, shrunken liver, and caudate/left lobe hypertrophy would be in favor of cirrhosis of the liver.

   In precirrhotic stage of α1-antitrypsin deficiency, the liver intensity is either normal or heterogeneous; it becomes similar to cirrhosis in later stages.

   In glycogen storage disease, there is enlargement of liver, spleen, and kidneys due to accumulation of glycogen metabolites. There is usually massive hepatomegaly sometimes with steatosis.

2. The signal increase on out-of-phase T1W GRE compared to in-phase T1W GRE is the most sensitive MR method to detect iron overload.

3. Hemochromatosis, Wilson disease, and amiodarone toxicity cause generalized increase in hepatic density. A liver density less than 40 HU or a liver density >10 HU less than the splenic density can be used as criteria for hepatic steatosis.

4. Biochemical tests are used to diagnose this condition, not MRI. For accurate measurement of iron overload liver biopsy is required. MRI can be used for estimating the hepatic iron overload noninvasively to avoid repeated biopsy. MRI is also useful as a screening tool to detect cirrhosis and hepatocellular carcinoma. MR elastography shows promise in quantitating fibrosis.

5. Complications of hemochromatosis are cirrhosis, HCC, diabetes, cardiomyopathy, arthropathy, and impotence. Destruction of endocrine cells in the pancreas leads to diabetes (bronze diabetes). The most common neoplasm in this population is hepatocellular carcinoma. Iron is directly toxic to hepatocytes and causes liver cirrhosis.

Pearls

- Imaging plays a limited role in diagnosis of primary hemochromatosis; MRI is used to estimate the iron load and monitor therapy.
- Biochemical and genetic tests are used for the diagnosis of primary hemochromatosis.
- In primary hemochromatosis, diffuse signal loss occurs first in the liver and then in the pancreas in more advanced cases; in cases of secondary hemochromatosis diffuse signal loss is seen in the liver and the spleen.
- T1W GRE in and out of phase is the most sensitive MRI sequence for detection of iron load.
- MRI quantification of hepatic iron can avoid multiple liver biopsies during the course of treatment.

Suggested Readings

Alústiza JM, Artetxe J, Castiella A, et al. MR quantification of hepatic iron concentration. *Radiology*. February 2004;230(2):479-484.

Emanuele D, Tuason I, Edwards QT. HFE-associated hereditary hemochromatosis: overview of genetics and clinical implications for nurse practitioners in primary care settings. *J Am Assoc Nurse Pract*. March 2014;26(3):113-122.

Queiroz-Andrade M, Blasbalg R, Ortega CD, et al. MR imaging findings of iron overload. *Radiographics*. October 2009;29(6):1575-1589.

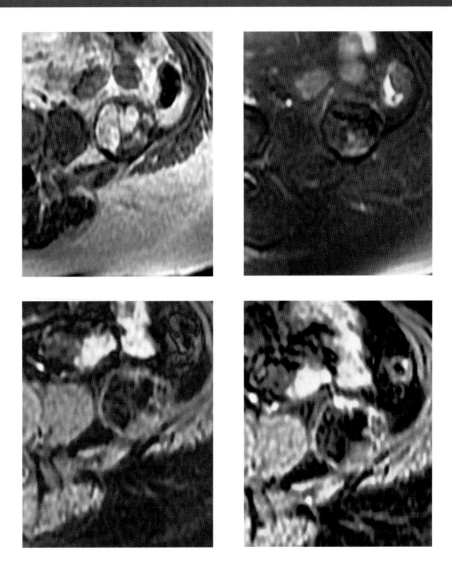

1. What is the most likely diagnosis?

2. What are the radiographic findings of encapsulated fat necrosis?

3. What are the differential diagnoses of this lesion?

4. What is the best treatment for encapsulating fat necrosis?

5. What are the imaging findings of primary omental infarct?

Case ranking/difficulty: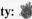

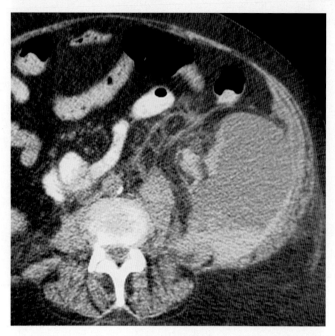

Noncontrast CT performed one-and-a-half years before MRI at the time of fall shows a left retroperitoneal hemorrhage (same patient as first page).

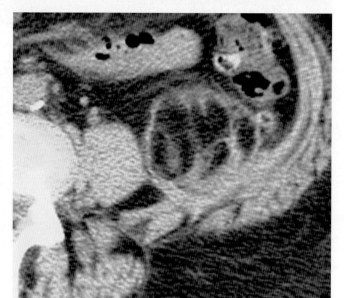

A 3-month follow-up CT after MRI shows a fat density left retroperitoneal mass lesion with intervening soft tissue strands and capsule.

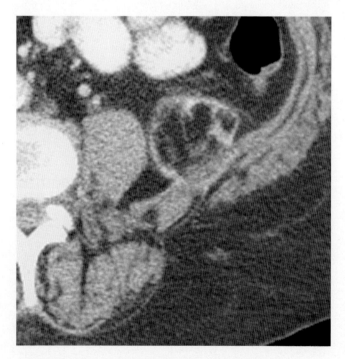

A 6-month follow-up CT after MRI shows interval diminution in size of the left retroperitoneal fat density mass lesion.

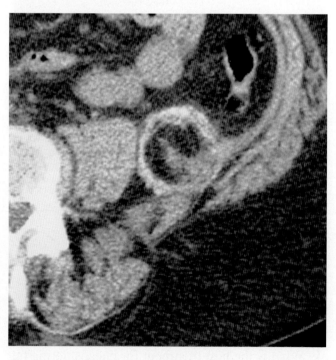

The 6-month follow-up CT after MRI at a different level: Note the peripheral calcification.

Answers

1. Subacute hematoma can show T1 high signal, but no signal suppression on fat sat images. Absence of enhancement makes the liposarcoma least likely and almost exclude the possibility of metastasis and hemangioma.

2. Interval increase in size raises the possibility of liposarcoma. On contrary, the encapsulated fat necrosis will decrease or disappear in subsequent follow-up. Central area of low density due to necrosis is a feature of malignant tumor, but there is central fat density or signal intensity in encapsulated fat necrosis.

3. The descending colon is well seen separately from the lesion. The abscess contains central fluid signal (low on T1W and high on T2W images) with peripheral contrast enhancement. In the absence of enhancement, the possibility of liposarcoma is least likely, but cannot be excluded.

4. It does not need any treatment. It resolves slowly in time.

5. Large fatty mass, right-sided involvement, and normal adjacent colonic wall thickening are the imaging findings of primary omental infarct.

Pearls

- Central globular fat signal intensity and linear marginal fibrous tissue with a history of trauma/surgery is characteristic of encapsulated fat necrosis.
- Other features are absence of contrast enhancement, interval decrease in size, and complete resolution.
- Differential diagnosis of T1 high signal lesion in MR imaging includes lipoma, liposarcoma, hematoma, and hemangioma.

Suggested Readings

Kamaya A, Federle MP, Desser TS. Imaging manifestations of abdominal fat necrosis and its mimics. *Radiographics.* 2011;31(7):2021-2034.

López JA, Saez F, Alejandro Larena J, Capelastegui A, Martín JI, Canteli B. MRI diagnosis and follow-up of subcutaneous fat necrosis. *J Magn Reson Imaging.* 1997;7(5):929-932.

Takao H, Yamahira K, Watanabe T. Encapsulated fat necrosis mimicking abdominal liposarcoma: computed tomography findings. *J Comput Assist Tomogr.* 2004;28(2):193-194.

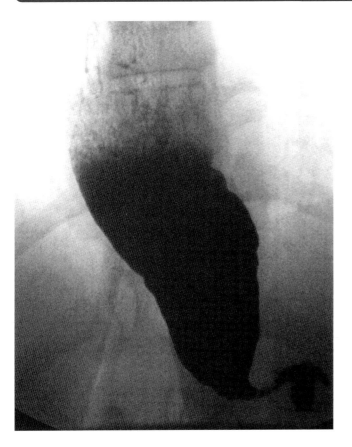 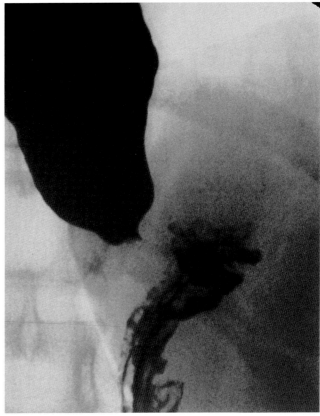

1. What is the most likely diagnosis?

2. What is the gold standard diagnostic test for this condition?

3. What are the radiographic findings of achalasia?

4. What are the possible complications in achalasia?

5. What is the most common symptom of esophageal achalasia?

Case ranking/difficulty:

Category: Esophagus

Answers

1. Reflux esophagitis with stricture is almost always associated with hiatus hernia. Scleroderma shows a wide and patulous gastroesophageal junction unless there is a superimposed stricture. In that case the barium will constantly dribble through as opposed to the start/stop of achalasia.

   Irregular stricture with shouldering is the classical finding in esophageal carcinoma. Even in the absence of these findings the possibility of carcinoma (pseudoachalasia) needs consideration, especially if the disease has its onset in the middle aged to elderly.

2. Manometric study is not only used as a diagnostic test, but also used to evaluate the treatment response. It involves the simultaneous continuous recording of pressure within the esophagus, lower esophageal sphincter, and stomach. Barium swallow is most commonly used initial noninvasive test.

3. Dilated esophagus, air fluid level within the mediastinum on plain radiography, absence of esophageal stripping wave on fluoroscopy, and absence or paucity of air within the stomach. Wide and patulous lower esophageal sphincter is a finding in favor of scleroderma.

4. Aspiration pneumonia, megaesophagus, and carcinoma of the esophagus. The risk of malignancy is 3% (a 50-fold increased risk). Megaesophagus can occur in 10% of cases and may require esophagectomy.

5. Progressive dysphagia is the typical symptom in most of the cases.

Pearls

- Failure of opening of lower esophageal sphincter gives rise to the bird-beak appearance of distal esophagus.
- Absence of primary peristalsis on fluoroscopy.
- The gold standard diagnostic test is the manometric study, which can also be used to evaluate treatment response.
- Normal barium esophagogram cannot exclude the diagnosis of achalasia.
- Endoscopic examination should be done to exclude pseudoachalasia due to malignancy.

Suggested Readings

Campo SM, Zullo A, Scandavini CM, Frezza B, Cerro P, Balducci G. Pseudoachalasia: a peculiar case report and review of the literature. *World J Gastrointest Endosc.* 2013 Sep;5(9):450-454.

O'Neill OM, Johnston BT, Coleman HG. Achalasia: a review of clinical diagnosis, epidemiology, treatment and outcomes. *World J Gastroenterol.* 2013 Sep;19(35): 5806-5812.

Vaezi MF, Pandolfino JE, Vela MF. ACG clinical guideline: diagnosis and management of achalasia. *Am J Gastroenterol.* 2013 Aug;108(8):1238-1249; quiz 1250.

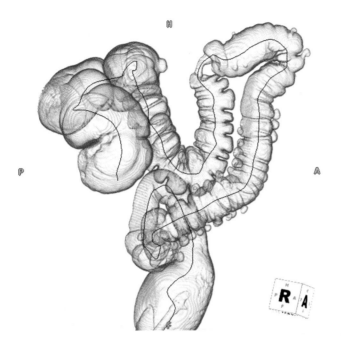

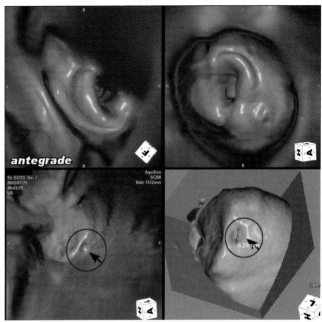

1. What is causing the narrowing of the distal transverse colon?

2. What are the most common and second most common causes of cancer death in the United States?

3. What are the drawbacks of optical colonoscopy for colorectal carcinoma screening?

4. What are the drawbacks of CT colonography for colorectal carcinoma screening?

5. As a cause of luminal narrowing, what favors carcinoma over diverticulitis?

Case ranking/difficulty: 🍂

Category: Colorectum

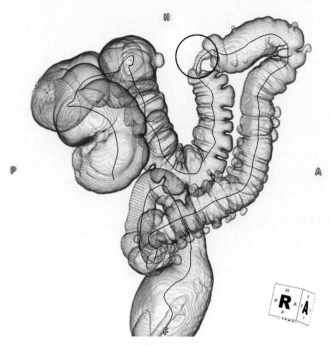

Right side down decubitus BE-like view from CTC shows annular narrowing distal transverse colon (*circle*).

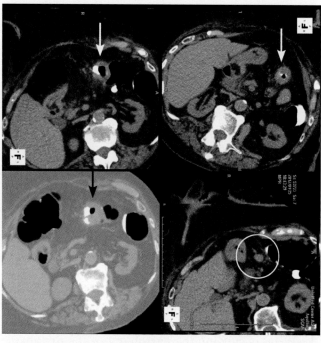

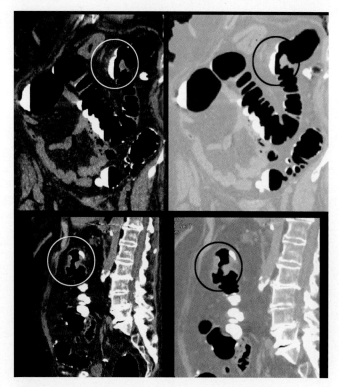

Right down decubitus coronal abdomen and polyp windows, top left and right, respectively, and right down decubitus sagittal abdomen and polyp windows, bottom left and right, respectively, show short segment narrowing, wall thickening, and overhanging edges (*circles*).

Right down decubitus (*top left*) and left down (*top right*) showing an abnormal thick-walled segment of transverse colon (*arrows*) corresponding to narrowed segment. Right down decubitus polyp window at almost the same level (*lower left*) shows the same thick-walled colonic segment (*arrow*). Right down decubitus adjacent slice (*lower right*) shows adenopathy (*circle*) in the gastrohepatic ligament.

Answers

1. The short segment narrowing, wall thickening, mucosal destruction, overhanging edges, and lymphadenopathy all point to the correct diagnosis of colonic carcinoma. The endoluminal views on the prior page are of the entrance to the cancer (top left antegrade, top right retrograde) and also show a small polyp (endoluminal view bottom left and cube view bottom right).

2. Approximately 4.8% of US men and women will be diagnosed with colorectal cancer at some point during their lifetime. Colorectal carcinoma is the second leading cause of US cancer death trailing only lung cancer.

3. Perforation rate is about 1/1000. Splenic rupture after colonoscopy is reported. The need for sedation translates into higher cost, loss of 1 day at work, and need for a driver to accompany the patient. Infections have been transmitted due to improper instrument cleaning.

4. "Prepless" CTC has been studied but is not yet validated. A prep is needed as of now but it is less unpleasant than the optical colonoscopy prep. X-rays are obviously needed but doses are about equivalent to 1 year's background

and patients are not young. Polyps cannot be removed. Detection rate for flat lesions is not really known compared to optical colonoscopy but most can be seen on CTC. Perforation during *screening* CTC is virtually unheard of.

5. Mass effect > fat infiltration favors CA.

Small lymph nodes no help.

Large lymph nodes favor CA.

Absence of diverticula in and adjacent to affected segment almost excludes diverticulitis.

Free air is uncommon in each condition. Any perforation is usually sealed off.

Blood in the stool can be seen in each condition.

Pearls

- Differential diagnosis of luminal narrowing or obstruction at CT colonography:
  - Most important—collapse or narrowing due to underinflation.
  - Needs to be suspected by the technologist or radiologist prior to concluding examination.
- Eliminate underinflation:
  - Inflate more.
  - Get decubitus scans in the appropriate position—air rises.
- Endoluminal view characterization of narrowed/obstructed segments:
  - Often limited as the camera can only show the entrance and exit.
  - As in this case some carcinomas will be obvious.
- 2D MPRs:
  - Wall thickening of carcinoma is usually greater than that of a collapsed segment and mucosal destruction of carcinoma is sometimes obvious.
  - Off-axis "spots" of a narrowed loop due to carcinoma may show an apple core lesion or a semiannular saddle-shaped lesion.
- Adjacent organ ca invading the colon: Source of the luminal narrowing is usually obvious on 2D.
- Diverticulitis (acute or chronic) versus CA:
  - Mass effect > fat infiltration = CA.
  - Small lymph nodes no help.
  - Large lymph nodes = CA.
  - Diverticula in affected segment: Almost required for diverticulitis but does not exclude CA.

Suggested Readings

Cash BD, Riddle MS, Bhattacharya I, et al. CT colonography of a Medicare-aged population: outcomes observed in an analysis of more than 1400 patients. *AJR Am J Roentgenol.* July 2012;199(1):W27-W34.

Hassan C, Pickhardt PJ. Cost-effectiveness of CT colonography. *Radiol Clin North Am.* January 2013;51(1):89-97.

Yee J, Keysor KJ, Kim DH. The time has arrived for national reimbursement of screening CT colonography. *AJR Am J Roentgenol.* July 2013;201(1):73-79.

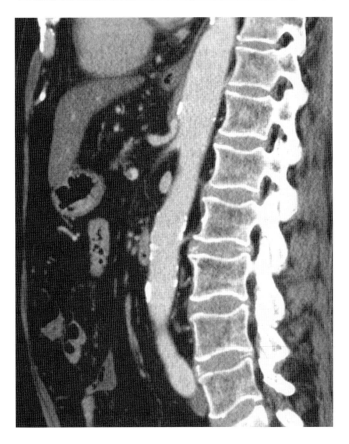 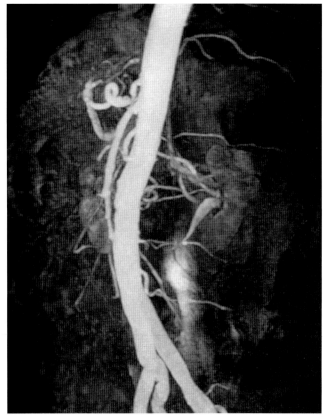

1. Where is the abnormality in the given images?

2. What is the diagnosis?

3. What is the classical triad of median arcuate ligament syndrome?

4. What are the radiological findings in favor of hemodynamically significant vascular compromise?

5. What are the predictors of better surgical treatment outcome?

Case ranking/difficulty: **Category:** Mesentery

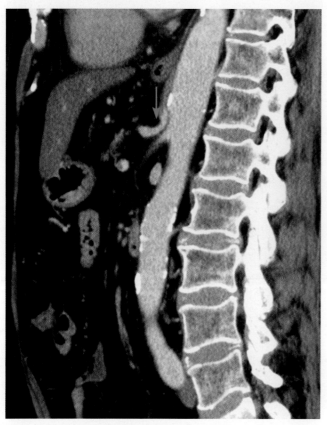

Sagittal reconstructed image of abdomen in portal venous phase shows caudal angulation of the celiac artery with anterior indentation (*green arrow*).

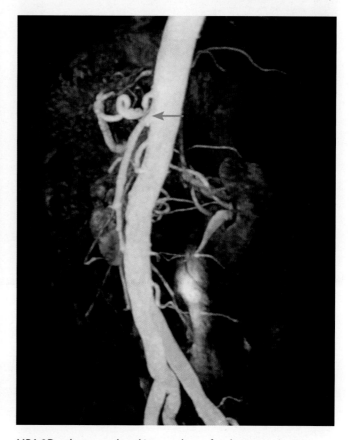

MRA 3D volume rendered image shows focal stenosis (*green arrow*) of the proximal celiac artery with poststenotic dilatation

Answers

1. There is anterior indentation and acute caudal angulation of the celiac artery.

2. Anterior indentation and acute caudal angulation along with poststenotic dilatation of the proximal celiac artery are consistent with median arcuate ligament (MAL) syndrome. Atherosclerotic stenosis is usually seen at the celiac artery origin and is associated with wall calcifications.

3. Postprandial abdominal pain, weight loss, and epigastric abdominal bruit is the triad. Pain is worse after a meal, during exercise, or when leaning forward. The mechanism is thought to be related to foregut vascular ischemia due to stenosis or midgut ischemia due to vascular steal through collaterals. Another possible explanation is irritation or direct compression of the celiac nerve plexus by the median arcuate ligament. Weight loss of more than 20 lb is significant. The celiac artery stenosis causes an epigastric bruit on auscultation.

4. Poststenotic dilatation is a reliable sign of vascular compromise. The prominent collaterals through gastroduodenal artery can be better seen on CTA/MRA than angiography. An anterior indentation over the celiac artery during expiration and caudal angulation of celiac artery can be seen in normal asymptomatic individuals with an anteriorly placed MAL, a normal anatomical variant.

   However, persistence of this impression during inspiration is a significant finding and implies a significant compression. Dynamic flow-related changes during different phases of respiration and changes of posture can be demonstrated on duplex color Doppler sonography.

5. Patients with weight loss more than 20 lb, presence of postprandial abdominal pain, and age 40 to 60 years are likely to have a favorable outcome after surgery.

Pearls

- Median arcuate ligament syndrome (MALS) is a controversial clinical and anatomic entity.
- Anterior indentation of the celiac artery is present in 10% to 24% of asymptomatic individuals. Only a small subset of these patients has a hemodynamically significant compromise.
- Duplex color Doppler US can be used as a diagnostic tool with functional information during different phases of respiration and change of posture.
- CTA/MRA sagittal 3D images are best to assess any indentation, configuration, or stenosis of the celiac artery.
- The goal of treatment is to restore blood flow and remove any compression/irritation over the celiac nerve plexus.

Suggested Readings

Gruber H, Loizides A, Peer S, Gruber I. Ultrasound of the median arcuate ligament syndrome: a new approach to diagnosis. *Med Ultrason*. 2012 Mar;14(1):5-9.

Horton KM, Talamini MA, Fishman EK. Median arcuate ligament syndrome: evaluation with CT angiography. *Radiographics*. 2005;25(5):1177-1182.

van Petersen A, Meerwaldt R, Beuk R, Kolkman J, Geelkerken R. "Re: Management of median arcuate ligament syndrome: a new paradigm." *Ann Vasc Surg*. 2010 Jul;24(5):699-700.

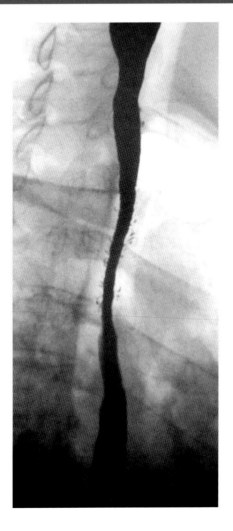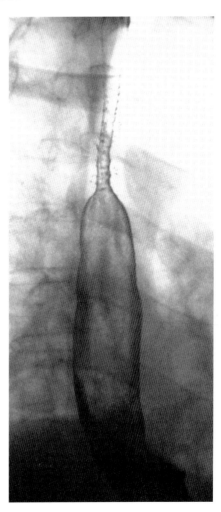

1. What is the most likely diagnosis?

2. What is the most sensitive diagnostic test for intramural pseudodiverticulosis (IMP)?

3. What are the differential diagnoses of upper or midesophageal stricture?

4. What are the conditions associated with IMP?

5. What is the best treatment for stricture associated with IMP?

Case ranking/difficulty:

Category: Esophagus

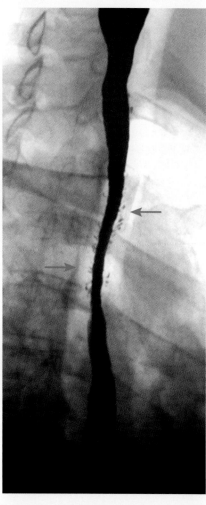

Single-contrast barium esophagogram shows multiple tiny outpouchings in the upper esophageal wall associated with long segmental stenosis, characteristic of esophageal IMP.

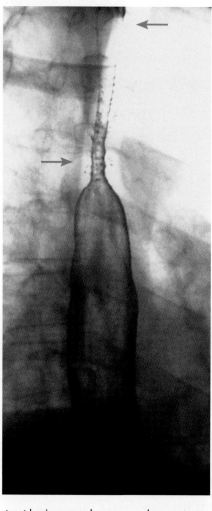

Double-contrast barium esophagogram demonstrates a stricture associated with segmental esophageal intramural pseudodiverticulosis.

Answers

1. Findings are characteristic of esophageal intramural pseudodiverticulosis (IMP). Malignant stricture is typically irregular with shouldering proximally and distally.

   The history is vital in cases of radiation and drug- or caustic substance–induced strictures. The radiation-induced stricture is usually smooth long segmental tapered narrowing at the radiation portal. Most commonly occurs at 4 to 8 months after high-dose radiation (5000 cGy or more).

Drug- or caustic substance–induced strictures are typically at the site of physiological extrinsic compression at aortic arch, left main bronchus, and enlarged left heart chamber. The stricture is usually extremely long and tread-like lumen. In addition, there are associated gastric changes.

Reflux-induced stricture is almost always associated with hiatus hernia (95%). It is typically ring-like narrowing in the distal esophagus and larger than Schatzki ring. In reflux esophagitis, there may be fixed incomplete transverse folds or pseudodiverticula. However, these pseudodiverticula show visible communication with esophageal lumen and much larger than IMP.

Mid- or upper esophageal stricture may be a feature of Barrett esophagus with changes in the distal esophagus. Barrett esophagus is a premalignant condition which need periodic surveillance.

2. Single-contrast barium is the most sensitive test to diagnose IMP and to detect early stricture. Occasionally, CT may demonstrate tiny gas collections within the pseudodiverticula of the thickened esophageal wall.

Endoscopy can identify the opening of pseudodiverticula in only about 20% of cases IMP. Thin, low-density barium used in single contrast can readily fill the pseudodiverticula. Practically, the double contrast can detect only about 1/4 of cases detected in the single-contrast barium study.

3. The differential diagnoses of upper or midesophageal stricture are congenital stenosis, pemphigoid, drug induced, and Barrett esophagus. Schatzki ring is usually seen about few centimeters above the GE junction, but never in the upper or midesophagus.

4. IMP can be associated with diabetes, alcoholism, reflux esophagitis, malignancy, and *Candida albicans*.

5. Balloon dilatation of the stricture. The clinical success rate of balloon dilatation is over 90%. However, the visible pseudodiverticula may persist even after therapy.

Pearls

- Single-contrast barium esophagogram is the most sensitive and diagnostic examination for IMP.
- Radiological findings are almost pathognomonic of this entity.
- IMP is associated with esophageal stricture in the proximal esophagus.
- An esophageal stricture is not always benign, and therefore, some authors recommend periodic surveillance to look for malignancy.

Suggested Readings

Arakawa A, Tsuchigame T, Ohkuma T, Takahashi M. Esophageal intramural pseudodiverticulosis. *AJR Am J Roentgenol*. 1989 Apr;152(4):893.

Attila T, Marcon NE. Esophageal intramural pseudodiverticulosis with food impaction. *Can J Gastroenterol*. 2006 Jan;20(1):37-38.

Eliakim R, Libson E, Rachmilewitz D. Diffuse intramural esophageal pseudodiverticulosis. *J Natl Med Assoc*. 1989 Jan;81(1):93, 96-98.

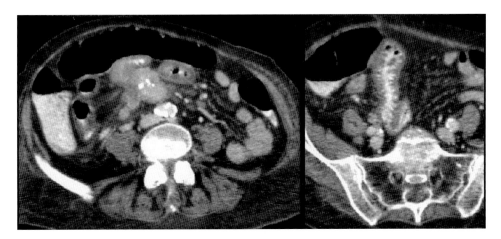

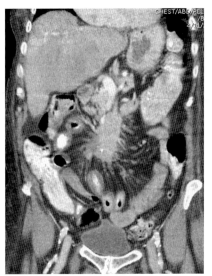

1. Based on the images what is the correct diagnosis?

2. What comprises the carcinoid syndrome?

3. What is the cause of carcinoid syndrome and which patients get it?

4. What is the frequency of calcification on CT and MR of carcinoid metastases in the mesentery?

5. What are good ways of imaging carcinoid liver metastases?

Case ranking/difficulty: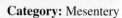

Category: Mesentery

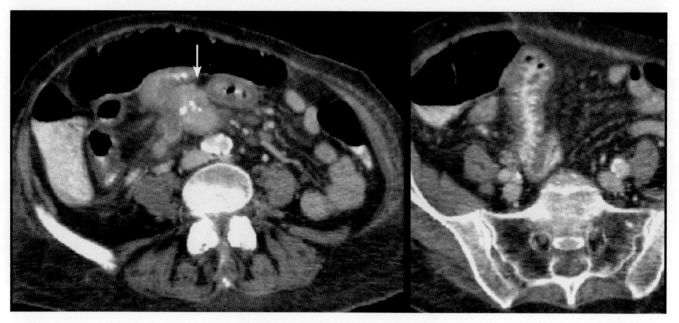

Partially calcified mesenteric mass (*arrow, left*) with adjacent small nodes and adjacent bowel wall thickening. On a more caudal slice (*right*) subjacent marked small bowel wall thickening is shown to advantage as well as mild mesenteric vascular nodular thickening.

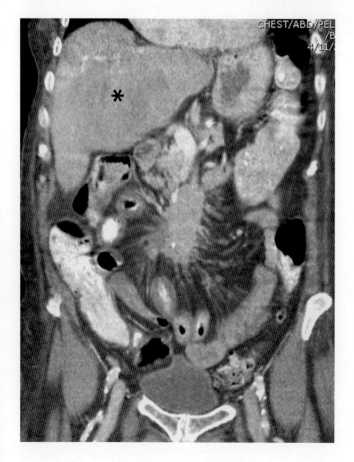

Coronal CT shows large mesenteric mass with a few calcifications. Thickened distorted vessels radiate into it consistent with desmoplasia. Regional bowel loops have thick walls. A large nearly isodense liver metastasis is visible (*asterisk*).

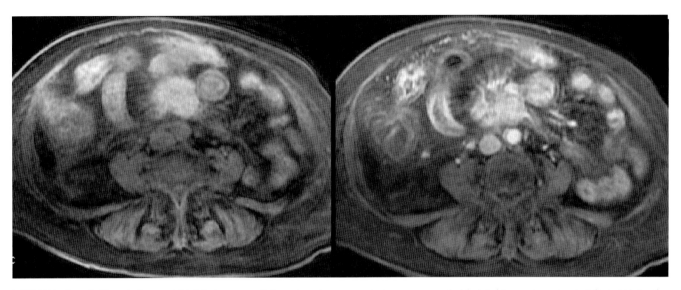

LAVA T1 before (*left*) and after gad (*right*) shows a mildly enhancing mesenteric mass remarkably bright on precontrast. Adjacent bowel is thick walled and mesenteric stranding is seen emanating from the mass on the postcontrast image.

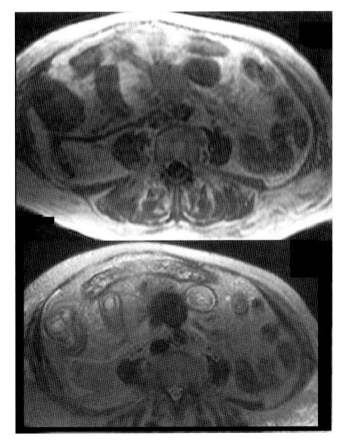

T1 top and SSFSE T2 bottom show a moderate intensity T1 mass with remarkably low signal intensity on T2. Again noted are radiating lines into the mesentery and regional bowel wall thickening.

Answers

1. The calcified mesenteric mass with radiating spicules, vascular distortion, and regionally thickened bowel loops is virtually pathognomonic of carcinoid.

2. Cutaneous flushing, sweating, bronchospasm, colicky abdominal pain, diarrhea, and right-sided cardiac valve fibrosis. Alcohol, stress, and exercise may precipitate/exacerbate symptoms. Fatality after liver metastasis biopsy reported.

3. Carcinoid syndrome affects <10% of patients with carcinoid tumors. Most common in patients with ileal carcinoids and hepatic or retroperitoneal metastases. The cause is vasoactive substances that enter circulation and bypass metabolic degradation in the liver. Carcinoid syndrome is virtually never seen in patients with pulmonary carcinoid tumors.

4. Calcification is detected in 70% of mesenteric lymph node metastases and may be faint and stippled, coarse and dense, or diffuse. This calcification is usually not depicted on MRI.

5. Liver metastases from carcinoid are generally hypervascular and best seen during the arterial phase of intravenous contrast material administration on CT and MRI. Some central necrosis is common. Octreotide scans are sometimes useful for imaging carcinoid tumors and their metastases.

Pearls

- Primary carcinoid tumor:
  - CT and MRI: Small solitary or multifocal primary carcinoids are often not seen; may be identified as small enhancing small bowel submucosal nodules.
  - The primary tumor may also manifest as asymmetric or concentric mural thickening.
  - CT and MRI: Transmural extension is depicted as fibrosis and desmoplasia, concentric mural thickening, and a focal soft-tissue mass of tumor located immediately adjacent to a thickened small intestinal wall.
  - Mesenteric fibrosis retracts, angulates, and kinks the involved intestine, which may cause intestinal obstruction.
  - Hairpin turn: Thickened, distorted segment of small intestine.
  - Mural thickening due to ischemia: low-attenuation circumferential mural thickening, target sign, and halo sign.
- Carcinoid in the mesentery:
  - Carcinoid mesenteric metastases: Enlarged lymph nodes or masses in the mesentery that have well-defined or spiculated, irregular margins, mesenteric retraction, and soft-tissue stranding within the mesentery radiating from the mesenteric mass on CT and MRI.
  - Fibrosis in the mesentery creates a "spoke-wheel" or "sunburst" arrangement of mesenteric vessels.
  - Calcification is depicted by CT in 70% of mesenteric lymph node metastases and may be faint and stippled, coarse and dense, or diffuse. This calcification is rarely seen on MRI.
  - Eventually extensive mesenteric and peritoneal disease produces miliary peritoneal implants, large masses, or mesenteric caking.

Suggested Readings

Horton KM, Lawler LP, Fishman EK. CT findings in sclerosing mesenteritis (panniculitis): spectrum of disease. *Radiographics*. April 2007;23(6):1561-1567.

Levy AD, Rimola J, Mehrotra AK, Sobin LH. From the archives of the AFIP: benign fibrous tumors and tumorlike lesions of the mesentery: radiologic-pathologic correlation. *Radiographics*. April 2007;26(1):245-264.

Martínez-Sapiña Llanas MJ, Ríos Reboredo A, Romay Cousido G, Romero González JA. Severe intestinal ischemia as a presenting feature of metastatic ileal carcinoid tumor: role of MDCT with coronal reformation in the early diagnosis. *Abdom Imaging*. August 2012;37(4):558-560.

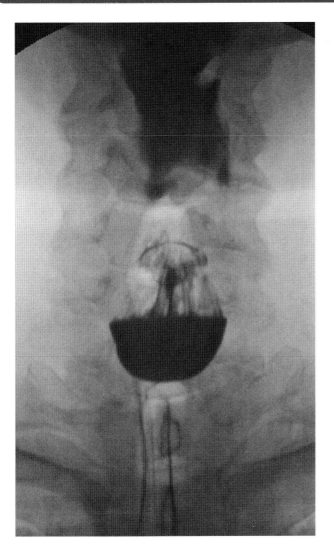 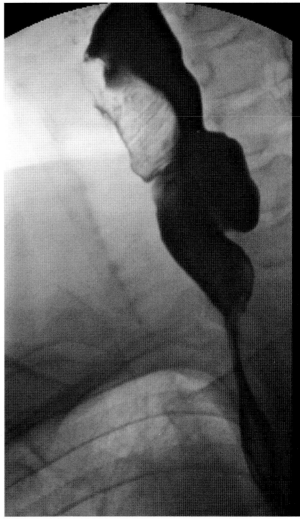

1. What is the diagnosis?

2. What is the best imaging modality for diagnosing the Zenker diverticulum?

3. What is the relationship of Zenker, lateral pharyngeal, and Killian-Jamieson diverticulum to the cricopharyngeal bar?

4. What is the site of weakness through which the Zenker diverticulum protrudes?

5. What are the complications of Zenker diverticulum?

Case ranking/difficulty:

Category: Esophagus

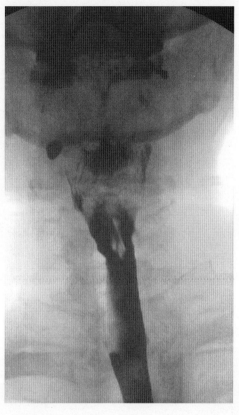

Barium swallow frontal projection demonstrates a lateral cervical diverticulum (different patient).

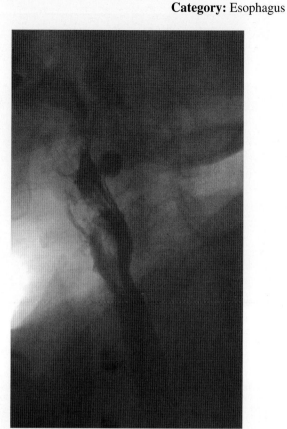

Barium swallow lateral view demonstrates a lateral cervical diverticulum (different patient).

Answers

1. Zenker diverticulum. Killian-Jamieson diverticulum is usually smaller than Zenker diverticulum and mostly asymptomatic. Lateral pharyngeal pouches are protrusions of the lateral pharyngeal wall through the thyrohyoid membrane. When it enlarged, it is called diverticulum.

2. Barium swallow is the best modality for diagnosing the Zenker diverticulum. It can clearly demonstrate the neck of the diverticulum. Additionally, barium swallow is also useful to demonstrate any associated hiatus hernia and gastroesophageal reflux.

3. Zenker diverticulum is above the cricopharyngeal bar. Killian-Jamieson diverticulum is below the cricopharyngeal bar. Lateral pharyngeal diverticulum is a protrusion through the thyrohyoid membrane (above the cricopharyngeus).

4. Between thyropharyngeus and cricopharyngeus of inferior constrictor (Killian triangle). Killian-Jamieson diverticulum arises from the anterolateral wall of esophagus below the upper esophageal sphincter.

5. Aspiration, esophageal obstruction, and rarely, squamous cell carcinoma are complications of Zenker diverticula.

Pearls

- Barium swallow is the diagnostic test for Zenker diverticulum.
- It is a disease of elderly, particularly in the sixth to eighth decade.
- Aspiration and esophageal obstruction are the most common complications; rare chances of malignancy (squamous cell carcinoma).

Suggested Reading

Grant PD, Morgan DE, Scholz FJ, Canon CL. Pharyngeal dysphagia: what the radiologist needs to know. *Curr Probl Diagn Radiol.* 2008 Dec;38(1):17-32.

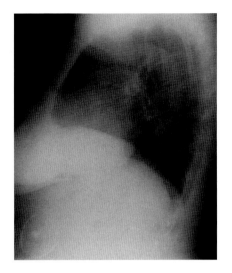
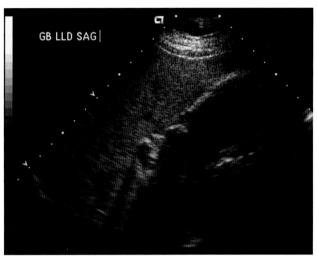

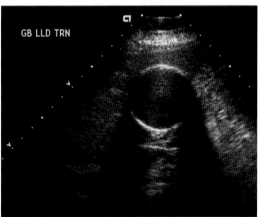

1. What is the best diagnosis based on the images and history?

2. What are the unusual causes of gallbladder wall calcification or high density on CT?

3. The development of what malignancy is associated with porcelain gallbladder?

4. In which portion of the gallbladder does schistosomal gallbladder wall calcification tend to occur?

5. What imaging modality can best help distinguish emphysematous cholecystitis from porcelain gallbladder?

Case ranking/difficulty:

Category: Gallbladder

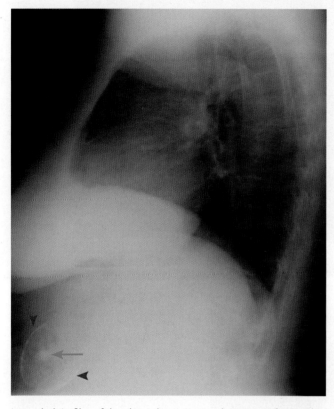

Lateral plain film of the chest shows incomplete circumferential calcification of the wall of the gallbladder (*red arrowheads*) and a calcified stone within the lumen of the gallbladder (*green arrow*).

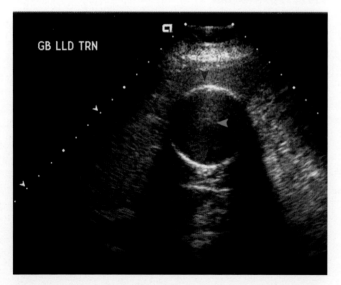

Transverse ultrasound image demonstrates the echogenic wall somewhat more clearly than the sagittal image (*red arrowheads*), and echogenic sludge within the gallbladder lumen (*green arrowhead*).

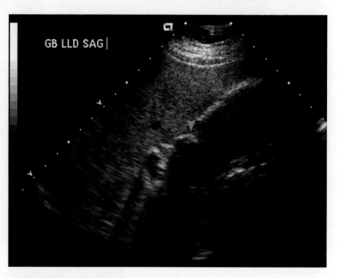

Sagittal ultrasound image shows echogenic wall of the gallbladder (*red arrowhead*) and an echogenic near wall of a gallstone within the gallbladder (*green arrowhead*).

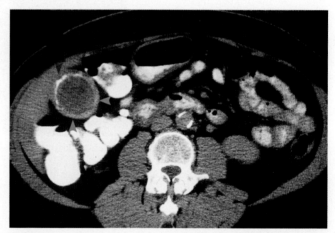

Axial CT from a companion case in a 52-year-old female scanned for left lower quadrant pain incidentally shows incomplete gallbladder wall calcification (*red arrowhead*) with a circumferentially thickened gallbladder wall (*green arrowheads*).

Answers

1. Based on the plain radiograph and ultrasound images the best diagnosis is porcelain gallbladder. Emphysematous cholecystitis could be considered, but the shadowing related to air is usually not as crisp and there may be reverberation artifact. The plain film makes it clear that there are calcifications in the wall of the gallbladder.

2. Porcelain gallbladder itself is likely the result of chronic cholecystitis and chronic bile stasis and obstruction. Unusual causes of calcification include schistosomal infection (at least in the US) and high density on CT can be caused iatrogenically by iodized oil introduced via vessels feeding the gallbladder wall. The other choices listed (hepatitis, acute cholecystitis, and pancreatitis) are not causes of gallbladder wall calcification or high density on CT.

3. Historically, porcelain gallbladder has been reported to carry a significant risk of developing gallbladder carcinoma (12%-61%). More recent studies suggest a weaker, although still present association (7% for a particular pattern of calcification in one study). Some of the decline in the strength of the association may be related to a greater number of cholecystectomies and earlier resection of diseased gallbladders. Essentially all patients with porcelain gallbladder have underlying gallbladder disease and most will proceed to cholecystectomy unless there are contraindications for surgery.

4. Schistosomal calcifications are related to calcified granulomas and tend to occur in the neck of the gallbladder. This can be considered if the patient is from or has traveled to an endemic area.

5. Sometimes it may be difficult to distinguish emphysematous cholecystitis from porcelain gallbladder on ultrasound since in both cases there will be hyperechoic foci seen within the gallbladder wall. With air, the shadowing is usually "dirty," whereas the shadowing is cleaner and sharper with calcifications. The clinical history will also usually be helpful, but CT or plain radiography is recommended if there is ambiguity as this can easily differentiate between the two entities.

Pearls

- Some association with gallbladder carcinoma, although weaker than previously suspected.
- Much more common in females.
- Schistosomal infection and iatrogenically introduced iodized oil are other etiologies of gallbladder wall calcification or high density, respectively.

Suggested Readings

Grand D, Horton KM, Fishman EK. CT of the gallbladder: spectrum of disease. *AJR Am J Roentgenol.* 2004 Jul;183(1):163-170.

Khan ZS, Livingston EH, Huerta S. Reassessing the need for prophylactic surgery in patients with porcelain gallbladder: case series and systematic review of the literature. *Arch Surg.* 2011 Oct;146(10):1143-1147.

Stephen AE, Berger DL. Carcinoma in the porcelain gallbladder: a relationship revisited. *Surgery.* 2001 Jun;129(6):699-703.

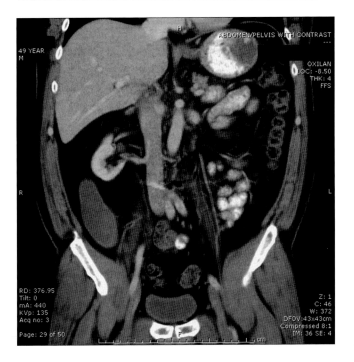
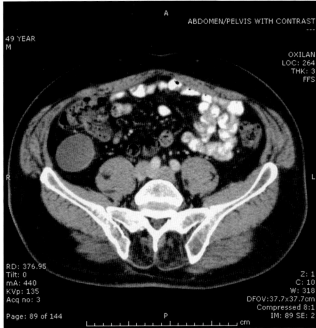

1. What is the best diagnosis?

2. Are most cases of mucocele of the appendix benign or malignant?

3. What imaging and epidemiologic features may suggest the diagnosis?

4. Name several causes of an appendiceal mucocele.

5. What are the possible complications of an appendiceal mucocele?

Case ranking/difficulty:

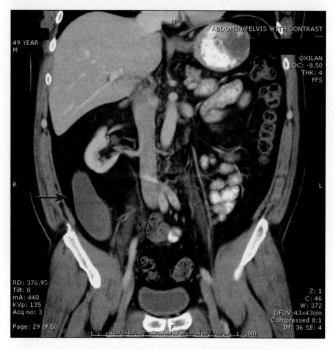

Coronal contrast-enhanced CT demonstrates a long tubular structure filled with relatively homogeneous low-density material within the distal portion of the appendix (*red arrow*). The connection to the appendix is not shown in the image.

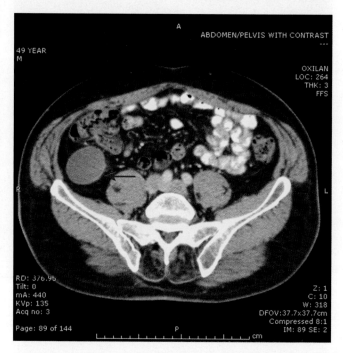

Axial contrast-enhanced CT shows the round structure with sharply defined margins and very little, if any, stranding of the surrounding fat (*red arrow*). The connection to the appendix is not shown.

Answers

1. Mucocele of the appendix is the best diagnosis given the large distended fluid/mucus-filled structure in the right lower quadrant.

   Mucocele is a descriptive term only. The etiology is variable and may be due to overproduction of mucus or due to blockage of the appendix by a mass.

   Some etiologies include cystadenoma, cystadenocarcinoma, carcinoid tumor, adenocarcinoma of the colon, mucous hyperplasia, simple mucocele, and endometriosis.

2. In the series cited, mucous hyperplasia and simple mucocele accounted for 63% of the cases.

3. Mucoceles often develop chronically, and the presentation is atypical for appendicitis. Thus, patients tend to be older (middle aged), and signs of inflammation are often absent.
   However, appendicitis can be a complication of an appendiceal mucocele.

4. Endometriosis, cystadenoma, cystadenocarcinoma, mucous hyperplasia, and adenocarcinoma of the colon have all been described as the cause of an appendiceal

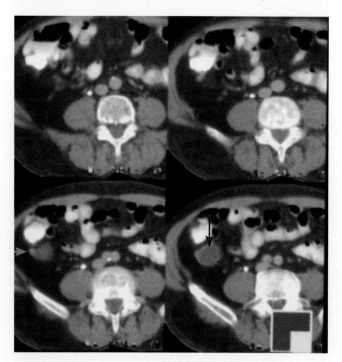

Second case: Contrast-enhanced axial CT collage showing a distended tubular structure in the right lower quadrant containing low-density material (*red arrow*). In this case, there is also a peripheral soft tissue component (*green arrow*).

mucocele. Any process that chronically obstructs the appendix or that results in the overproduction of mucus can cause a mucocele.

5. Appendicitis, pseudomyxoma peritonei, intussusception, and ureteral obstruction are all potential complications of an appendiceal mucocele. Appendicitis results from superinfection and obstruction; pseudomyxoma peritonei is caused by an underlying tumor and seeding of the peritoneal cavity. Intussusception has been described, and the mass effect can cause ureteral obstruction.

Pearls

- Mucocele is a descriptive term referring to the accumulation of material within the appendix.
- Etiology may be benign or malignant.
- May result in pseudomyxoma peritonei.
- Presentation is atypical for appendicitis in that patients are older, often asymptomatic, and there frequently will be no periappendiceal fat stranding or edema.

Suggested Readings

Bartlett C, Manoharan M, Jackson A. Mucocele of the appendix—a diagnostic dilemma: a case report. *J Med Case Rep*. 2007 ;1(1):183.

Pickhardt PJ, Levy AD, Rohrmann CA, Jr., Kende AI. Primary neoplasms of the appendix: radiologic spectrum of disease with pathologic correlation. *Radiographics*. 2003;23(3):645-662. Epub 2003/05/13. doi: 10.1148/rg.233025134.

Ruiz-Tovar J, Teruel DG, Castiñeiras VM, Dehesa AS, Quindós PL, Molina EM. Mucocele of the appendix. *World J Surg*. 2007;31(3):542-548. Epub 2007/02/24. doi: 10.1007/s00268-006-0454-1.

77-year-old male with history of liver disease presenting with acute abdominal pain

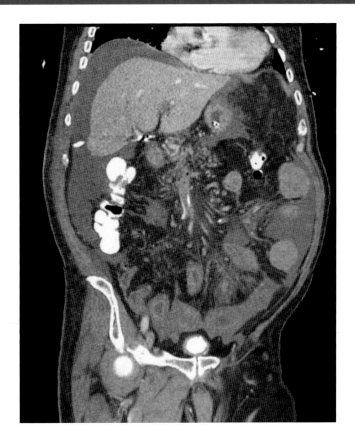

1. What complication of cirrhosis is seen here that explains the presentation?

2. In what percentage of cases is portomesenteric venous gas idiopathic?

3. Among steroid therapy, cytostatic therapy, seizures, ischemia, and COPD, which one is not a benign cause of portal venous gas?

4. Which modalities are the primary recommended modalities for the evaluation of suspected mesenteric ischemia?

5. Among anticoagulation, surgical thrombectomy, percutaneous thrombectomy, thrombolysis and TIPS, which are treatment options of portomesenteric thrombosis?

Case ranking/difficulty: 🔥

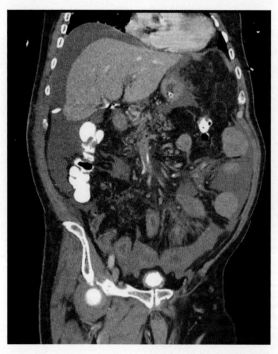

Contrast-enhanced coronal CT shows intermediate-density material within the superior mesenteric vein with tram tracking (one side is the catheter) of contrast around the thrombus and distention of the vein (*red arrow*). Also noted are the interventional catheter and bowel wall thickening.

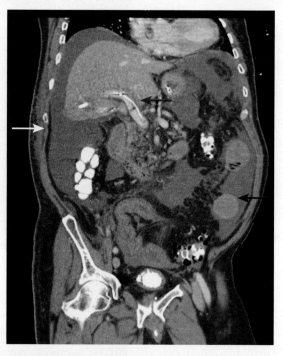

Contrast-enhanced coronal CT shows a percutaneous interventional catheter within the right and main portal veins and extending inferiorly (*red arrow*). There are ascites (*white arrow*), and there is bowel wall thickening (*blue arrow*).

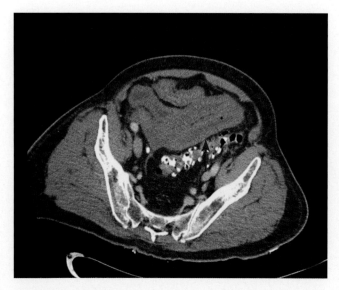

Contrast-enhanced axial CT shows bowel thickening involving the small bowel (*red arrow*).

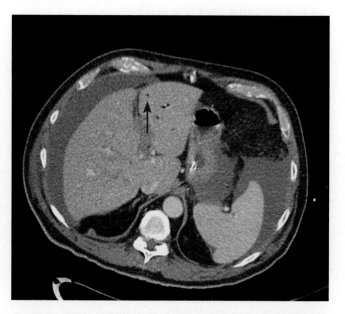

Contrast-enhanced axial CT shows air within the nondependent left lobe of the liver (*red arrow*), extending peripherally within the liver.

Answers

1. There is acute appearing thrombus noted in the superior mesenteric vein with tram tracking of contrast around the thrombus. This is causing bowel wall edema involving the served portion of small bowel and likely accounts for the acute abdominal pain.

2. Portal venous gas can be related to infection, inflammatory change, ischemia, bowel distention, interventional procedures, trauma, and transplantation. In approximately 15% of cases it is thought to be idiopathic, so there are benign causes.

3. All of the choices listed, except for ischemia, have been associated with the finding of portomesenteric gas without bowel complication.

4. MDCT angiography and 3D gadolinium enhanced MR angiography are the preferred modalities for evaluation, although CT may afford a better evaluation of the bowel and superior detection of air.

   Plain radiography is insensitive when compared to CT and MRI for the detection of portomesenteric venous gas and for the evaluation of bowel abnormalities.

   Doppler US is a good modality for the evaluation of the central portal venous system, but it does not evaluate peripheral mesenteric vessels as well, and it is more difficult to evaluate bowel with ultrasound examination.

   Nuclear medicine plays little role in the evaluation of bowel ischemia.

5. All of the answers are correct. A TIPS does not really directly treat the thrombus, but it can increase hepatopetal flow within the portal venous system and therefore indirectly help lyse thrombus. It will also ameliorate the portal hypertension.

Pearls

- Although frequently an ominous finding, portomesenteric gas can be "benign" in approximately 15% of cases.
- Therapies for portomesenteric thrombosis include thrombectomy, thrombolysis, and anticoagulation. A TIPS procedure may also be helpful.
- Cirrhosis represents a significant public health problem in the United States and worldwide, being the 12th leading cause of death in the United States for 2009.
- Major predisposing conditions for portal vein thrombosis include underlying cirrhosis and portal hypertension, hepatic malignancy, hypercoagulable states.

Suggested Readings

Bradbury MS, Kavanagh PV, Bechtold RE, Chen MY, Ott DJ, Regan JD, et al. Mesenteric venous thrombosis: diagnosis and noninvasive imaging. *Radiographics*. 2002 Nov;22(3):527-541.

Hidajat N, Stobbe H, Griesshaber V, Felix R, Schroder RJ. Imaging and radiological interventions of portal vein thrombosis. *Acta Radiol*. 2005 Jul;46(4):336-343.

Sebastià C, Quiroga S, Espin E, Boyé R, Alvarez-Castells A, Armengol M. Portomesenteric vein gas: pathologic mechanisms, CT findings, and prognosis. *Radiographics*. 2000;20(5):1213-1224; discussion 24-6. Epub 2000/09/19. doi: 10.1148/radiographics.20.5.g00se011213.

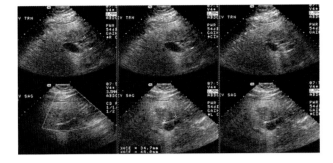

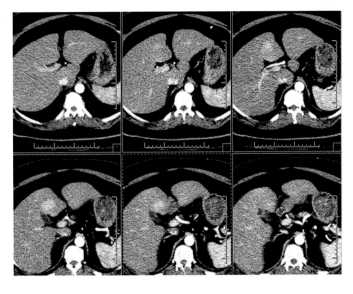

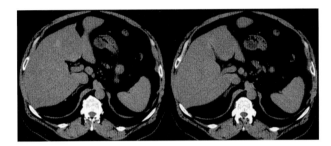

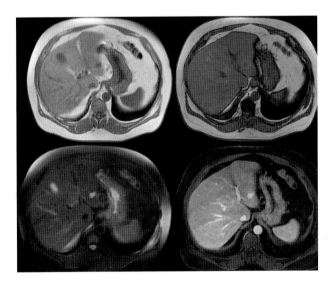

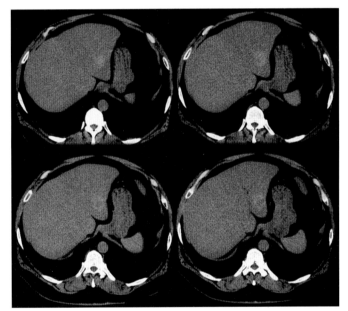

1. Looking at top-left and top-right figures, what is in your differential diagnosis?

2. What is the best test to clinch the correct diagnosis?

3. What is your diagnosis after looking at bottom-left and bottom-right figures?

4. What are the most common places in the liver to get focal sparing?

5. What is another type of focal sparing?

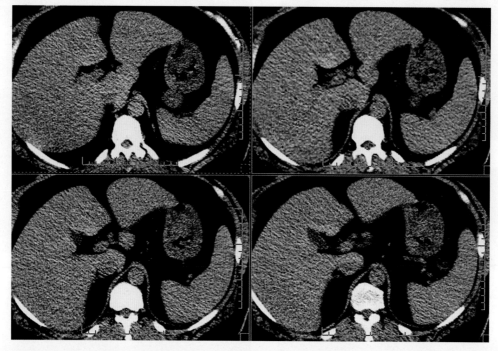

The area in question adjacent to the GB has increased density on noncontrast CT compared to the rest of the liver, which is slightly less dense than the spleen. Therefore, the area in question is not an enhancing mass, rather it is focal sparing in a fatty liver.

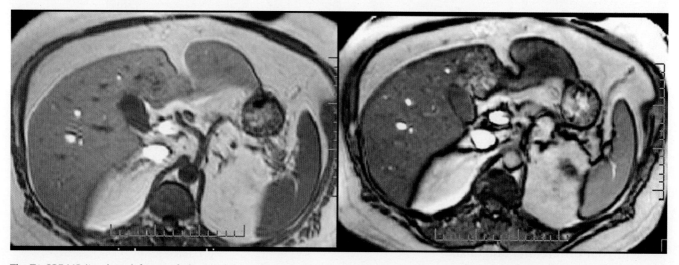

The T1 GRE MR (*in-phase left, out-of-phase right*) proves unequivocally the diagnosis of fatty sparing. The region is isointense in-phase and is the only part of the liver that does not drop in signal on the out-of-phase image.

Answers

1. Focal sparing in hepatic steatosis is the most likely diagnosis. Hemangioma, focal nodular hyperplasia, hepatocellular carcinoma, and hypervascular metastasis are in the differential.

2. By demonstrating a region of no drop out on the out-of-phase images (with the rest of the liver losing signal) that corresponds to the hypoechoic region on US, dense area on CT and hyperintensity on chemical shift MR can clinch the diagnosis of focal sparing. Noncontrast CT will also work.

3. Both the increased density on the unenhanced CT and the failure to drop in signal on the out-of-phase MR are diagnostic of focal sparing.

4. Focal sparing characteristically occurs in the porta hepatis and the gallbladder fossa. Reasons for this

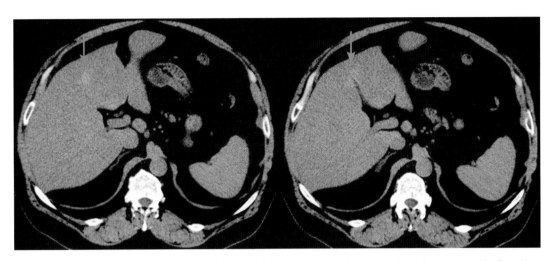

Peritumoral sparing: noncontrast stone CT shows subtle pericholecystic and periportal sparing and a fatty liver.

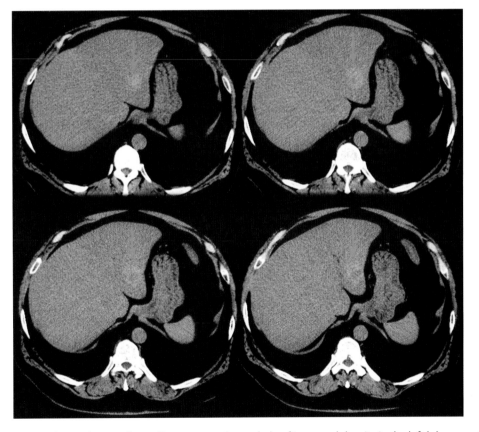

Peritumoral sparing: same patient as Image above. *Green arrows* show a halo of increased density in the left lobe more inferiorly due to peritumoral sparing. The tumor itself is isodense to the fatty liver.

distribution are not known but have been attributed to anomalous venous circulation.

5. Peritumoral sparing of fatty infiltration can occur surrounding focal hepatic mass lesions in patients with hepatic steatosis. It is manifested as a hypoechoic halo on US, a radiodense halo on CT, or a hyperintense halo on out-of-phase chemical shift MRI. This case is peritumoral sparing around a flash hemangioma.

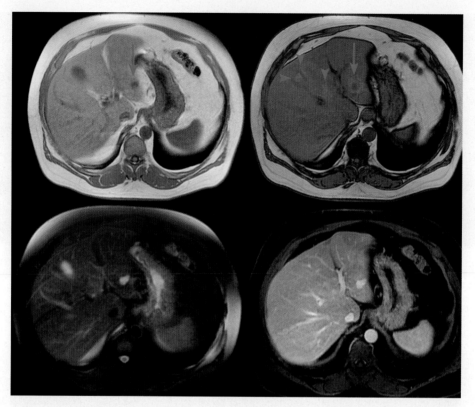

Peritumoral sparing: same patient as in prior set of CT images. Top row: in-phase GRE T1 left, out of phase right. Bottom row: T2 left, early postcontrast T1 right. There is diffuse signal drop on the opposed image except for pericholecystic and periportal sparing (*arrowheads*). The hemangioma (*arrow*) is hypointense on the in-phase image, surrounded by a halo of preservation on the opposed image (*arrow*), very hyperintense on T2, and exhibits flash filling on the early postgadolinium T1.

Pearls

- Imaging findings suggestive of focal sparing rather than true mass are:
  - Echopenic ellipsoid mass adjacent to the gallbladder or porta hepatis.
  - Lack of mass effect on traversing vessels.
  - Density near that of normal liver with the rest of the liver hypodense.
  - Contrast enhancement similar to or less than normal liver.
  - MRI is diagnostic: Focally spared area fails to lose signal on opposed images, remainder of liver does.
- When a radiologist gets used to the appearance of focal sparing on US and CT it not only becomes easy but it actually assists in making the diagnosis of fatty liver.
- An unusual type of focal sparing is peritumoral sparing of fatty infiltration surrounding focal hepatic mass lesions in patients with hepatic steatosis.

Suggested Readings

Bhatnagar G, Sidhu HS, Vardhanabhuti V, Venkatanarasimha N, Cantin P, Dubbins P. The varied sonographic appearances of focal fatty liver disease: review and diagnostic algorithm. *Clin Radiol*. April 2012;67(4):372-379.

Kim KW, Kim MJ, Lee SS, et al. Sparing of fatty infiltration around focal hepatic lesions in patients with hepatic steatosis: sonographic appearance with CT and MRI correlation. *AJR Am J Roentgenol*. April 2008;190(4):1018-1027.

Lawrence DA, Oliva IB, Israel GM. Detection of hepatic steatosis on contrast-enhanced CT images: diagnostic accuracy of identification of areas of presumed focal fatty sparing. *AJR Am J Roentgenol*. July 2012;199(1):44-47.

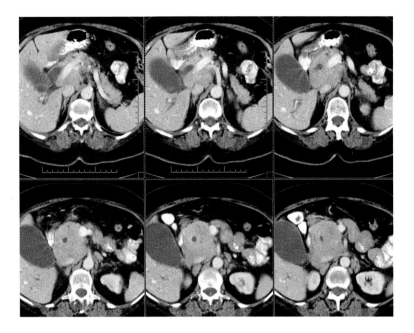

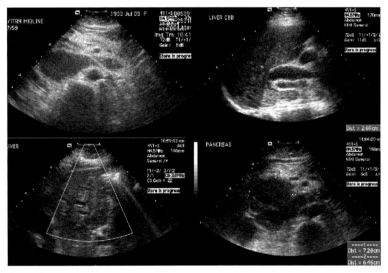

1. What is the most likely diagnosis?

2. Compared to adenocarcinoma of the pancreas, what is the prognosis of pancreatic lymphoma?

3. What imaging features suggest lymphoma rather than carcinoma when there is a mass in the head of the pancreas?

4. What imaging features distinguish pancreatic lymphoma from peripancreatic adenopathy?

5. Second set of images on the answer page are of a 60-year-old man. What are likely diagnoses?

Case ranking/difficulty:

Category: Pancreas

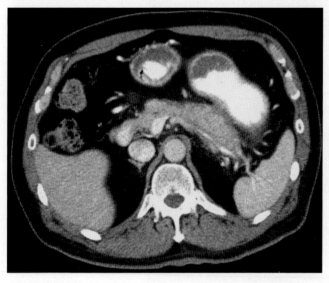

A 60-year-old man with diffuse mild pancreatic swelling and heterogeneity with mild peripancreatic fat infiltration due to pancreatic NHL.

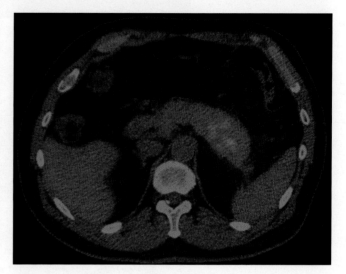

A 60-year-old man with marked diffusely increased pancreatic metabolic activity due to pancreatic NHL.

Answers

1. The large homogeneous pancreatic head mass producing biliary dilatation, no pancreatic duct dilatation, and associated retroperitoneal adenopathy favor pancreatic lymphoma. Carcinoma of the pancreas should be hypodense with upstream pancreatic ductal dilatation. A neuroendocrine tumor should be hyperenhancing. Sarcoid and tuberculosis are possible but unlikely.

2. Chemotherapy and radiation therapy are much more effective treating pancreatic lymphoma than they are in treating pancreatic carcinoma, so the prognosis is much better for lymphoma.

3. A bulky localized tumor in the pancreatic head with CBD dilatation and no or only mild main pancreatic duct (MPD) dilatation is characteristic of lymphoma. CBD dilatation is more common than MPD dilatation in lymphoma.

   Vascular invasion or encasement is more characteristic of carcinoma than lymphoma.

   Neither adenocarcinoma of the pancreas nor untreated pancreatic lymphoma is likely to have intratumoral calcification.

   Pancreatic lymphoma can infiltrate the mesentery, retroperitoneal or upper abdominal organs, and the GI tract.

   Lymphadenopathy below the level of the renal vein is uncommon in pancreatic adenocarcinoma.

4. Anterior displacement of the pancreas and/or an intact fat plane between the pancreas and adjacent disease is

seen in peripancreatic lymphadenopathy distinguishing it from pancreatic lymphoma. Vascular occlusion is seen in neither peripancreatic adenopathy nor pancreatic lymphoma. Common bile duct dilatation can be seen in either.

5. Neuroendocrine tumor is not likely to produce diffuse swelling of the pancreas and mild peripancreatic fat infiltration. The patient was asymptomatic with normal lipase. This eliminates pancreatitis and autoimmune pancreatitis. CBC was normal, making leukemia highly unlikely. This is a case of low-grade follicular B-cell pancreatic lymphoma, diffuse type. Diffuse pancreatic lymphoma has diffuse glandular enlargement and poor definition with infiltration of adjacent fat simulating the appearance of acute pancreatitis on imaging.

Pearls

- Although pancreatic lymphoma represents <0.5% of pancreatic masses, it is treatable so correct diagnosis is important.
- Can encase vessels but does not occlude them.
- Often bulky.
- Pancreatic and biliary ductal dilatation is lesser than seen in a comparably sized adenocarcinoma.
- Two morphologic patterns of pancreatic lymphoma: focal and diffuse forms.

- Focal: In the pancreatic head in 80% with a mean size of 8 cm (range, 2-15 cm). Typically hypoechoic on sonography and uniform low attenuation at CT. MRI shows low SI on T1WI and higher SI than the pancreas but lower SI than fluid on T2WI, and mild contrast enhancement on postgad T1WI.
- Diffuse: Infiltrative, glandular enlargement, and poor definition, infiltration of adjacent fat simulating the appearance of acute pancreatitis on US and CT.
- MR shows low SI on T1- and T2WI and with homogeneous contrast enhancement.
- Clinical differentiating clue: Patients with typical diffuse pancreatic lymphoma that looks like pancreatitis will *not* have pain.

Suggested Readings

Coakley FV, Hanley-Knutson K, Mongan J, Barajas R, Bucknor M, Qayyum A. Pancreatic imaging mimics: part 1, imaging mimics of pancreatic adenocarcinoma. *AJR Am J Roentgenol*. August 2012;199(2):301-308.

Holalkere NS, Soto J. Imaging of miscellaneous pancreatic pathology (trauma, transplant, infections, and deposition). *Radiol Clin North Am*. May 2012;50(3):515-528.

Low G, Panu A, Millo N, Leen E. Multimodality imaging of neoplastic and nonneoplastic solid lesions of the pancreas. *Radiographics*. July-August 2011;31(4):993-1015.

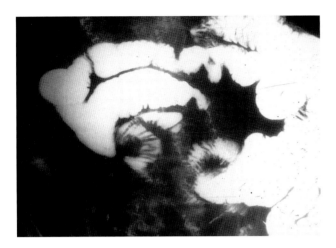 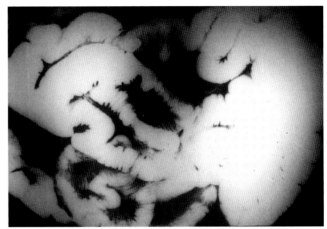

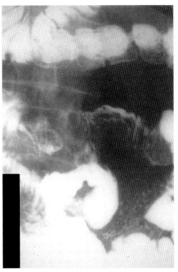

1. What is the most likely diagnosis?

2. Why is surgical resection of bowel lymphoma usually performed before chemotherapy or radiation therapy?

3. What is the most common site of GI tract lymphoma? What is the most common site of lymphoma in the small bowel?

4. Why does lymphoma of the small bowel usually not obstruct?

5. What are the different forms of small bowel lymphoma?

Case ranking/difficulty:

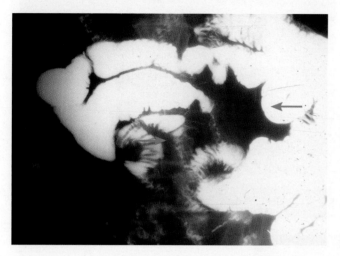

Overhead 1: Some separation of loops centrally which are not well filled.

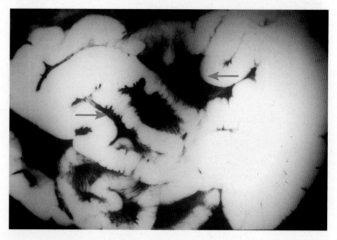

Overhead 2: Despite better filling later in examination these central loops are still separated and distorted, folds mildly thickened but intact (*arrows*). Mesenteric nodal form.

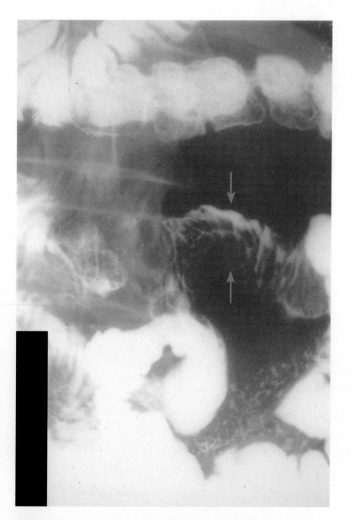

Later in the examination (colon filled) a spot film again shows a distorted loop (*arrows*) with distorted but intact folds.

Answers

1. Separation of loops indicating mesenteric mass and adjacent fold and loop distortion without obstruction are highly suggestive of lymphoma. Bleeding into the bowel wall and mesentery is possible but not likely absent a history of bleeding diathesis or overanticoagulation or trauma. Tuberculosis is possible but not likely. There is insufficient kinking to suggest carcinoid although it is possible. A foreign body perforation with focal inflammatory mesenteric mass is possible but less likely than lymphoma.

2. The bowel wall can be completely replaced by lymphoma so that perforation may occur after response to chemotherapy or radiation therapy.

3. Small bowel is second most frequent site of GI tract involvement by lymphoma after the stomach. The ileum is most common site and the duodenum is the least frequent. The ileum has most lymphoid tissue. Almost all cases of small bowel lymphoma are non-Hodgkin. Most small bowel NHLs are of B-cell origin but most cases of lymphoma complicating celiac disease are of T-cell origin.

4. Obstruction is uncommon because the infiltrating tumor weakens the muscularis propria of the bowel wall and does not elicit a desmoplastic response.

5. Five classic forms: multiple nodules, infiltrating, polypoid, endoexoenteric +/− cavitation or fistula, and invasive mesenteric form with large extraluminal masses.

This has been modified to:

Primary intestinal

Mesenteric nodal

Complicating sprue (celiac disease)

Diffuse nodular

Pearls

- Five classic forms of small bowel lymphoma:
  - Multiple nodules
  - Infiltrating
  - Polypoid
  - Endoexoenteric +/− cavitation or fistula
  - Invasive mesenteric form with large extraluminal masses
- This has been modified to:
  - Primary Intestinal
  - Mesenteric nodal
  - Complicating celiac disease
  - Diffuse nodular

Suggested Readings

Gollub MJ. Imaging of gastrointestinal lymphoma. *Radiol Clin North Am*. March 2008;46(2):287-312, ix.

Johnson PT, Horton KM, Fishman EK. Nonvascular mesenteric disease: utility of multidetector CT with 3D volume rendering. *Radiographics*. 2009;29(3):721-740

Minordi LM, Vecchioli A, Mirk P, Filigrana E, Poloni G, Bonomo L. Multidetector CT in small-bowel neoplasms. *Radiol Med*. October 2007;112(7):1013-1025.

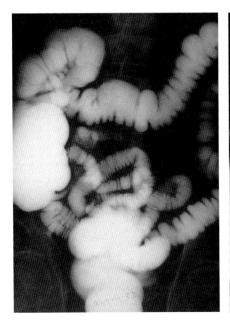 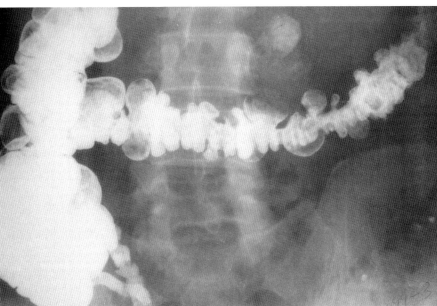

1. What is the most likely diagnosis?

2. What are the UGI/small bowel findings in scleroderma shown in the bottom 2 images on next page?

3. What are the colonic findings in scleroderma?

4. The colon is affected in approximately what percentage of scleroderma patients?

5. What are characteristics of pseudosacculations of scleroderma?

Case ranking/difficulty: **Category:** Colorectum

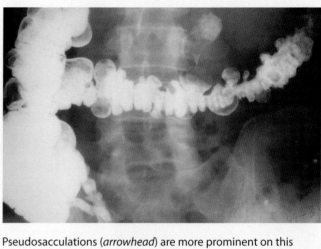

Pseudosacculations (*arrowhead*) are more prominent on this post-evacuation radiograph.

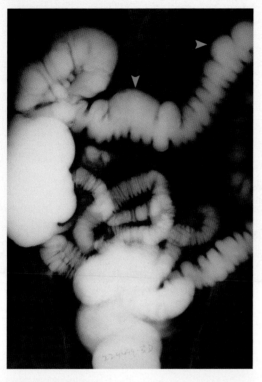

Filled single-contrast barium enema shows multiple transverse colon pseudosacculations (*arrowheads*).

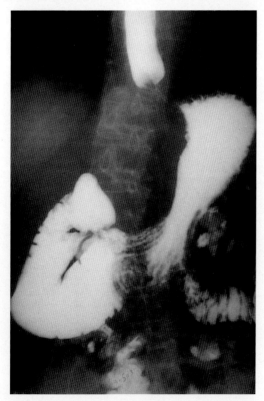

Overhead radiographs from an UGI series show marked duodenal dilatation without obstruction, a typical finding in scleroderma.

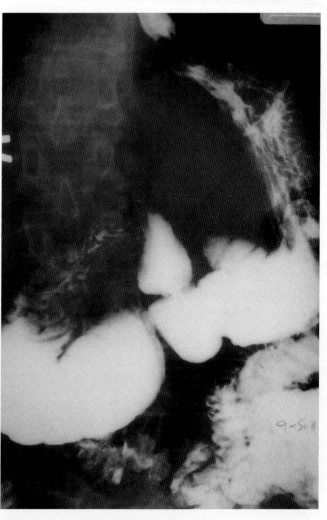

Overhead radiographs from an UGI series show marked duodenal dilatation without obstruction, a typical finding in scleroderma.

Answers

1. Pseudosacculations in the colon are typical of scleroderma. In Crohn colitis or ischemic colitis there should be mucosal disease and/or scarring opposite the pseudosacculation. In intestinal pseudoobstruction there is usually small and large bowel dilatation without pseudosacculation. Cathartic colon exhibits loss of haustration without foreshortening but not pseudosacculation.

2. The bottom 2 images on previous page show a dilated duodenum without obstruction and more barium in the esophagus than is usually seen on UGI overheads consistent with reflux and/or poor clearing of the esophagus. Carcinoma of the GE junction, hidebound small bowel, and malabsorption pattern can be seen in scleroderma but are not shown in these figures.

3. Colonic findings in scleroderma include:

   1) Pseudosacculation

   2) Loss of haustration

   3) Colonic dilatation

   4) Prolonged colonic transit time

   5) Incontinence due to poor sphincter tone

4. The colon is affected in ~40% of scleroderma patients and may cause constipation or diarrhea.

5. The pseudosacculations of scleroderma are not brought about by peristaltic abnormality and are due to muscle atrophy and replacement by collagen. They are wide mouthed, may contain fecaliths, and do not contract on postevacuation films. They are usually antimesenteric.

Pearls

- The colonic pseudosacculations of scleroderma are:
  - Not brought about by peristaltic abnormality
  - Due to muscle atrophy and replacement by collagen
  - Wide mouthed, may contain fecaliths, and do not contract on postevacuation films
  - Usually antimesenteric

Suggested Readings

Martel W, Chang SF, Abell MR. Loss of colonic haustration in progressive systemic sclerosis. *AJR Am J Roentgenol.* April 1976;126(4):704-713.

Sanderson AJ, Elford J, Hayward SJ. Case report: volvulus of the splenic flexure in a patient with systemic sclerosis. *Br J Radiol.* May 1995;68(809):537-539.

Schulte-Brinkmann W, Pöttgen W. [Radiographic symptoms in progressive scleroderma]. *Radiologe.* July 1971;11(7):250-258.

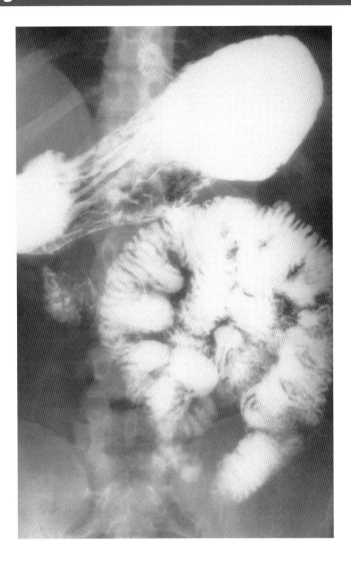

1. What is the most likely diagnosis?

2. What are the complications of scleroderma?

3. What are characteristics of scleroderma
   involvement of the GI tract?

4. How does gastric involvement by scleroderma
   manifest?

5. How does colonic involvement by scleroderma
   manifest?

Case ranking/difficulty: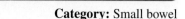

Category: Small bowel

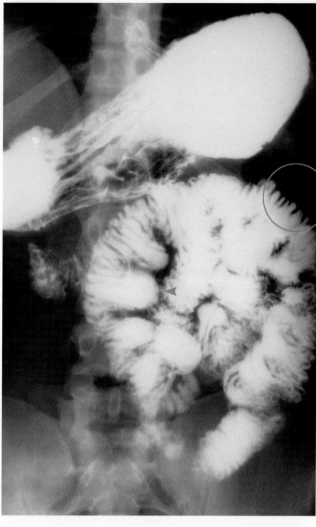

Overhead from a small bowel follow through shows markedly dilated small bowel. There are regions with too many folds per inch, the hidebound small bowel (*circle*). Pseudosacculation on the antimesenteric border is seen as well (*arrowhead*).

Answers

1. The findings of a dilated, hidebound small bowel with pseudosacculation are virtually pathognomonic of scleroderma. This is confirmed by the dilated aperistaltic esophagus. Celiac disease will diminish, not increase, the folds per inch. Neither intestinal pseudoobstruction nor mechanical obstruction will increase folds per inch or cause pseudosacculation. Crohn disease can cause pseudosacculation but not increased folds per inch.

2. The prognosis for patients with diffuse rather than local cutaneous disease generally is worse because of frequent renal, cardiac, and pulmonary involvement.

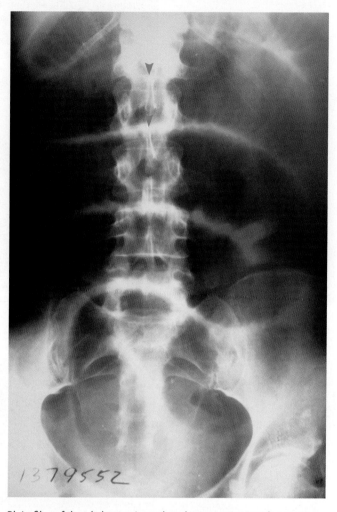

Plain film of the abdomen is a scleroderma patient with nausea. Marked diffuse small bowel dilatation (*arrowheads*) raised the possibility of small bowel obstruction.

3. Although any portion of the gut may be affected, esophageal disease is the most common affecting 50% to 90% of patients with scleroderma. The small bowel is the next most common site of involvement; disease in this region is present in up to 50% of cases. Colonic and gastric findings are less frequent.

4. Gastric manifestations of scleroderma include delayed gastric emptying with or without gastric dilatation and gastric antral vascular ectasia (dilated submucosal capillaries; aka watermelon stomach), which can be a cause of GI bleeding.

5. The colon is affected in ~40% of scleroderma patients and may cause constipation or diarrhea. There can be reduced anal sphincter tone causing incontinence. The colon may be dilated and ahaustral with or without pseudosacculation, and transit time may be prolonged.

Pearls

- The hidebound bowel sign is seen on small bowel series in patients with scleroderma. The sign refers to a decreased separation between normally thick valvulae conniventes despite luminal dilatation (too many folds per inch, normal = 5).
- Scleroderma affects the small bowel in about 50%. Hypomotility from smooth muscle atrophy and fibrosis leads to stasis, dilatation, and pseudoobstruction. Plain film findings of small bowel dilatation and air-fluid levels in patients with scleroderma can require barium studies to exclude mechanical obstruction. Radiographic small bowel findings in scleroderma:
  - Luminal dilatation—reduced peristalsis/delayed transit
  - Smooth mucosal folds
  - Hidebound bowel sign (crowding of folds): thought to be pathognomonic of scleroderma
  - Accordion sign: Well seen evenly spaced mucosal folds in duodenum
  - Pseudosacculation (antimesenteric border)
- Esophageal dysmotility and dilation and gastric dilation with delayed emptying may be present.
- Basilar peripheral predominant interstitial pulmonary fibrosis is a serious, sometimes fatal, complication of scleroderma.

Suggested Readings

Pickhardt PJ. The "hide-bound" bowel sign. *Radiology.* December 1999;213(3):837-838.

Rohrmann CA, Ricci MT, Krishnamurthy S, Schuffler MD. Radiologic and histologic differentiation of neuromuscular disorders of the gastrointestinal tract: visceral myopathies, visceral neuropathies, and progressive systemic sclerosis. *AJR Am J Roentgenol.* November 1984;143(5):933-941.

Shanks MJ, Blane CE, Adler DD, Sullivan DB. Radiographic findings of scleroderma in childhood. *AJR Am J Roentgenol.* October 1983;141(4):657-660.

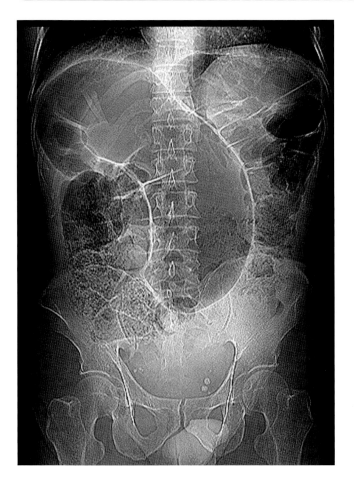 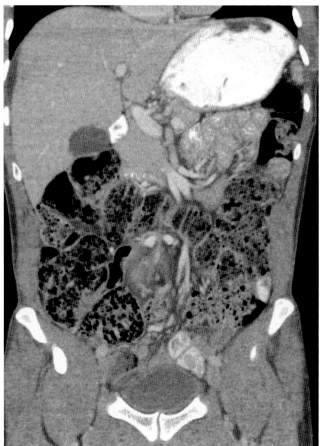

1. What is the best diagnosis?

2. What are the conditions that predispose to sigmoid volvulus?

3. What are some plain film radiographic findings in sigmoid volvulus?

4. What is the differential diagnosis of sigmoid volvulus on plain films?

5. What are the CT findings of sigmoid volvulus?

Case ranking/difficulty:

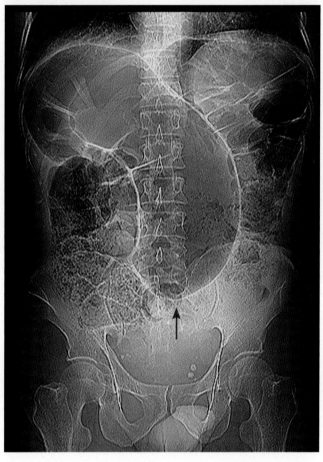

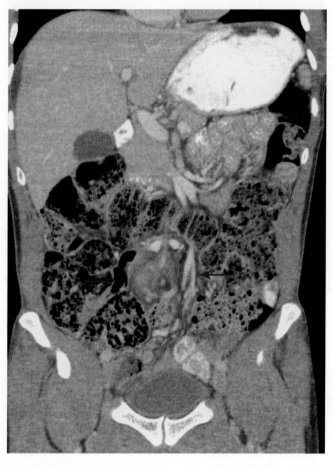

There is a markedly dilated loop of colon (*arrow*) rising out of the pelvis to the RUQ in a coffee bean shape and there is no distal colonic gas. The splenic flexure is dilated. Findings are diagnostic of sigmoid volvulus.

The whirl sign on the coronal CT (*arrows*) confirms the diagnosis of sigmoid volvulus.

Answers

1. The scoutview findings of a markedly dilated loop of colon rising out of the pelvis to the RUQ in a coffee bean shape and absence of distal colonic and rectal gas with splenic flexure dilatation are diagnostic of sigmoid volvulus. The whirl sign on CT with proximal colonic dilatation confirms the diagnosis.

2. Chagas disease, constipation and laxative abuse, pregnancy, neuropsychiatric disorders, and a high fiber diet are risk factors for sigmoid volvulus.

3. Small bowel obstruction is a feature commonly seen in cecal volvulus but rarely in sigmoid volvulus. One or two large air fluid levels on upright or decubitus films, absence of rectal gas, coffee bean–shaped distention of the sigmoid, and proximal colonic dilatation are radiographic findings of sigmoid volvulus.

4. Colonic pseudoobstruction causes colonic dilatation that may look like sigmoid volvulus. Presence of rectal

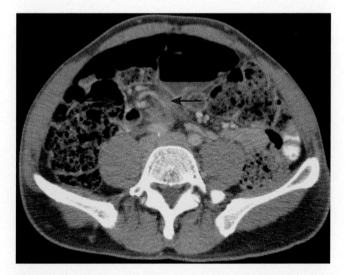

The whirl sign on the axial CT (*arrows*) confirms the diagnosis of sigmoid volvulus.

gas (in the absence of digital rectal examination) favors pseudoobstruction. Cecal volvulus may be confused with sigmoid volvulus. The dilated cecum is often in the LUQ whereas the dilated sigmoid is more likely to be in the RUQ. SBO is more often present in cecal volvulus. Two air-fluid levels are more often seen in sigmoid volvulus. A distended and redundant transverse colon may look like sigmoid volvulus but it does not originate in the pelvis and rectal gas should be present. Ulcerative colitis and small bowel obstruction should not be confused with sigmoid volvulus.

5. CT signs that model the pathophysiologic characteristics of volvulus (X-marks-the-spot sign for more complete twisting and split-wall sign for less severe twisting) may improve diagnostic confidence compared to plain radiography. Inverted U sign refers to the appearance of the distended sigmoid loop and can be seen on plain film as well. The whirl sign is diagnostic of volvulus but not specific to sigmoid volvulus.

Pearl

- Radiographic findings of sigmoid volvulus:
  - Marked distention of an ahaustral sigmoid colon that assumes a coffee bean–like configuration.
  - Air-fluid level may be seen in each segment of dilated bowel on upright and decubitus radiographs. The loop is classically described as pointing to the right upper quadrant but may lie to the left or right of the midline.
  - Single-contrast BE: Abrupt termination of the barium column at the twist in the form of a bird beak.
  - CT signs: (X-marks-the-spot sign for more complete twisting and split-wall sign for less severe twisting) may improve diagnostic confidence compared to plain radiography. The whirl sign is diagnostic of volvulus but not specific to sigmoid volvulus.

Suggested Readings

Levsky JM, Den EI, DuBrow RA, Wolf EL, Rozenblit AM. CT findings of sigmoid volvulus. *AJR Am J Roentgenol.* January 2010;194(1):136-143.

Macari M, Spieler B, Babb J, Pachter HL. Can the location of the CT whirl sign assist in differentiating sigmoid from caecal volvulus? *Clin Radiol.* February 2011;66(2):112-117.

Salati U, McNeill G, Torreggiani WC. The coffee bean sign in sigmoid volvulus. *Radiology.* February 2011;258(2):651-652.

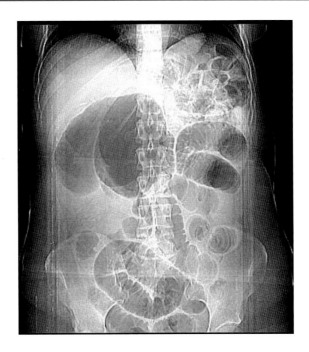

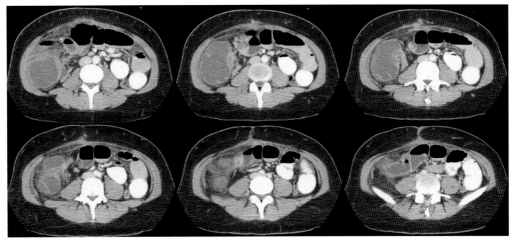

1. What is the most likely diagnosis?

2. What are the types of cecal volvulus?

3. On plain films, where is the dilated cecum located?

4. What are the contraindications to barium enema in patients with suspected cecal volvulus?

5. What are the CT signs of cecal volvulus?

Case ranking/difficulty: 🥦

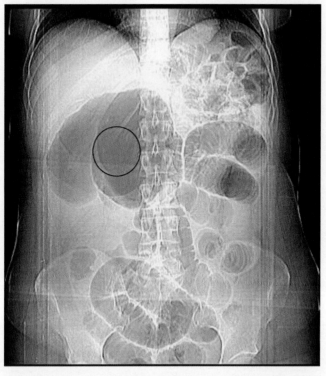

Scout film from a CT scan showing multiple dilated loops of small bowel and a coffee bean–shaped distended cecum (*circle*) in the right upper quadrant.

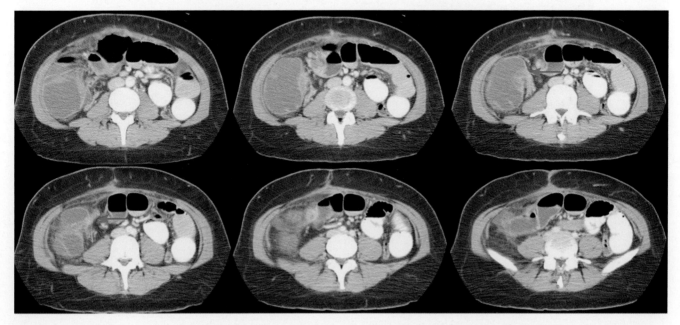

The obstructed dilated small bowel is seen proximal to the dilated cecum. Two transition points (*arrows*) have a characteristic crossing configuration centered on a single point, termed the X-marks-the-spot sign representing a complete winding of the twisted bowel loop limbs onto each other.

Answers

1. The presence of small bowel obstruction, a dilated loop of colon consistent with cecum in the LUQ, empty RLQ, and the "X marks the spot sign" on CT are diagnostic of cecal volvulus. A giant sigmoid diverticulum would not have haustral markings and should not cause SBO. The cecum would be between the stomach and the pancreas if it were herniated through the foramen of Winslow. Sigmoid volvulus is associated with colonic, not small bowel, obstruction. The small bowel would not be dilated in gastric outlet obstruction.

2. The two types of cecal volvulus are axial torsion and cecal bascule.

   Axial torsion, the most common form, involves the development of a twist of 180° to 360° along the longitudinal axis of the ascending colon. The small bowel is usually obstructed. The volvulus is associated with vascular compromise.

   In cecal bascule (up to 1/3 of cecal volvulus) the cecum folds anteromedial to the ascending colon, with the production of a flap-valve occlusion at the site of flexion. This form of torsion occurs in a transverse plane and is associated with marked distention of the cecum, which is often displaced into the center of the abdomen. The ileum may passively twist with the cecum and not be obstructed. A constant feature of cecal bascule is the presence of a constricting band across the ascending colon. Vascular compromise is less common.

3. Typical plain film findings of cecal volvulus are a markedly distended loop of large bowel with its long axis extending from the right lower quadrant to the epigastrium or left upper quadrant. The latter is the most common site to which the cecum is displaced. Small bowel obstruction usually is present.

4. The contraindications for a barium enema are signs and symptoms of peritonitis, rectal bleeding, radiologic signs of gas in the bowel wall, and pneumoperitoneum.

   BE reduction is particularly successful in the rare cecal volvulus that occurs in the postpartum patient; postpartum state is not a contraindication.

5. Cecal volvulus is often a closed-loop obstruction and CT scans characteristically demonstrate a U-shaped distended bowel segment sometimes with signs of ischemia (mural thickening, infiltration of the mesenteric fat, and pneumatosis intestinalis).

   At least one transition point is identified in the majority of cases. In a minority of cases, there are two well-defined transition points.

Most cases with two transition points have a characteristic crossing configuration centered on a single point, termed the X-marks-the-spot sign representing a complete winding of the twisted bowel loop limbs onto each other.

The split-wall appearance of a twisted loop caused by invagination of surrounding pericolic fat is noted in about ½ of patients with cecal volvulus.

The whirl is a well-recognized sign of intestinal volvulus identified in the majority of patients with cecal volvulus. The whirl represents tight torsion of the mesentery that is caused by a twist between the afferent and efferent loops. The whirl sign on CT scans is not specific for cecal volvulus and may also occur in other types of volvulus, including sigmoid volvulus.

Invagination of mesenteric fat into distended bowel is a sign of intussusception.

Pearls

- Cecal volvulus is a misnomer because in most patients the torsion is located in the ascending colon above the ileocecal valve.
- Two types of cecal volvulus are described: axial torsion type (2/3) and the cecal bascule type (1/3).
- Axial torsion, the most common form of volvulus, occurs with the development of a twist of 180° to 360° along the longitudinal axis of the ascending colon. The obstructive process is associated with vascular compromise.
- In the cecal bascule type of volvulus, the cecum folds anteromedial to the ascending colon, with the production of a flap-valve occlusion at the site of flexion. Vascular compromise is less common.
- Plain film: Typically a markedly distended loop of large bowel with its long axis extending from the right lower quadrant to the epigastrium or left upper quadrant, the most common site to which the cecum is displaced. Accompanying SBO usually present.
- BE: Bird-beak obstruction.
- CT: X-marks-the-spot sign, whirl sign.

Suggested Readings

Macari M, Spieler B, Babb J, Pachter HL. Can the location of the CT whirl sign assist in differentiating sigmoid from caecal volvulus? *Clin Radiol.* February 2011;66(2):112-117.

Rosenblat JM, Rozenblit AM, Wolf EL, DuBrow RA, Den EI, Levsky JM. Findings of cecal volvulus at CT. *Radiology.* July 2010;256(1):169-175.

Salati U, McNeill G, Torreggiani WC. The coffee bean sign in sigmoid volvulus. *Radiology.* February 2011;258(2):651-652.

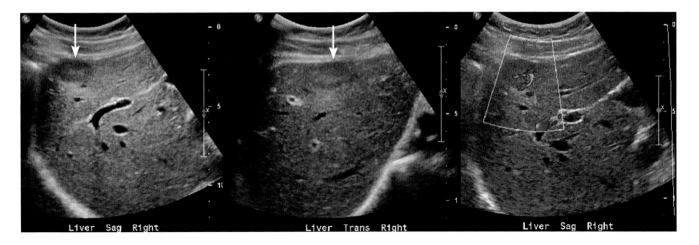

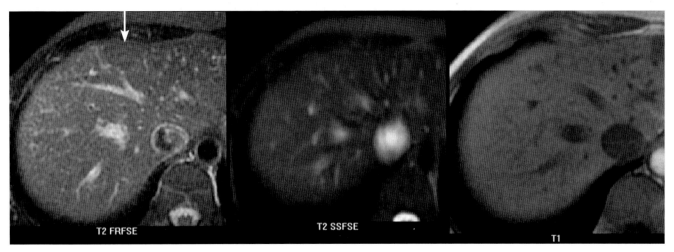

1. Based on the gray scale and color Doppler examination (top figure), what is the most likely diagnosis and why?

2. Based on the bottom figure of the first page of this case and the images on the second page of this case, what diagnosis is certain?

3. What are the histologic components of focal nodular hyperplasia (FNH)?

4. What are the characteristics of FNH on noncontrast MRI?

5. What are the characteristics of FNH on sulfur colloid and hepatobiliary nuclear medicine examinations?

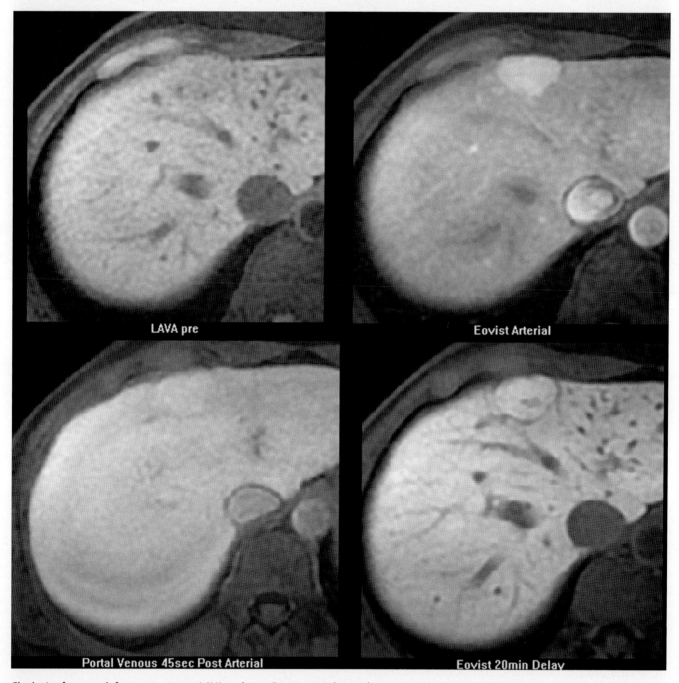

Clockwise from top left are precontrast LAVA and post-Eovist arterial, portal venous, and 20-minute delay images. The mass is barely visible before contrast, enhances briskly in the arterial phase, is nearly isointense in the portal venous phase, and is enhanced in the hepatogram phase except for an unenhanced central scar and capsule.

Answers

1. There is a suggestion of a central echogenic scar and there is peripheral curvilinear vascularity with radiation toward the center—a partial spokewheel. These findings are most compatible with FNH. Hemangiomas are usually not hypoechoic although they can be. The spokewheel vascular pattern is not common in adenomas. The patient's age is against fibrolamellar carcinoma. The lack of cirrhosis speaks against HCC.

2. The appearance on the 20-minute delayed post-Eovist scan of a slightly hyperintense mass with a central scar is pathognomonic for focal nodular hyperplasia.

3. FNH is a polyclonal proliferation of hepatocytes, Kupffer cells, vascular structures, and biliary ductules. However, there is no connection to the biliary tree since no bile ducts are formed. It has a complex architecture, with well-differentiated hepatocytes forming nodules subdivided by fibrous septa. The latter coalesce to form a characteristic central stellate vascular scar.

4. FNH is usually homogeneous and nearly isointense on both T1- and T2-weighted images. If visible the scar is usually hypointense on T1WI and hyperintense on T2WI due to its watery myxomatous tissue.

5. Sulfur colloid imaging: Normal uptake in 60% to 75% of FNH due to the presence of Kupffer cells. Remaining FNH show either increased or decreased radionuclide accumulation compared to normal liver. Normal or increased uptake distinguishes FNH from hepatic adenoma and malignant liver masses.

   Hepatobiliary scintigraphy: Increased uptake with delayed excretion is shown in 90% of FNH due to uptake by functioning hepatocytes and excretion since intratumoral biliary ductules do not communicate normally with larger ducts.

Pearls

- FNH appears similar to normal liver on imaging and may be inapparent except for mass effect on adjacent structures.
- The central scar often aids mass identification on US or unenhanced CT or MRI.
- Feeding vessels from the hepatic artery cause arterial phase contrast enhancement greater than that of normal liver.
- The scar, composed of myxomatous stroma, often demonstrates some delayed enhancement with renally excreted gadolinium.
- On delayed hepatocyte phase imaging with hepatobiliary MR agents FNHs may be:
  - Homogeneously hyperintense
  - Hyperintense with scattered 1 to 5 mm areas of diminished signal
  - Isointense and visible due to mass effect and/or central scar
  - Nonenhancing, spherical center surrounded by a thin peripheral rim of high signal intensity
- A hypointense scar (sometimes with hypointense septa) is usually visible and almost always so if the FNH is >3 cm.

Suggested Readings

Adeyiga AO, Lee EY, Eisenberg RL. Focal hepatic masses in pediatric patients. *AJR Am J Roentgenol*. October 2012;199(4):W422-W440.

Grieser C, Steffen IG, Seehofer D, et al. Histopathologically confirmed focal nodular hyperplasia of the liver: gadoxetic acid-enhanced MRI characteristics. *Magn Reson Imaging*. June 2013;31(5):755-760.

Kim MJ, Rhee HJ, Jeong HT. Hyperintense lesions on gadoxetate disodium-enhanced hepatobiliary phase imaging. *AJR Am J Roentgenol*. November 2012;199(5):W575-W586.

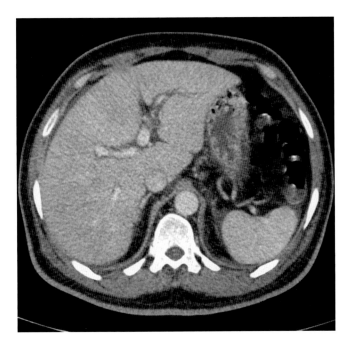 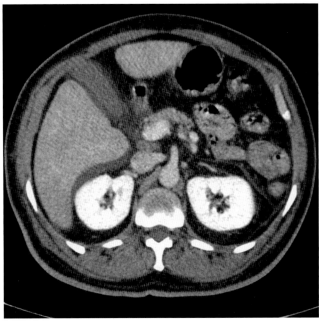

1. What is in your differential diagnosis?

2. What symptoms or signs may be present in acute viral hepatitis?

3. What types of viral acute hepatitis may progress to chronic?

4. What drugs can cause acute hepatitis?

5. What diseases can produce imaging findings similar to acute viral hepatitis?

Case ranking/difficulty: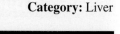

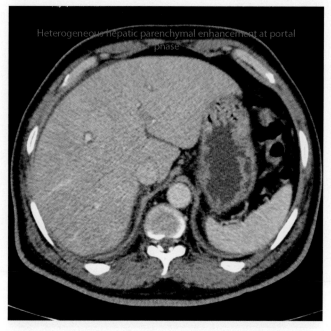

Heterogeneous hepatic parenchymal enhancement at portal phase.

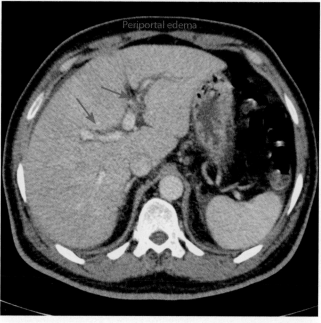

Periportal edema presented by hypodense cuffing (*arrow*) of the portal vein trunk and branches.

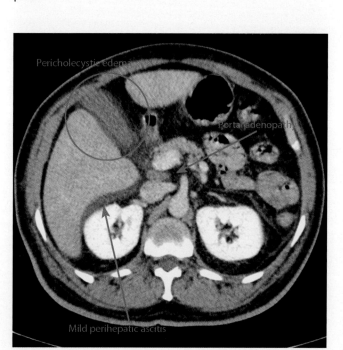

Additional findings including mild perihepatic ascites, pericholecystic edema, and portal adenopathy (*arrow* and *circle*).

Answers

1. Differential might include sarcoid, lymphoma, acute hepatitis, and passive congestion. Sarcoid can infiltrate the liver usually accompanied by splenomegaly and periportal adenopathy. The above are true of lymphoma as well so sarcoid and lymphoma are unlikely but possible. Vigorous rehydration in the ER can cause periportal edema but not hepatomegaly and ascites. Both acute hepatitis and congestive heart failure can enlarge the liver and cause heterogeneous diminished parenchymal enhancement and periportal edema. The correct diagnosis of acute viral hepatitis was made clinically.

2. Loss of appetite, aversion to smoking, splenomegaly, lymphadenopathy, and tender hepatomegaly may be present in acute hepatitis.

3. Hepatitis A does not cause chronic hepatitis. Hepatitis B, C, D, and E do.

4. Acetaminophen, isoniazid, NSAIDs, allopurinol, and oral contraceptives are some of the drugs that can cause acute hepatitis.

5. Alcoholic hepatitis, veno-occlusive disease, and ischemic hepatitis are correct. Wilson disease and α1-antitrypsin disease are causes of chronic, not acute, hepatitis.

Pearls

- There are no imaging signs specific for acute viral hepatitis. Differential diagnosis includes passive congestion, veno-occlusive diseases, and infiltrative diseases such as granulomatous disease and lymphoma.
- US findings: Parenchymal heterogeneity and mild hepatomegaly, accentuation of the portal triads, multilayered GB wall thickening, and GB contraction.
- CT and MRI: Periportal edema, and heterogeneous diminished arterial phase perfusion resolving or improving in the portal phase.
- All modalities commonly show mild ascites and periportal adenopathy.

Suggested Readings

Cakir B, Kirbas I, Demirhan B, et al. Fulminant hepatic failure in children: etiology, histopathology and MDCT findings. *Eur J Radiol*. November 2009;72(2):327-334.

Kim SW, Shin HC, Kim IY. Diffuse pattern of transient hepatic attenuation differences in viral hepatitis: a sign of acute hepatic injury in patients without cirrhosis. *J Comput Assist Tomogr*. March 3, 2011;34(5):699-705.

Suk KT, Kim CH, Baik SK, et al. Gallbladder wall thickening in patients with acute hepatitis. *J Clin Ultrasound*. March 3, 2011;37(3):144-148.

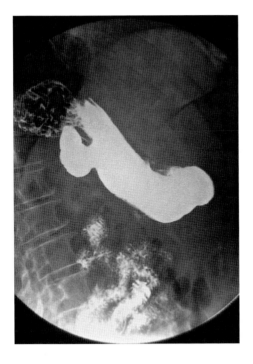
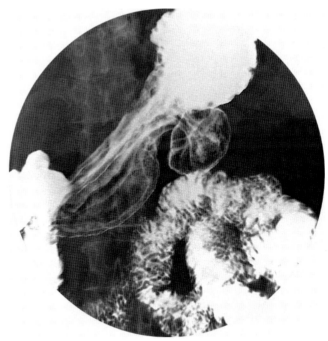

1. What is the most likely diagnosis?

2. What are the possible signs and symptoms of gastric diverticula?

3. What are the features of gastric diverticulum on a UGI series?

4. What are the features of other types of gastric diverticula?

5. What can gastric diverticula be confused with on CT or MRI, especially without oral contrast?

Case ranking/difficulty:

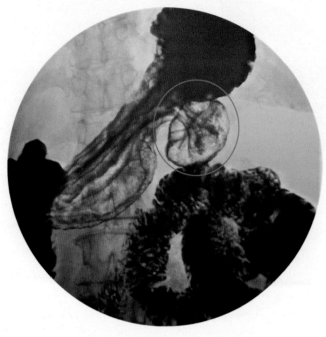

AP inverted double-contrast film shows normal gastric folds extending from the stomach into the diverticulum (*circle*).

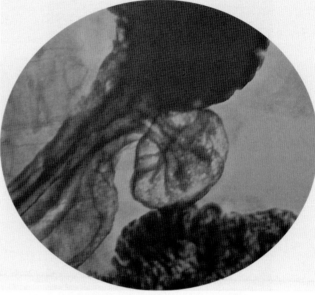

Magnification of image on the left.

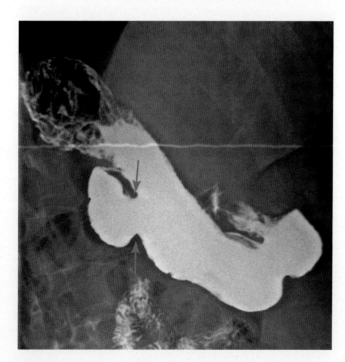

Steep oblique view delineating the neck of the diverticulum (*arrows*).

Answers

1. This is a pretty classic appearance for gastric diverticulum, maybe a little further south of the GE junction than usual. Normal folds and mucosa exclude ulcer; lack of any mass or wall thickening excludes carcinoma and leiomyosarcoma.

2. Food rarely collects within a gastric diverticulum. Occasionally, bleeding and/or ulceration may occur. Carcinoma is rare within a gastric diverticulum but can occur. Most are asymptomatic.

3. On upper GI series, changes in the size and configuration of the diverticulum will be observed. Identification of mucosal folds and a neck communicating with the rest of the stomach suggest the diagnosis.

4. A partial gastric diverticulum is a very rare (0.5% of population) protrusion of mucosa into the muscular wall of the stomach. Most are along greater curvature of the antrum. Their neck is narrow and they change shape during fluoroscopy. Partial gastric diverticula are difficult to differentiate from penetrating ulcer and ectopic pancreas.

   Intramural/intraluminal gastric diverticula were reported but are probably nonexistent and "caused" by poor mixing of barium and retained secretions.

5. Gastric diverticula can be confused with solid or cystic adrenal masses, gastric masses, gastric ulcers, or abscesses on CT or MR. Gastric diverticula are correctly diagnosed on CT or MR when they fill with gas and/or oral contrast and show no central enhancement.

Pearls

- Gastric diverticula are generally asymptomatic incidental findings, although bleeding sometimes occurs.
- Gastric diverticula can be confused with solid or cystic adrenal masses, gastric masses, gastric ulcers, or abscesses on CT or MR. Gastric diverticula are correctly diagnosed on CT or MR when they fill with gas and/or oral contrast and show no central enhancement.

Suggested Readings

Chaulin B, Damoo B, Verdeil C, Laurent F, Drouillard J.[Gastric diverticulum mimicking adrenal mass. X-ray computed tomographic aspect]. *J Radiol*. October 1992;73(6-7):389-393.

Gokan T, Ohgiya Y, Nobusawa H, Munechika H. Commonly encountered adrenal pseudotumours on CT. *Br J Radiol*. February 2005;78(926):170-174.

Silverman PM. Gastric diverticulum mimicking adrenal mass: CT demonstration. *J Comput Assist Tomogr*. September 1989;10(4):709-710.

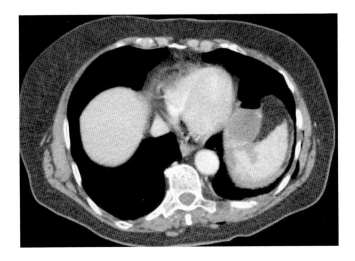
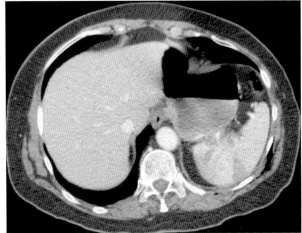
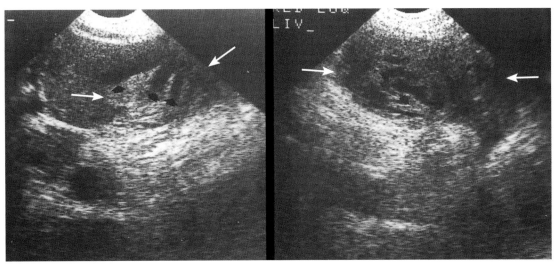

1. What is the most likely diagnosis based on the above CT and ultrasound?

2. What is the finding with the arrow in lower right image next page?

3. What is free fluid in the abdominal cavity in the ER trauma patient detected by emergency sonography considered to be?

4. How is splenic injury treated?

5. What are the characteristics of splenic injury grading?

Case ranking/difficulty: 🔥

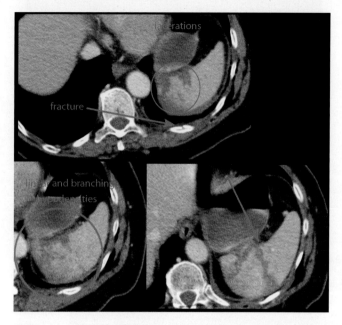

CECT top and bottom left show a left rib fracture (*arrow*) with splenic upper pole lacerations (*circle*). Bottom right is a splenic fracture (*arrow*), a liner hypodensity through the entire spleen. All images are of the same patient but a different patient than on the previous page.

Answers

1. The wedge-shaped and linear lucencies with perisplenic fluid are most consistent with splenic lacerations and perisplenic hematoma. The spleen is not completely disrupted as in shattered spleen. The history also suggests splenic trauma.

2. A through and through laceration is called a splenic fracture.

3. Focused abdominal sonography for trauma (FAST) scanning is used to detect intraperitoneal fluid assumed to be blood in the trauma setting and has largely replaced diagnostic peritoneal lavage.

4. Patients in unstable condition are not referred for imaging. Instead, they usually undergo emergency sonography or peritoneal lavage and are referred for surgery or sometimes embolization. Patients with blunt abdominal trauma who are hemodynamically stable generally undergo CT scanning. Diagnosing splenic injury before the patient becomes significantly symptomatic is important so that treatment can be initiated before systemic compromise and patients at risk for delayed rupture are identified. Conservative treatment of splenic injuries has gained favor over recent years.

5. Grade I—Subcapsular hematoma of less than 10% of surface area. Capsular tear of less than 1 cm in depth.

Grade II—Subcapsular hematoma of 10% to 50% of surface area. Intraparenchymal hematoma of less than 5 cm in diameter. Laceration of 1 to 3 cm in depth and not involving trabecular vessels.

Grade III—Subcapsular hematoma of greater than 50% of surface area or expanding and ruptured subcapsular or parenchymal hematoma. Intraparenchymal hematoma of greater than 5 cm or expanding. Laceration of greater than 3 cm in depth or involving trabecular vessels.

Grade IV—Laceration involving segmental or hilar vessels with devascularization of more than 25% of the spleen.

Grade V—Shattered spleen or hilar vascular injury.

Advance one grade for multiple injuries up to grade III.

Pearls

- CT: Splenic hematomas-hyperdense relative to splenic parenchyma on unenhanced CT and usually hypodense on contrast-enhanced CT. Splenic fractures-lacerations that extend completely across the splenic parenchyma and commonly involve the splenic hilum. Severe disruption of the splenic parenchyma results in a shattered spleen.
- Sonography is less sensitive than CT for acute splenic injuries (hematomas, lacerations with clotted blood) because they are nearly isoechoic to normal spleen. Fresh (unclotted) and chronic hemorrhage can appear hypoechoic. However, significant splenic injuries usually have hemoperitoneum that is detectable by focused abdominal sonography for trauma (FAST).

Suggested Readings

Cathey KL, Brady WJ, Butler K, et al. Blunt splenic trauma: characteristics of patients requiring urgent laparotomy. *Am Surg*.1998;64:450-454.

Gralla J, Spycher F, Pignolet C, et al. Evaluation of a 16-MDCT scanner in an emergency department: initial clinical experience and workflow analysis. *AJR*. 2005;185:232-238.

Rhea JT, Garza DH, Novelline RA. Controversies in emergency radiology. CT versus ultrasound in the evaluation of blunt abdominal trauma. *Emerg Radiol*. 2004;10:289-295.

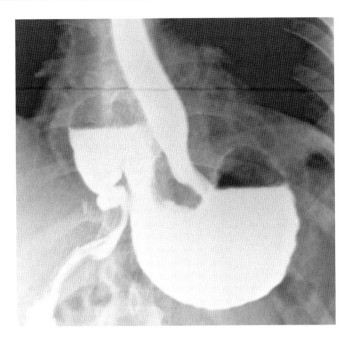 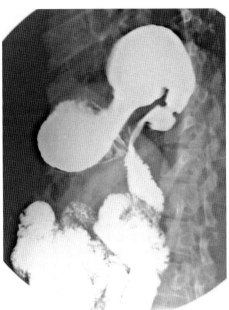

1. What is the most likely diagnosis based on both figures?

2. Paraesophageal gastric hiatal hernia accounts for what percentage of hiatal hernias?

3. What are clinical characteristics of paraesophageal hernias?

4. What are some serious complications of paraesophageal hernia?

5. How are paraesophageal hernias treated?

Case ranking/difficulty: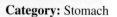

Category: Stomach

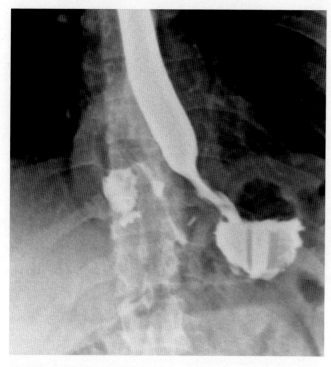

Erect film from early in the UGI shows a normally located gastroesophageal junction.

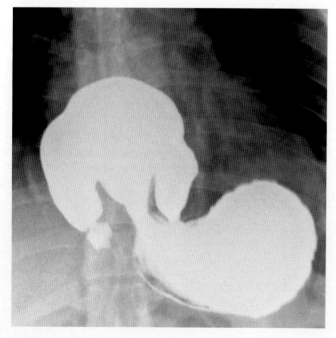

AP view clearly identifies paraesophageal hernia with gastric antrum located above the diaphragm.

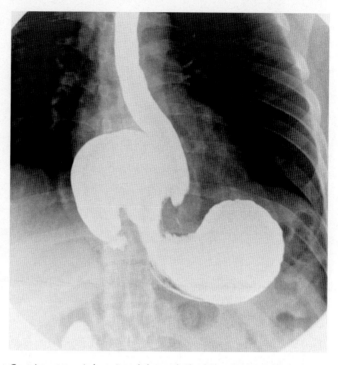

Gastric antrum is herniated through the hiatus above the diaphragm.

Answers

1. The gastroesophageal junction is normally situated below the diaphragm and the antrum and duodenum are herniated into the chest. If this were a sliding hernia, the gastroesophageal junction would be displaced into the chest. There is no evidence of gastric or duodenal ulcer or obstruction.

2. Paraesophageal gastric hiatal hernia is uncommon, representing only about 5% of all hiatal hernias.

3. Patients with a small paraesophageal hernia are usually asymptomatic. In patients with larger hernias, food and air may distend the herniated gastric segment, causing discomfort and chest pain usually postprandial, relieved by belching and retching. As opposed to sliding hiatal hernia, dysphagia and symptoms of reflux esophagitis are uncommon. Respiratory symptoms may be prominent, especially postprandially. Anemia from occult bleeding gastric ulcerations in the herniated stomach may be a presenting clinical feature.

4. Serious complications such as volvulus, incarceration, strangulation, obstruction, gangrene, perforation, and recurrent pneumonia may occur. There is no known predisposition toward malignancy.

5. Treatment of a symptomatic patient with a paraesophageal hernia is usually surgery. Emergency surgery is indicated in obstruction or symptomatic volvulus. Elective surgery in asymptomatic paraesophageal hernia patients in the absence of comorbidities/contraindications should be considered in view of the high morbidity and mortality rates of complications. Open laparotomy is standard, but laparoscopic repair is increasingly used.

Pearls

- On plain film examination paraesophageal hiatal hernia appears as a retrocardiac mass with or without an air-fluid level.
- A paraesophageal hiatal hernia is diagnosed by the position of the gastroesophageal junction.
- In patients with paraesophageal hernias, the gastroesophageal junction remains in its normal position below the diaphragm, and only the stomach herniates into the thorax, adjacent to the normally placed gastroesophageal junction. In patients with the more common sliding hiatal hernia the gastroesophageal junction is above the diaphragm.

Suggested Readings

Abbara S, Kalan MM, Lewicki AM. Intrathoracic stomach revisited. *AJR Am J Roentgenol.* August 2003;181(2): 403-414.

Eisenberg RL. Miscellaneous abnormalities. In: Gore RN, Levine MS, Laufer I, eds. *Textbook of Gastrointestinal Radiology*, Philadelphia, PA: WB Saunders; 1994.

Gerson DE, Lewicki AM. Intrathoracic stomach: when does it obstruct? *Radiology.* 1976;119:257-264.

Gore RM, Levine SL. *Textbook of Gastrointestinal Radiology.* 2nd ed. Philadelphia, PA: WB Saunders; 2000.

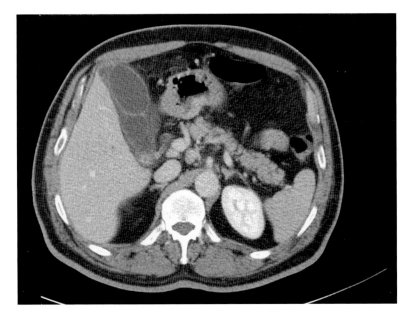 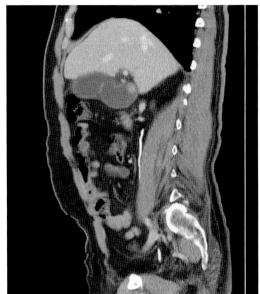

1. What is the most likely diagnosis?

2. What is the abnormality of the gallbladder fundus best shown on the first image next page?

3. In what conditions is gallbladder wall thickening seen?

4. What are sonographic findings in acute cholecystitis?

5. What are CT findings in acute cholecystitis?

Case ranking/difficulty:

Category: Gallbladder

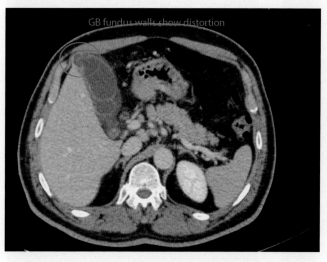

Fundal distortion with intramural lucencies (*circle*) due to an incidental fundal adenomyoma.

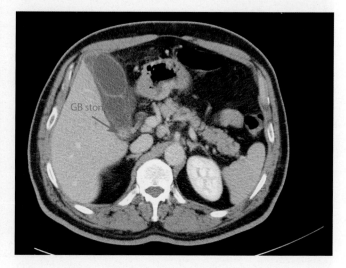

Stones (*arrow*) impacted in gallbladder neck.

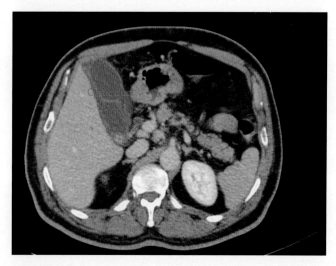

Cystic duct (*arrow*) with enhanced walls.

Answers

1. The distended gallbladder with stones in its neck and discontinuous mucosal enhancement point to a diagnosis of acute cholecystitis.

2. The abnormality of the gallbladder fundus best shown on the top left is a small mass with tiny intramural cysts characteristic of fundal adenomyoma.

3. Isolated gallbladder wall thickening is a nonspecific finding that can be seen in acute or chronic cholecystitis, nonfasting state, liver disease including hepatitis, low protein states, congestive heart failure, portal hypertension, and AIDS cholangiopathy.

4. Sonographic findings in acute cholecystitis include gallstones, gallstone impacted in the GB neck or cystic duct, diffuse gallbladder wall thickening (>3 mm), gallbladder distention, hepatocholecystic space sonolucency, intraluminal membranes, intraluminal debris, and pericholecystic fluid (in the absence of ascites). If at least two of these are present, the diagnosis is likely. The more of these that are present, the more likely the diagnosis. The presence of gallbladder hyperemia on power or color Doppler and the sonographic Murphy sign are adjunctive findings.

5. CT findings in acute cholecystitis are GB wall thickening in the presence of gallbladder distention, gallstones, cystic duct dilatation, cystic duct stone, discontinuous contrast enhancement of the gallbladder mucosa, and edema of pericholecystic fat. True "pericholecystic fluid" in the absence of ascites is an uncommon finding usually due to a sealed off gallbladder perforation. Other additional features include the presence of intraluminal membranes, an irregular wall, and increased hepatic enhancement (rim sign) surrounding the gallbladder. A hyperdense gallbladder wall on unenhanced CT has been reported as a sign of acute gangrenous cholecystitis.

Pearls

- Diffuse gallbladder wall thickening (>3 mm), edema of the hepatocholecystic space and gallstones in the presence of a sonographic Murphy sign and/or increased Doppler flow to the gallbladder is virtually diagnostic for acute cholecystitis. The presence of isolated gallbladder wall thickening on ultrasound, CT, or MRI is a nonspecific finding that can be seen in acute and chronic cholecystitis, nonfasting state, liver disease including hepatitis, low protein states, congestive heart failure, portal hypertension, and AIDS cholangiopathy.

- Discontinuous and irregular mucosal enhancement and/or the rim sign on contrast-enhanced CT suggests gangrenous cholecystitis.

Suggested Readings

Kiewiet JJ, Leeuwenburgh MM, Bipat S, Bossuyt PM, Stoker J, Boermeester MA. A systematic review and meta-analysis of diagnostic performance of imaging in acute cholecystitis. *Radiology*. September 2012;264(3):708-720.

Soyer P, Hoeffel C, Dohan A, ct al. Acute cholecystitis: quantitative and qualitative evaluation with 64-section helical CT. *Acta Radiol*. February 2013;54(5):477-486.

Teefey SA, Dahiya N, Middleton WD, et al. Acute cholecystitis: do sonographic findings and WBC count predict gangrenous changes? *AJR Am J Roentgenol*. February 2013;200(2):363-369.

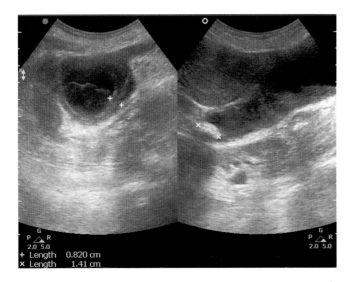
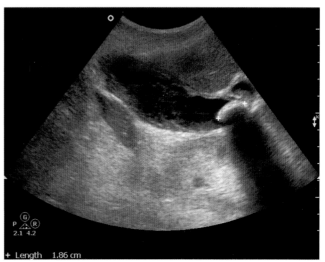

1. What is the most likely diagnosis?

2. What are gray scale ultrasound findings in acute cholecystitis?

3. What are the causes of gallbladder wall thickening?

4. What is edema of the hepatocholecystic space?

5. What is the role of the sonographic Murphy sign?

Case ranking/difficulty:

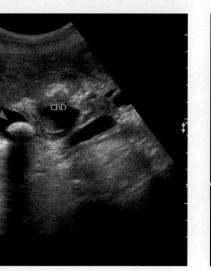

Transverse scan shows a dilated CBD with echogenic sludge medial to the gallbladder neck which contains the stone (*arrow*). A minority of patients with acute cholecystitis will have stones and/or sludge within the common bile duct.

Answers

1. Gallbladder wall thickening, stone impacted in the gallbladder neck, gallbladder distention, and intraluminal debris are four findings consistent with acute cholecystitis, so that diagnosis is highly likely.

2. Sonographic findings in acute cholecystitis include gallstones, gallstone impacted in the GB neck or cystic duct, diffuse gallbladder wall thickening (>3 mm), gallbladder distension, hepatocholecystic space sonolucency, intraluminal membranes, intraluminal debris, and pericholecystic fluid (in the absence of ascites). If at least two of these are present, the diagnosis is likely. The more of these that are present the more likely the diagnosis.

3. Isolated GB wall thickening can be seen in acute or chronic cholecystitis, nonfasting state, liver disease including hepatitis, low protein states, congestive heart failure, portal hypertension, AIDS cholangiopathy, and other etiologies. In the presence of pericholecystic ascites the gallbladder wall can be artifactually thickened on US due to side lobe artefacts.

4. Edema of the hepatocholecystic space is often called pericholecystic fluid. True pericholecystic fluid is seen in the absence of ascites as fluid adjacent to the gallbladder due to a sealed perforation. It is uncommon. Edema of the hepatocholecystic space is layered sonolucency between the liver and GB and usually indicates acute cholecystitis or hepatitis. It can be seen in any regional inflammation such as pancreatitis. Congestive failure causes diffuse GB wall thickening.

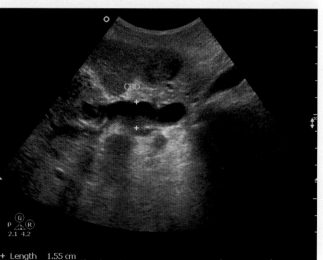

RAO parasagittal scan shows a 1.6-cm dilated common duct with a fluid debris level. A minority of patients with acute cholecystitis will have stones and/or sludge within the common bile duct.

5. The presence of a gallbladder hyperemia on power or color Doppler and the sonographic Murphy sign are findings adjunctive to gray scale findings. The sonographic Murphy sign is prone to false positives and may be falsely negative in cases of gangrenous cholecystitis (hyperemia by Doppler can be absent as well). This is due to destruction of pain fibers and ischemia in gangrenous cholecystitis. The sonographic Murphy sign suffers from subjectivity by the examiner. False positives abound since patients are being scanned because they have RUQ pain and/or tenderness.

Pearls

- Gray scale sonographic findings in acute cholecystitis:
  - Gallstones
  - Gallstone impacted in the GB neck or cystic duct
  - Diffuse gallbladder wall thickening >3 mm
  - Gallbladder distension
  - Hepatocholecystic space sonolucency
  - Intraluminal debris and/or membranes
  - Pericholecystic fluid (in the absence of ascites)
- Two or more of the above present suggests the diagnosis. The more that are present, the more likely the diagnosis.
- Adjunctive findings:
  - GB wall hyperemia on power or color Doppler (may be falsely negative in gangrenous cholecystitis).
  - Sonographic Murphy sign (prone to false positives) and may also be falsely negative in cases of gangrenous cholecystitis.

Suggested Readings

Bree RL, Ralls PW, Balfe DM, et al. Evaluation of patients with acute right upper quadrant pain. American College of Radiology. ACR appropriateness criteria. *Radiology*. 2000;215(suppl):153.

Paulson EK. Acute cholecystitis: CT findings. *Semin Ultrasound CT MR*. 2000;21:56-63.

Schiller VL, Turner RR, Sarti DA. Color Doppler imaging of the gallbladder wall in acute cholecystitis: sonographic-pathologic correlation. *Abdom Imaging*. 1996;21:233.

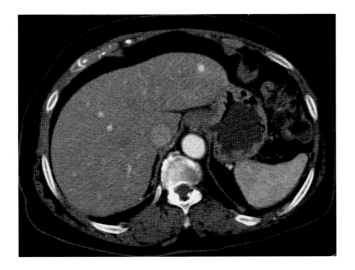 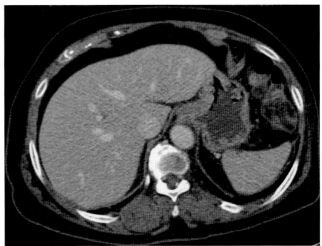

1. What is the best diagnosis?

2. What is the best diagnosis in a different patient (second CT next page)?

3. Differentiation of flash hemangiomas from vascular metastasis is best made by what modality and what phase/sequence?

4. What factors/conditions predispose toward hemangioma?

5. What other abnormalities/masses enhance strongly in the arterial phase?

Case ranking/difficulty:

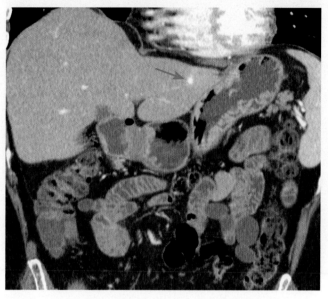

Coronal curved reformatted image demonstrating "flash" enhanced hepatic mass (*arrow*) in the arterial phase.

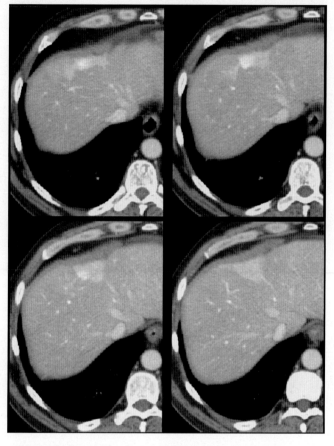

Composite of four CT images of a different patient in the arterial phase showing an intensely enhancing flash hemangioma (density greater than aorta) with perilesional enhancement. This perilesional enhancement disappeared in the portal venous phase (THAD).

Answers

1. The enhancement equal to the aorta in the arterial phase and equal to the blood pool in the portal venous phase is typical of flash hemangioma. Without any history of a primary a metastasis is unlikely. Without evidence of cirrhosis and without greater washout an HCC is unlikely. Most arterioportal shunts give peripheral geographic transient arterial enhancement.

2. Transient areas of enhancement of liver parenchyma during arterial phase imaging (THAD) are diffuse or focal areas of homogeneous arterial phase enhancement either from nontumorous arterioportal shunts or from focal obstruction of distal parenchymal portal venous flow (commonly due to HCC or cholangiocarcinoma). Wedge/geographic shape, peripheral location, nondisplaced internal vasculature, and absence of mass the same size as the THAD on T1- and T2-weighted noncontrast MRI are diagnostic. Flash hemangiomas often exhibit transient perilesional enhancement probably due to arterioportal shunting.

3. Vascular metastases can exhibit an enhancement pattern very similar to that of flash hemangioma. Both may be hyperintense on T2-weighted MR but metastases lose signal on heavily T2-weighted images whereas hemangiomas retain their hyperintensity.

4. Female gender, estrogens, presence of FNH elsewhere in the liver, Klippel-Trenaunay-Weber syndrome, Osler-Weber-Rendu disease, and/or von Hippel-Lindau disease make hepatic hemangioma more likely.

5. Small arteriovenous shunts and pseudoaneurysms (sometimes due to a previous biopsy) can enhance strongly in the arterial phase and exhibit enhancement = to the blood pool in later phases the same as flash hemangiomas. They are benign so confusion with flash hemangioma is of no consequence.

Transient areas of enhancement of liver parenchyma during arterial phase imaging, either from nontumorous arterioportal shunts or from focal obstruction of distal parenchymal portal venous flow can cause focal or diffuse areas of homogeneous arterial phase enhancement that may simulate flash hemangioma. Wedge/geographic shape, peripheral location, nondisplaced internal vasculature, and absence of mass on T1- and T2-weighted noncontrast MRI are diagnostic.

FNH and HCC enhance strongly in the arterial phase but wash out in the portal venous phase to a greater degree than flash hemangioma.

Pearls

- Flash hemangiomas: Rapid "flash" contrast enhancement at arterial phase CT (or MR) with contrast attenuation similar to the aorta in the arterial phase and the blood pool in the portal venous phase. Many show fading with enhancement less than the blood pool in the portal venous phase. Many show transient arterial phase perilesional enhancement.
- Strongly hyperintense at T2W MR imaging even on heavily T2WI.

Suggested Readings

Alturkistany S, Jang HJ, Yu H, Lee KH, Kim TK. Fading hepatic hemangiomas on multiphasic CT. *Abdom Imaging.* October 2012;37(5):775-780.

Prasanna PM, Fredericks SE, Winn SS, Christman RA. Best cases from the AFIP: giant cavernous hemangioma. *Radiographics.* November 2010;30(4):1139-1144.

Silva AC, Evans JM, McCullough AE, Jatoi MA, Vargas HE, Hara AK. MR imaging of hypervascular liver masses: a review of current techniques. *Radiographics.* May 2010;29(2):385-402.

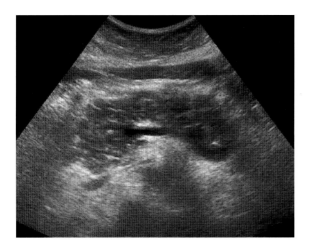 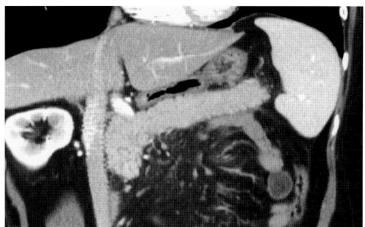

1. Based on the two images above (you can peek at the two images on the next page if you want) as well as the clinical information what is the most likely diagnosis?

2. What are some of the causes of acute pancreatitis?

3. What is the best imaging modality for diagnosis and staging of pancreatitis?

4. What are some clinical signs/symptoms of acute pancreatitis?

5. What are some laboratory abnormalities in acute pancreatitis?

Case ranking/difficulty: **Category:** Pancreas

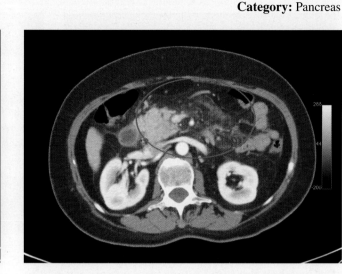

Enlarged enhanced pancreas (*arrows*) with minimal peripancreatic fat infiltration.

More caudal image shows infiltration of the mesenteric fat (*circle*).

Answers

1. The imaging findings as well as the history are consistent with acute pancreatitis. Lymphoma of the pancreas is possible but unusual and the patient usually would not present with acute symptoms.

2. Ethanol abuse and biliary tract stones are the most common causes of acute pancreatitis, accounting for 60% to 80% of cases (about 65% ethanol in the United States). Post-ERCP pancreatitis is the third most common cause of pancreatitis, but usually has a mild course.

   Other causes are trauma, autoimmune, metabolic (hypertriglyceridemia, hypercalcemia, renal failure, pregnancy), infection (mumps, coxsackie, viral hepatitis, mycoplasma, ascariasis), drugs, familial pancreatitis, any ampullary obstruction, idiopathic, vasculitis, pancreatic malignancy, and postcardiac bypass.

3. CT: the imaging modality of choice for diagnosis and staging of acute pancreatitis and its complications
   US: best for gallstones
   MRI: as sensitive as CT, but not as practical or accessible. MRCP best for gallstone pancreatitis and structural pancreaticobiliary ductal anomalies
   ERCP with sphincterotomy and stone extraction: should only be used if a patient has biliary pancreatitis and signs of biliary obstruction

4. Clinical presentation: epigastric pain, often radiating to the back with tenderness, fever, nausea and vomiting
   Grey Turner sign: bluish discoloration of flanks
   Cullen sign: periumbilical discoloration

5. Laboratory abnormalities are:

   Increased serum amylase and lipase

   Hyperglycemia, increased lactate dehydrogenase, hypocalcemia (poor prognostic sign)

   Leukocytosis, fall in hematocrit, rise in blood urea nitrogen

Pearls

- CT is the modality of choice for acute pancreatitis imaging.
- Nonnecrotizing pancreatitis (Balthazar score A-C) means that no fluid collections and no pancreatic parenchymal necrosis develops.
- Normal contrast enhancement of the pancreas on CT scan means absence of necrosis.
- Imaging characteristics:
  - Diffuse or focal enlargement of pancreas.
  - Homogeneous normal or diminished or heterogeneous enhancement; nonenhancing necrotic areas.
  - Infiltration of peripancreatic fat, peripancreatic phlegmons.
  - Rim enhancement of acute fluid collections, abscesses, and pseudocysts.
  - Look for cholelithiasis and choledocholithiasis.
  - Severity and necrosis are best assessed by CT done about 72 hours after symptom onset.

Suggested Readings

Balthazar EJ. Acute pancreatitis: assessment of severity with clinical and CT evaluation. *Radiology*. June 2002;223(3):603-613.

Lenhart DK, Balthazar EJ. MDCT of acute mild (nonnecrotizing) pancreatitis: abdominal complications and fate of fluid collections. *AJR*. March 2008;190(3):643-649.

O'Connor OJ, McWilliams S, Maher MM. Imaging of acute pancreatitis. *AJR Am J Roentgenol*. August 2011;197(2):W221-W225.

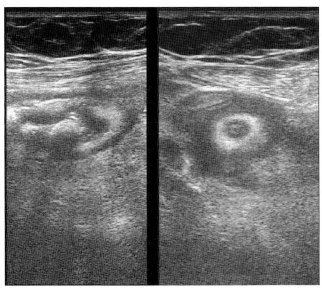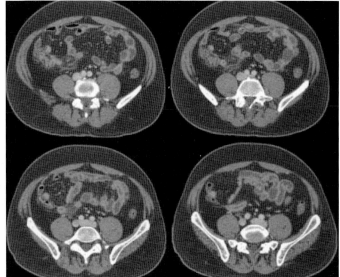

1. Based on both images what is the correct diagnosis?

2. Why is imaging needed for acute appendicitis?

3. What is the cause of acute appendicitis?

4. What are some pluses and minuses of US in appendicitis?

5. What are the US findings of appendicitis?

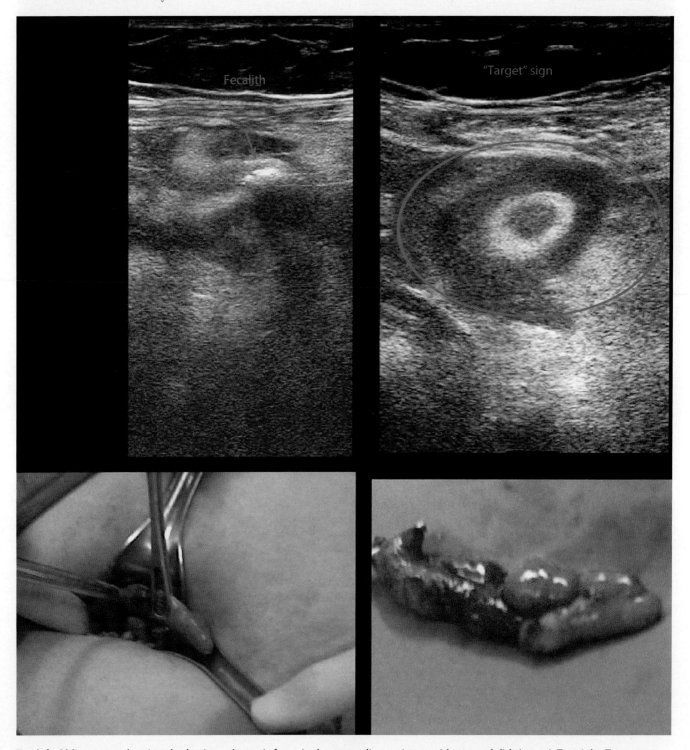

Top left: Oblique scan showing shadowing echogenic focus in the appendix consistent with appendolith (*arrow*). Top right: Transverse scan again showing target or pseudokidney sign signifying abnormal bowel (*circle*). Bottom left is surgical extraction of the appendix and bottom right is the specimen.

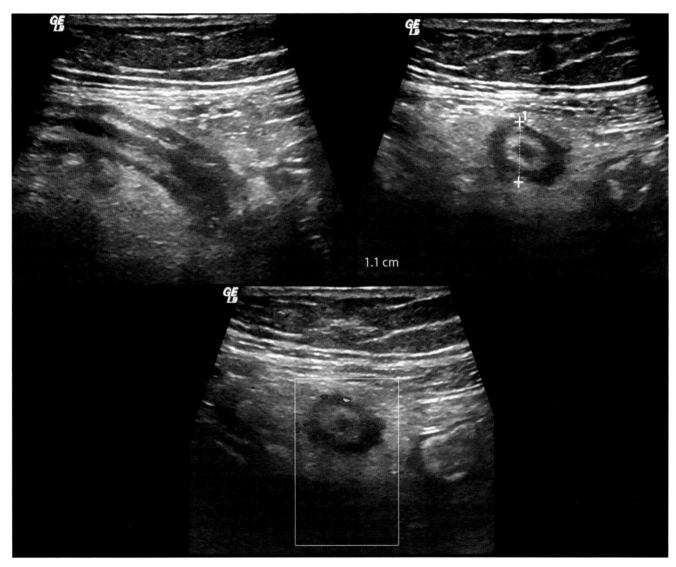

Same diagnosis. A 19-year-old female, severe abdominal pain. Scan over point of maximal tenderness. The appendix is enlarged, thick walled, incompressible, and possesses more than normal Doppler flow. Top left: sagittal. Top right: transverse. Bottom: Doppler.

Answers

1. The pseudokidney appearance on US (indicates abnormal bowel) with the central shadowing echogenic focus consistent with a fecalith or stone is consistent with acute appendicitis or, less likely, Meckel diverticulitis. The CT is diagnostic of appendicitis.

2. Imaging is needed because if clinical features are relied on without imaging a false-negative laparotomy rate of 20% is needed to avoid underdiagnosis and its attendant increased risk of complications.

3. Acute appendicitis is caused by lumen obstruction most frequently by a fecalith (found in up to 35% of cases), leading to distension and infection. Lymphoid hyperplasia is another cause of obstruction. Miscellaneous causes include carcinoma of the appendix or cecum, carcinoid of the appendix, and fibrous strictures.

4. US used by some as initial imaging tool in all patients with suspected appendicitis.

   US used for virtually all children and pregnant women with suspected appendicitis.

   US used in many women of child bearing age with suspected appendicitis due to possibility of GYN disease.

   Graded compression US is the most wide used technique.

   Obesity and surrounding gut contents may result in poor visualization of the region of interest.

Sensitivity varies from 44% to 94%, some of which is due to operator dependence.

5. US classic findings: Distended incompressible tubular structure arising from the cecal base filled by hypoechoic fluid, with an overall diameter greater than 6 mm.

Transverse imaging—target sign—hypoechoic muscular and hyperechoic mucosal layers with a hypoechoic center due to fluid/pus.

Intraluminal echoes with distal acoustic shadowing may be seen due to fecaliths.

Loss of normal appendiceal wall layers suggests gangrene.

Color Doppler may demonstrate increased flow in the appendiceal wall.

Ancillary findings: Hyperechoic inflamed surrounding fat, free fluid, and adenopathy. The site of appendiceal perforation and surrounding abscess(es) may be identifiable in complicated cases.

Pearls

- US of acute appendicitis: Incompressible blind-ending tubular structure measuring more than 6 mm in diameter. Echogenic shadowing fecalith(s) within the lumen is a common additional finding. Loss of normal appendiceal wall echogenicity may indicate developing gangrene. Additional signs include echogenic periappendiceal fat, regional free fluid, thickened cecal base, and adenopathy.
- CT is very sensitive and highly specific for acute appendicitis.
- Typical CT presentation of acute appendicitis is enlarged enhancing appendix >6 mm in diameter and infiltrated adjacent fat.

Suggested Readings

Kim MS, Park HW, Park JY, et al. Differentiation of early perforated from nonperforated appendicitis: MDCT findings, MDCT diagnostic performance, and clinical outcome. *Abdom Imaging*. June 2014;39(3):459-466.

Orth RC, Guillerman RP, Zhang W, Masand P, Bisset GS 3rd. Prospective comparison of MR imaging and US for the diagnosis of pediatric appendicitis. *Radiology*. July 2014;272(1):233-240.

Trout AT, Towbin AJ, Zhang B. Journal club: the pediatric appendix: defining normal. *AJR Am J Roentgenol*. May 2014;202(5):936-945.

Motor vehicle accident with blunt abdominal trauma

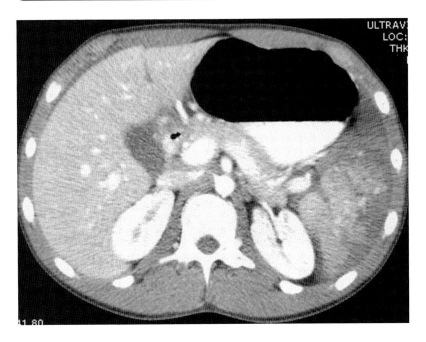 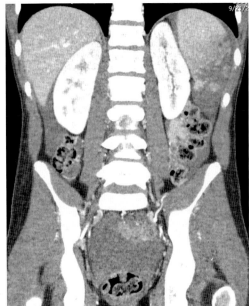

1. What is the correct diagnosis based on both images?

2. What conditions predispose to spontaneous splenic rupture?

3. What procedures cause iatrogenic splenic injury?

4. Where does splenosis occur?

5. What imaging modalities are useful for imaging splenic trauma?

Case ranking/difficulty:

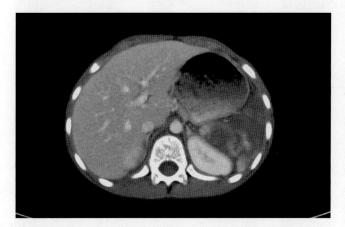

Second case. Motor vehicle accident with blunt abdominal trauma, an 8-year-old boy. Fragmented upper pole with adjacent blood. Lower pole was intact.

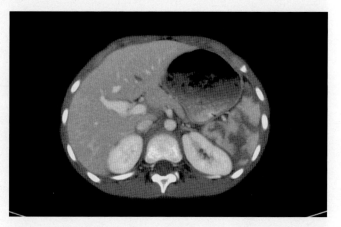

Second case. Motor vehicle accident with blunt abdominal trauma, an 8-year-old boy. Fragmented upper pole with adjacent blood. Lower pole was intact.

Answers

1. The complete disruption of the lower pole of the spleen with islands of enhanced parenchyma and large hemoperitoneum is diagnostic of shattered spleen.

2. Infectious or inflammatory diseases of the spleen such as mononucleosis, sarcoidosis and other granulomatous diseases, and rheumatoid arthritis predispose to nontraumatic splenic rupture. Splenic neoplasms, splenic abnormalities seen in hemolytic anemias, vascular abnormalities of the spleen, and splenic storage diseases also predispose toward nontraumatic splenic rupture.

3. Between 10% and 40% of adult splenectomies are done for iatrogenic injury. During abdominal surgery or colonoscopy traction on splenic peritoneal attachments can injure the spleen. Wayward needles may injure the spleen during left thoracentesis or left renal biopsy. Paracentesis is usually done in the lower parts of the abdominopelvic cavity so the spleen is not injured.

4. Splenosis is autotransplantation of splenic tissue usually after traumatic splenic rupture. Most nodules implant on the small bowel mesentery but they may implant on any intraperitoneal structure. If there has been a diaphragmatic tear intrathoracic splenosis may occur.

5. CT, sonography, MRI, radionuclide scanning, and angiography are all fairly sensitive and specific for depicting splenic injury. CT is fast and accurate and overall the best. Its drawbacks are radiation dose and lack of portability. US is best for detecting hemoperitoneum at the bedside and inferring splenic injury. Actually seeing the acute splenic injury can be tricky. MRI is very accurate but rarely used due to limited access and relatively long imaging time.

It has occasional use for splenic injury evaluation in pregnant patients and children. Radionuclide scanning was pretty good in its day but has been superseded by CT. Angiography is used today to control bleeding in patients with injured spleens and no longer used solely for diagnosis.

Pearls

- Findings in splenic trauma:
  - Acute hematoma: hyperdense on noncontrast CT; a low-attenuation area between the splenic capsule and parenchyma on contrast-enhanced CT
  - Laceration: linear or branching areas of low attenuation
  - Vascular injuries: pseudoaneurysms and arteriovenous fistulas
  - Posttraumatic infarction

Suggested Readings

Boscak A, Shanmuganathan K. Splenic trauma: what is new? *Radiol Clin North Am*. January 2012;50(1):105-122.

Boscak AR, Shanmuganathan K, Mirvis SE, et al. Optimizing trauma multidetector CT protocol for blunt splenic injury: need for arterial and portal venous phase scans. *Radiology*. July 2013;268(1):79-88.

Yu J, Fulcher AS, Turner MA, Halvorsen RA. Multidetector computed tomography of blunt hepatic and splenic trauma: pearls and pitfalls. *Semin Roentgenol*. October 2012;47(4):352-361.

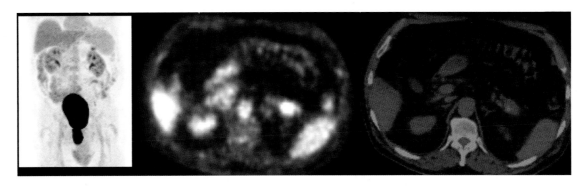

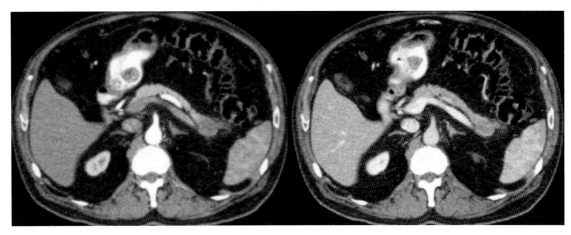

1. What is the most likely diagnosis based on the above figures?

2. Based on the above figures, is the duct cell adenocarcinoma (DCA) likely to be cured?

3. What is the significance of gastroduodenal artery encasement?

4. What determines local resectability for cure of ductal adenocarcinoma of the pancreas?

5. In what ways do DCAs of the pancreas spread beyond the gland?

Case ranking/difficulty: **Category:** Pancreas

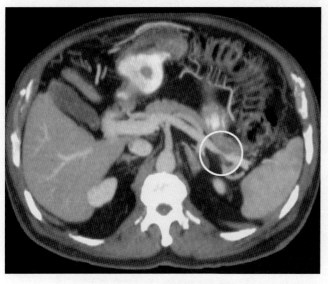

Axial MIP shows splenic vein encasement (*circle*).

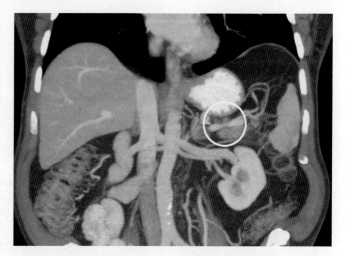

Coronal MIP shows splenic vein encasement (*circle*).

Answers

1. The most likely diagnosis is duct cell adenocarcinoma (DCA) of the tail of the pancreas in addition to rectal carcinoma. Rectal carcinoma metastasizing to the pancreas is rare. Neuroendocrine tumor is less common than DCA. The mass is not cystic so mucinous cystic neoplasm is unlikely. Mass-like pancreatitis limited to the tail would be very unusual.

2. In figures on first page of this case there is subtle nodular infiltration of fat anterolateral to the mass in the tail of the pancreas and in the figures on this page there is unequivocal encasement of the splenic vein. These indicate spread of the DCA beyond the gland and resection for cure is unlikely. The mass is not inoperable; a distal pancreatectomy can be done but the patient is unlikely to be cured.

3. The gastroduodenal artery (GDA) is sometimes hard to evaluate on CT but rarely the only sign of extrapancreatic spread. Some surgeons will resect (Whipple) if only the GDA involved. Efficaciousness of this approach is unproven.

4. Local resectability of DCA is determined by:

   • Whether the tumor involves major arterial structures (celiac axis, superior mesenteric artery, splenic artery, hepatic artery, gastroduodenal artery, left gastric artery)

   • Whether long segment involvement or occlusion of major venous structures (superior mesenteric, splenic, portal, left renal vein, and inferior vena cava) is present

5. Features of spread beyond the gland determining unresectability for cure are:

   • Vascular encasement, occlusion, contiguity, thick vessel

   • Liver metastases

   • Intraperitoneal spread

   • Invasion of contiguous structures, fat plane obliteration

   • Lymphadenopathy

   • Lung and distant metastases

Pearls

• Most DCA patients are not resectable for cure.
• Local resectability determined by:
  • Tumor extension to major arterial structures (celiac axis, superior mesenteric artery, splenic artery, hepatic artery, gastroduodenal artery, left gastric artery)
  • Presence/absence of long segment involvement or occlusion of major venous structures (superior mesenteric, splenic, portal, left renal vein, and inferior vena cava).
• Gastroduodenal artery (GDA) may be hard to evaluate on CT but rarely the only sign of extrapancreatic spread. Some surgeons will resect if only the GDA is involved.
• Features of spread beyond the gland determining unresectability for cure are:
  • Vascular encasement, occlusion, contiguity, thick vessel
  • Liver metastases

- Intraperitoneal spread
- Invasion of contiguous structures, fat plane obliteration
- Lymphadenopathy
- Lung and distant metastases
- Chest CT not needed for staging since lung mets will preferentially involve the lung bases and be seen on abdominopelvic CTs.

Suggested Readings

Sai M, Mori H, Kiyonaga M, Kosen K, Yamada Y, Matsumoto S. Peripancreatic lymphatic invasion by pancreatic carcinoma: evaluation with multi-detector row CT. *Abdom Imaging*. April 2010;35(2):154-162.

Vikram R, Balachandran A, Bhosale PR, Tamm EP, Marcal LP, Charnsangavej C. Pancreas: peritoneal reflections, ligamentous connections, and pathways of disease spread. *Radiographics*. July 2009;29(2):e34.

Zhang XM, Mitchell DG, Witkiewicz A, Verma S, Bergin D. Extrapancreatic neural plexus invasion by pancreatic carcinoma: characteristics on magnetic resonance imaging. *Abdom Imaging*. April 2010;34(5):634-641.

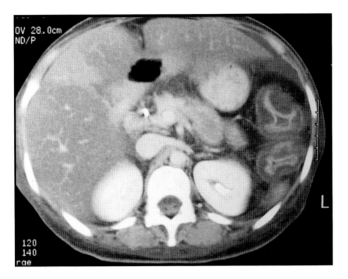
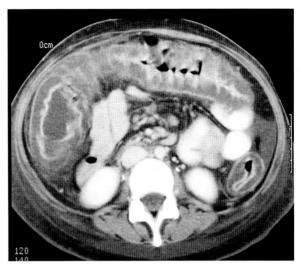
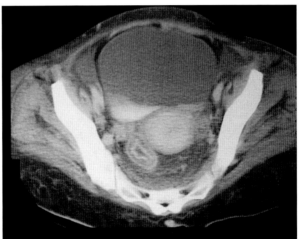

1. What is the most likely diagnosis?

2. What are common findings in infectious colitis?

3. What laboratory test(s) are usually required to make the diagnosis of cytomegalovirus (CMV) colitis?

4. What disease caused by Epstein-Barr virus can be mimicked by CMV?

5. What are treatments for uncomplicated CMV colitis?

Case ranking/difficulty:

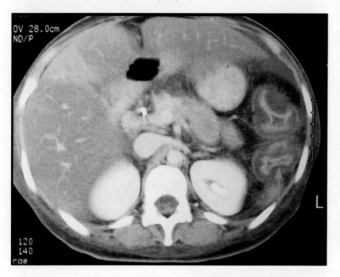

Portal venous phase CT shows bowel wall thickening (*red arrow*), mucosal enhancement (*green arrow*), ascites (*red arrowhead*), and pericolic edema.

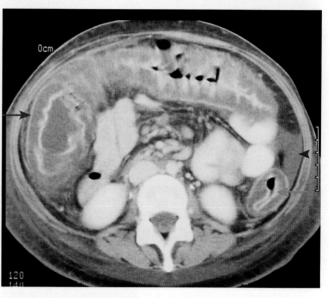

Portal venous phase CT shows marked bowel wall thickening (*red arrow*), mucosal enhancement (*green arrow*), ascites (*red arrowhead*), and pericolic edema.

Answers

1. Generally speaking, it is difficult to give a specific diagnosis based on CT findings alone. History can be helpful. There may be a travel history or other history (such as an outbreak of foodborne illness or a history of HIV).

   Cytomegalovirus infection is the most common cause of infectious colitis in patients with HIV/AIDS. Cryptosporidiosis, *Mycobacterium avium-intracellulare*, spirochetosis, and bacteria also cause disease, but they rank behind CMV colitis.

2. In general, it is difficult to distinguish infectious colitides based on imaging alone. Ulcerations, mural thickening, pericolic edema, and ascites can be seen in most causes of infectious colitides, as in CMV colitis. It is unusual to have ascites related to uncomplicated inflammatory bowel disease. The clinical history and the distribution may help narrow the diagnosis, but laboratory confirmation is required for a definitive diagnosis.

3. Serology can be helpful in establishing past or recent infection, but it cannot make a diagnosis of CMV colitis. Colon biopsy along with either histopathology or immunohistochemistry is required to make a definitive diagnosis.

4. A small proportion of cases of infectious mononucleosis like syndromes are actually caused by cytomegalovirus infection. Numerous other viruses can cause a similar syndrome, so-called heterophile-negative infectious mononucleosis because the heterophile antibody test/monospot test is negative but the signs and symptoms are similar to infectious mononucleosis.

5. Treatment is with intravenous ganciclovir for the CMV infection. In HIV/AIDS patients the HIV infection can also be treated in an effort to improve the CD4 count and boost host immunity.

Pearls

- Herpesviridae family virus infection that results from either reactivation or primary infection, usually in an immunocompromised host, although it can complicate inflammatory bowel disease or rarely occur in an immunocompetent host.
- Most common cause of infectious colitis in patients with HIV/AIDS.
- Definitive diagnosis usually requires examination of biopsy specimens from the bowel.
- Typical findings are mural thickening, ulcerations, pericolic edema, and ascites.

Suggested Readings

Al-Zafiri R, Gologan A, Galiatsatos P, Szilagyi A. Cytomegalovirus complicating inflammatory bowel disease: a 10-year experience in a community-based, university-affiliated hospital. *Gastroenterol Hepatol* (NY). 2012;8(4):230-239. Epub 2012/06/23.

Balthazar EJ, Megibow AJ, Fazzini E, Opulencia JF, Engel I. Cytomegalovirus colitis in AIDS: radiographic findings in 11 patients. *Radiology*. 1985;155(3):585-589. Epub 1985/06/01. doi: 10.1148/radiology.155.3.2988010.

Thoeni RF, Cello JP. CT imaging of colitis. *Radiology*. 2006;240(3):623-638. Epub 2006/08/24. doi: 10.1148/radiol.2403050818.

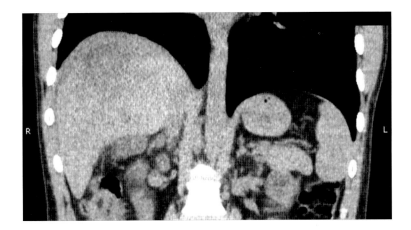
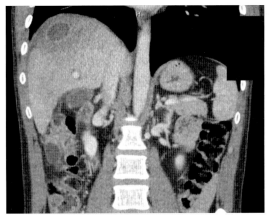
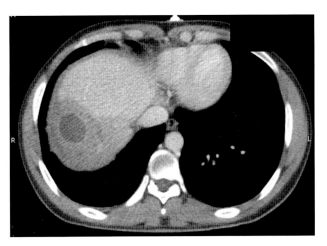
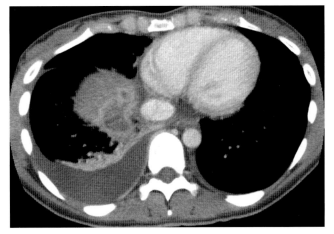

1. What is the most likely diagnosis?

2. What is the standard treatment for amebic abscess?

3. What demographic features suggest amebic abscess rather than pyogenic abscess?

4. After adequate time for an effective host response (7-10 days), how often are serologies positive in amebic liver abscess?

5. What is the appearance of hepatic abscesses on diffusion-weighted MRI?

Case ranking/difficulty:

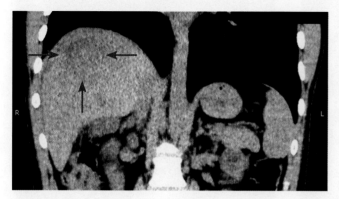

Noncontrast coronal CT shows a relatively inconspicuous area of low attenuation in the right hepatic lobe near the dome of the liver (*red arrows*).

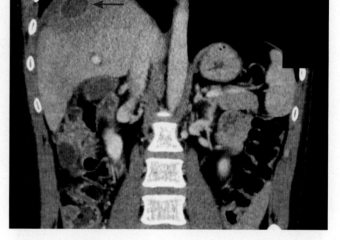

Contrast-enhanced CT shows the lesion more clearly. There is a faintly enhancing wall (*red arrow*), and the surrounding hepatic parenchyma has decreased density.

Answers

1. The clinical history would be important.

    In a patient with a fever and elevated white blood cell count one would consider primarily pyogenic abscess or amebic abscess.

    Pyogenic abscesses are frequently multiple when compared to amebic abscess, and the demographics are usually different with pyogenic abscesses occurring in an older population and without the high M:F ratio. Amebic abscess is the best choice.

    Cystic or necrotic tumors would be a consideration, but are uncommon and the history is most often contributory.

    An infarct is more often peripheral and wedge shaped, although they can be round and more central. It could develop necrosis and could have gas with or without infection.

2. Amebic abscesses can usually be treated successfully with Metronidazole or other agents alone. Aspiration or drainage is reserved for cases in which there is diagnostic uncertainty, no improvement with treatment or concern for rupture. Surgery is usually not required unless there are complications. Penicillin is ineffective.

3. In general, a solitary right hepatic lobe lesion in a young male patient that looks like an abscess is more likely to be an amebic abscess rather than a pyogenic abscess, although history is still important. Multiple lesions in an older patient are more likely to be pyogenic.

4. Serologies are quite sensitive in the detection of amebic abscess, being positive in over 90% of immunocompetent patients who have had enough time to mount an immune response. Notably, stool analysis in the same patient population is positive in only a minority of patients.

5. Diffusion-weighted (DW) imaging can be useful in the evaluation of suspected amebic abscesses. Benign lesions such as cysts, hydatid cysts, and hemangiomas have low intensity (high ADC values), abscesses have intermediate hyperintensity and intermediate ADC values, and malignant lesions have higher hyperintensity and low ADC values.

    Pyogenic abscesses tend to have higher signal intensity when compared to amebic abscesses.

Pearls

- History and demographics are important in suggesting the diagnosis. Typically in younger males when compared to older age group for pyogenic abscess.
- Solitary, peripheral round/oval lesion in the right hepatic lobe with travel history and typical demographic is suggestive.
- Serologies are positive in over 90% of immunocompetent patients 1 week after the onset of symptoms and are usually sufficient to make the diagnosis along with other clinical data.
- Treatment with Metronidazole or other agents is usually effective.

Suggested Readings

Chan JH, Tsui EY, Luk SH, Fung AS, Yuen MK, Szeto ML, et al. Diffusion-weighted MR imaging of the liver: distinguishing hepatic abscess from cystic or necrotic tumor. *Abdom Imaging*. 2001;26(2):161-165. Epub 2001/02/15.

Demir OI, Obuz F, Sağol O, Dicle O. Contribution of diffusion-weighted MRI to the differential diagnosis of hepatic masses. *Diagn Interv Radiol*. (Ankara, Turkey). 2007;13(2):81-86. Epub 2007/06/15.

Mortelé KJ, Segatto E, Ros PR. The infected liver: radiologic-pathologic correlation. *Radiographics*. 2004;24(4):937-955. Epub 2004/07/17. doi: 10.1148/rg.244035719.

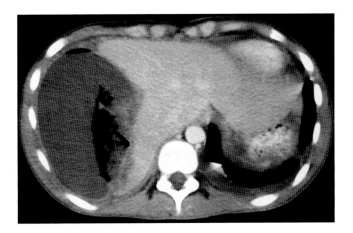

1. What is the most likely diagnosis?

2. What is the most common vascular complication of orthotopic liver transplant?

3. In a pregnant patient what etiology of hepatic infarction should specifically be considered?

4. On contrast-enhanced CT, what are various appearances of hepatic infarction?

5. Name four potential complications of hepatic infarction.

Case ranking/difficulty:

Category: Liver

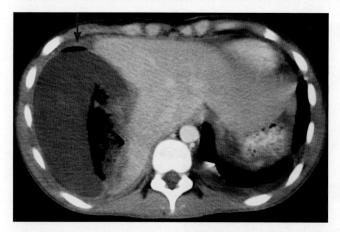

46-year-old male with diabetes, atherosclerosis, and hypercoagulable state. Axial portal venous phase CT shows a large avascular portion of the right hepatic lobe (*red arrow*) with bubbly gas and air fluid level. The liver capsule still slightly enhanced.

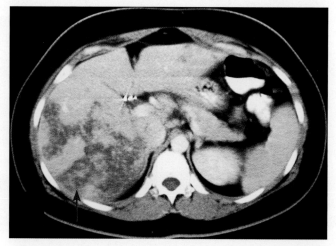

33-year-old female postpartum with HELLP syndrome (hemolysis, elevated liver enzymes, and low platelet count). Irregular areas of low density and infarction in the right hepatic lobe (*red arrow*).

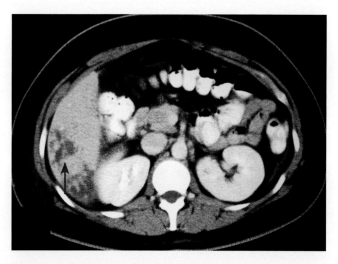

33-year-old female postpartum with HELLP syndrome (hemolysis, elevated liver enzymes, and low platelet count). Irregular areas of low density and infarction in the right hepatic lobe (*red arrow*).

Answers

1. The most likely diagnosis is hepatic infarct. The liver is somewhat unique in that it has a dual blood supply via the hepatic artery (25%) and the portal vein (75%), and infarction usually requires hepatic artery thrombosis with or without portal vein thrombosis. Infarction is often a peripheral wedge-shaped area of hypoattenuation in a vascular territory on CT, although it can have other appearances.

Focal fat is hypoattenuating, but it does not produce necrosis or air fluid levels, and the vessels and ducts are undistorted in the area of fatty change.

Abscess is hypoattenuating, and there may be satellite lesions, and the patients are usually ill with a fever and elevated WBC count.

Traumatic lacerations are usually linear and extend to the liver capsule, and may be associated with subcapsular hematomas, parenchymal hematomas, or active bleeding. There would be a history of trauma.

Hydatid cysts occur in patients who live in or who have traveled to an endemic area. There may be daughter cysts and other findings to suggest the diagnosis.

2. Hepatic artery thrombosis is the most severe and most common vascular complication of orthotopic liver transplant, occurring in around 3% of adult patients, and it is much more common in the pediatric population.

3. Trauma, hypercoagulability, sickle cell disease, and arteriosclerosis are all possible etiologies of hepatic artery thrombosis, but the HELLP syndrome (hemolysis, elevated liver enzymes, and low platelets) is specifically related to pregnancy.

4. The appearance of infarction on contrast-enhanced CT is variable but classically appears as peripheral wedge-shaped areas of low attenuation. Other appearances include round or geographic areas of low attenuation, or areas of low attenuation parallel to the bile ducts.

5. If detected early enough, hepatic artery thrombosis can be treated with thrombectomy or revascularization (or retransplant if possible). If a large portion of the liver is infarcted liver failure may ensue, and abscess formation and bilomas/bile lakes are recognized complications. Biliary strictures can also occur from infarction or from chronic ischemia and are a recognized issue in orthotopic liver transplant patients.

Pearls

- Hepatic infarction is somewhat rare because of the dual vascular supply to the liver.
- Serious potential complication of orthotopic liver transplant, usually monitored for by serial ultrasound or CT examinations.
- Variety of appearances, although classically a peripheral wedge-shaped area of decreased perfusion and edema (hypoechoic on US, low attenuation on CT, low signal on T1W MRI, and high signal on T2W MRI).
- Differential diagnosis can include fatty liver or abscess. In fatty liver the vessels in the affected portion are normal, and MRI could be used for verification. Abscess should have some mass effect and usually has some peripheral enhancement, whereas infarct should not.

Suggested Readings

Bishehsari F, Ting PS, Green RM. Recurrent gastrointestinal bleeding and hepatic infarction after liver biopsy. *World J Gastroenterol.* 2014;20(7):1878-1881. Epub 2014/03/04. doi: 10.3748/wjg.v20.i7.1878.

Boll DT, Merkle EM. Diffuse liver disease: strategies for hepatic CT and MR imaging. *Radiographics.* 2009;29(6):1591-1614. Epub 2009/12/05. doi: 10.1148/rg.296095513.

Giovine S, Pinto A, Crispano S, Lassandro F, Romano L. Retrospective study of 23 cases of hepatic infarction: CT findings and pathological correlations. *Radiol Med.* 2006;111(1):11-21. Epub 2006/04/21.

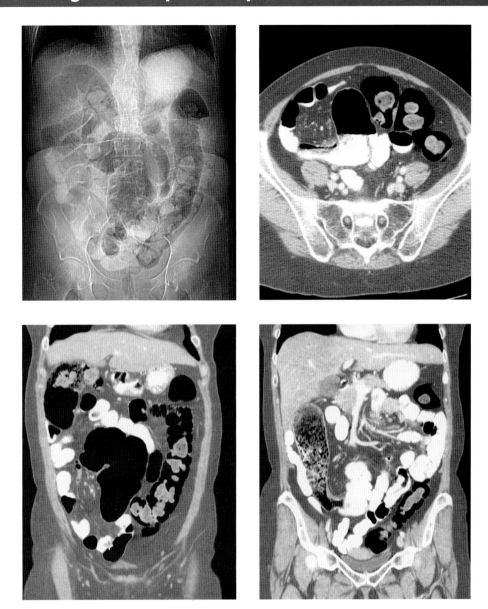

1. What is the most likely diagnosis?

2. What is the mechanism of obstruction in this condition?

3. What are the differentiating features of cecal bascule from cecal volvulus?

4. What is the best test for confirmation?

5. What is the treatment of choice?

Case ranking/difficulty:

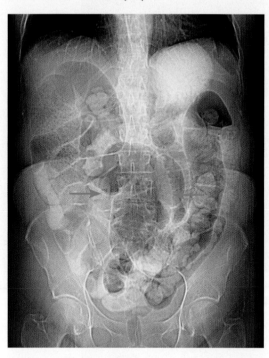

CT scanogram in frontal projection shows disproportionately more distended gas filled cecum (*arrows*) in the center of the abdomen. However, colon is normally distended (nonobstructed).

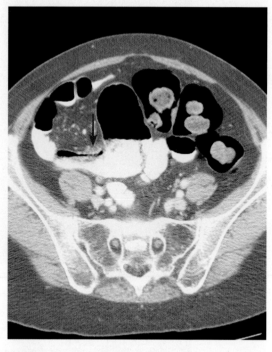

Axial CT scan at the level of folded cecum shows minimal soft tissue stranding (*arrow*), suggesting band or inflammation.

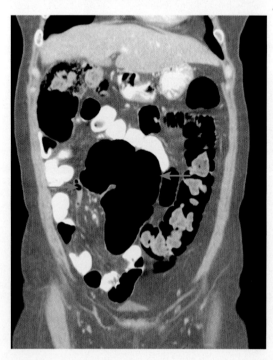

Coronal CT shows gas distended cecum (*arrows*) anteromedial to ascending colon.

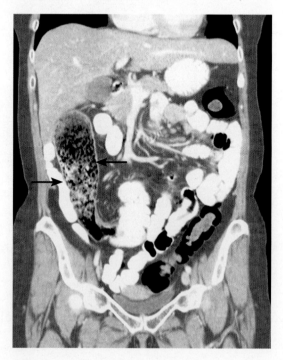

Coronal CT shows site of fold with soft tissue stranding and ascending colon with fecal residue (*arrows*).

Answers

1. Cecal bascule is the best diagnosis to explain the gas distended folded cecum anteromedial to the ascending colon. There is no bowel wall thickening to suggest typhlitis.

2. Fold acts like valve causing intermittent obstruction.

3. No twisting of cecum, no whirl sign, and cecum anteromedial to ascending colon are the features of cecal bascule. While intermittent obstruction can occur in cecal bascule, acute complete/incomplete obstruction is the rule in axial cecal volvulus.

4. Barium enema. It demonstrates the relationship of the cecum to the ascending colon, shows any obstruction, and rules out the possibility of axial volvulus.

5. Cecopexy is the definitive treatment.

Pearls

- Intermittent obstruction due to valve-like mechanism
- No twisting as seen in axial cecal volvulus
- Not an acute emergency

Suggested Readings

Oza V, Johnson A, Pfeil S. Cecal bascule: an unusual pathology of cecal dilation. Case report and brief review. *J Interv Gastroenterol*. October 2013;3(4):143-144.

Rozycki GS. Special feature: image of the month. Cecal bascule. *Arch Surg*. July 2001;136(7):835-836.

Yang SH, Lin JK, Lee RC, Li AF. Cecal volvulus: report of seven cases and literature review. *Zhonghua Yi Xue Za Zhi (Taipei)*. June 2000;63(6):482-486.

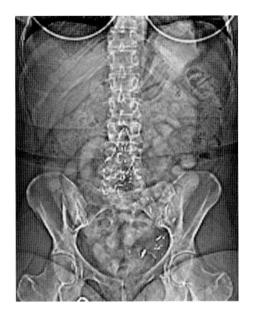
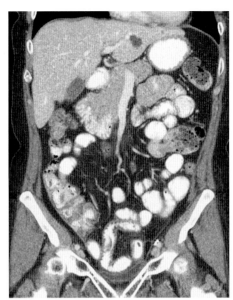
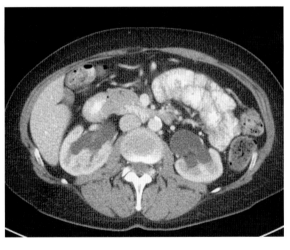
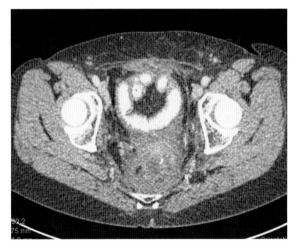

1. What is the most likely diagnosis?

2. What are the risk factors for the development of radiation enteritis?

3. What is the most common site of radiation enteritis?

4. What are the radiologic manifestations of chronic radiation enteropathy?

5. What radiotherapy techniques can reduce the chances of radiation enteritis?

Case ranking/difficulty:

Category: Small bowel

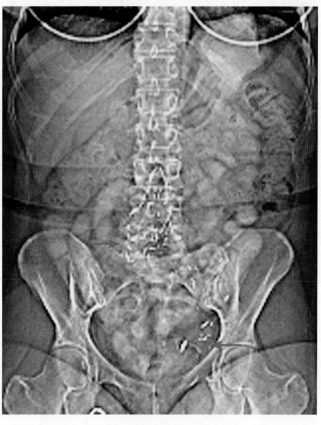

CT scanogram in frontal projection shows numerous surgical clips (*arrows*) along the course of the pelvic vessels, consistent with extensive lymph nodal dissection. It is a clue to the prior malignancy.

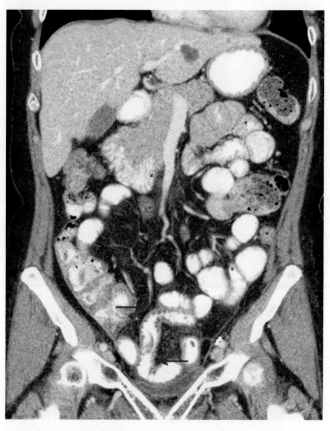

Coronal CT scan in portal venous phase demonstrates the diffuse bowel wall thickening (*arrows*) localized to the pelvic bowel loops. Incidental, liver cysts are noted.

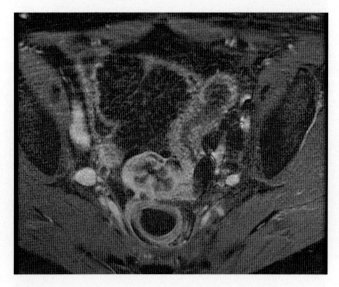

Circumferential segmental bowel wall thickening in the rectosigmoid, a proved second primary colonic neoplasm.

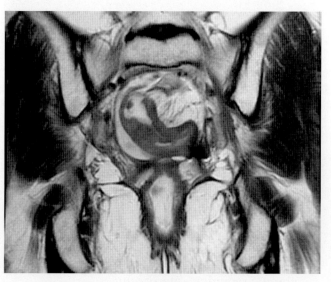

Coronal T2W MR image shows the bowel wall thickening with signal intensity higher than muscles, suggesting malignancy rather than radiation fibrosis (T2 low intensity).

Answers

1. Radiation enteritis is the best diagnosis. Ischemia can show similar findings. Identification of thrombus within the mesenteric vessels would favor the diagnosis of ischemia.

   Infiltrative lymphoma has similar bowel findings but is usually accompanied by lymphadenopathy.

   Angioedema has associated findings of laryngeal and cutaneous edema and previous episodes or family history. It usually involves a long segment of jejunum and is reversible after the acute episode.

   Crohn disease usually involves the terminal ileum and can have a halo sign and/or other signs of active inflammation.

2. Previous surgery, peritonitis, adhesions, high radiation dose, concomitant chemotherapy, diabetes, hypertension, and atherosclerosis are risk factors for radiation enteritis.

3. The ileum is the most common site of radiation enteritis.

4. Bowel wall thickening, stricture, adhesions, and small bowel obstruction are all radiologic findings in chronic radiation enteropathy.

5. Reducing the radiation field, using intensity modulated radiotherapy, using modern imaging guidance, evening radiation sessions, using a probiotic, an ACE inhibitor, and/or a statin can all diminish the incidence of radiation enteritis.

Pearls

- Disease within the radiation portal and history of irradiation are keys to the diagnosis.
- It is very important to look for tumor recurrence as it is common at the same site.
- Patients with radiation changes are more prone to have fistula or abscess after surgery, especially at the anastomosis site.
- Intensity modulated radiotherapy (IMRT) decreases the radiation dose to the bowel by up to 40%.

Suggested Readings

Harb AH, Abou Fadel C, Sharara AI. Radiation enteritis. *Curr Gastroenterol Rep.* May 2014;16(5):383.

Schembri J, Azzopardi M, Ellul P. Small bowel radiation enteritis diagnosed by capsule endoscopy. *BMJ Case Rep.* 6 March 2014; doi:10.1136/bcr-2013-202552.

Stacey R, Green JT. Radiation-induced small bowel disease: latest developments and clinical guidance. *Ther Adv Chronic Dis.* January 2014;5(1):15-29.

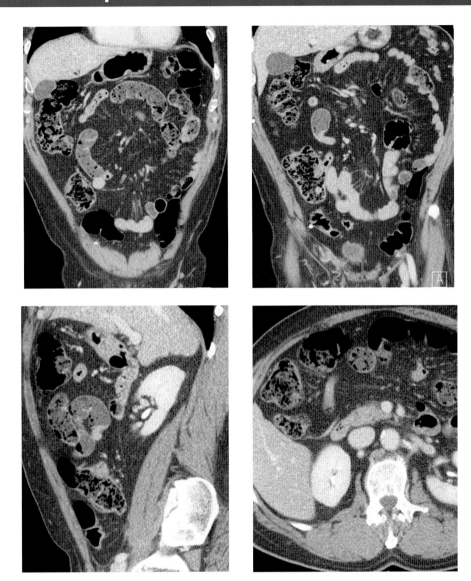

1. Name the sign demonstrated in the small bowel segment on CT.

2. What is the use of small bowel feces sign?

3. What are the possible mechanisms for development of small bowel feces sign?

4. What are the mimickers of small bowel feces sign?

5. What is the management of the patient with small bowel feces sign?

Case ranking/difficulty:

Category: Small bowel

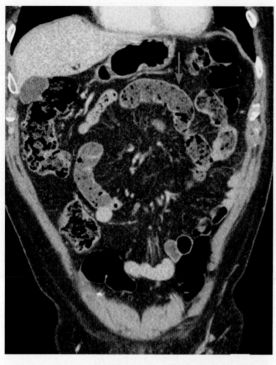

Coronal CT image shows fecal-like material with air bubbles within the dilated small bowel segments (*green arrow*) in the center of the abdomen, consistent with small bowel feces sign.

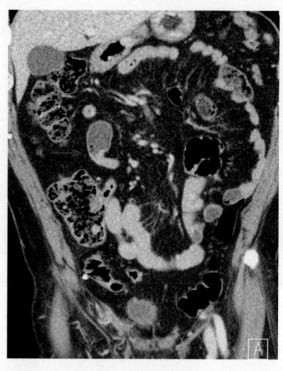

Coronal CT image shows a sudden change of caliber in the right upper quadrant (*red arrow*).

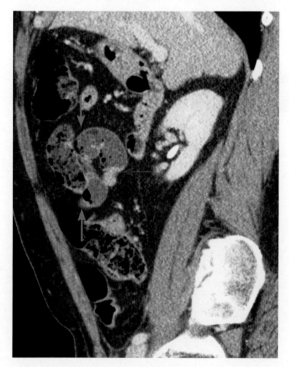

CT sagittal image shows small bowel feces sign (*green arrows*) proximal to transition zone (*red arrow*).

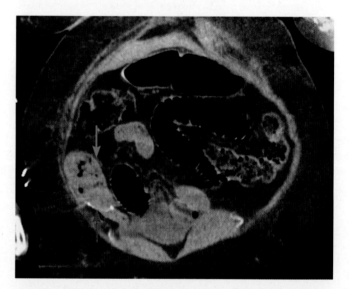

Different patient with known breast cancer and prior history of ileoileal anastomosis (*red arrow*). Note the small bowel feces sign (*green arrow*) localized to the stricture at the anastomotic site.

Answers

1. Small bowel feces sign. Presence of fecal-like material within the dilated small bowel segment.

2. Small bowel feces sign is useful to diagnose the presence of small bowel obstruction and to localize the transition point in difficult cases of small bowel obstruction.

3. Slow transit time, increased resorption of water, and accumulation of undigested food materials are the possible mechanisms for development of "small bowel feces" sign.

4. Bezoar, undigested food particles, rapid entry of food through jejunal feeding, and reflux of cecal contents, all can mimic the small bowel feces sign.

5. The management of the patient with small bowel feces sign is to treat the underlying cause of obstruction.

Pearls

- This sign is a reliable indicator of small bowel obstruction when proximal dilatation is >3 cm.
- This sign is useful to locate the transition zone in difficult cases.

Suggested Readings

Fuchsjäger MH. The small-bowel feces sign. *Radiology.* 2002 Nov;225(2):378-379.

Delabrousse E, Lubrano J, Sailley N, Aubry S, Mantion GA, Kastler BA. Small-bowel bezoar versus small-bowel feces: CT evaluation. *AJR Am J Roentgenol.* 2008 Nov;191(5):1465-1468.

Yadav MK, Lal A, Nagi B. Gossypiboma: stretched feces sign. *AJR Am J Roentgenol.* 2010 Nov;195(5):W375.

Early satiety, chronic left upper quadrant pain, nausea, and regurgitation of food

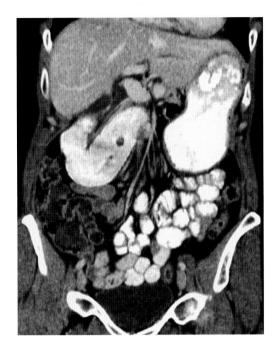 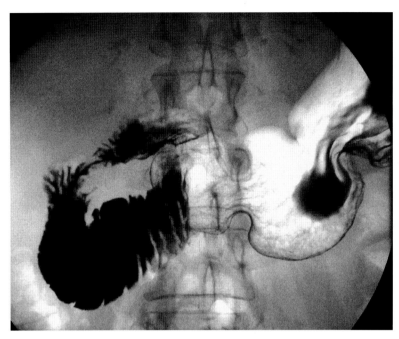

1. What is the most likely diagnosis?

2. What are the risk factors for this condition?

3. What is the best test for confirming the superior mesenteric artery syndrome?

4. What is the critical aorto-mesentric angle?

5. What is the position in which this finding may disappear?

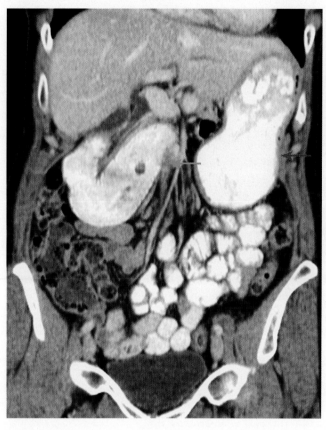

Coronal CT image in portal venous phase shows grossly distended stomach (*red arrow*) and duodenum (*green arrow*) proximal to SMA.

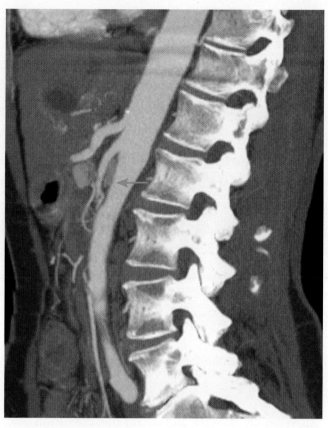

SMA aortic angle (*arrow*) measure about 15° in these sagittal MIP CTA images of aorta.

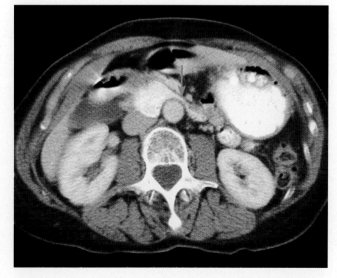

Axial CT image in portal venous phase demonstrates markedly narrowed distance between SMA and aorta compressing the third part of duodenum (*green arrow*) and distension of proximal duodenum.

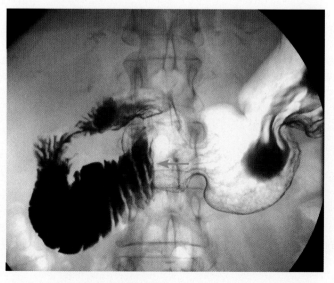

Upper GI series: characteristic linear extrinsic impression (*green arrow*) over the third part of duodenum at the level of SMA, consistent with SMA syndrome in the appropriate clinical setting.

Answers

1. Sudden linear cutoff in the midtransverse duodenum is the characteristic finding of superior mesenteric artery syndrome.

2. Prolonged bedridden patients due to spinal injury or scoliotic surgery, sudden weight loss, anorexia nervosa, and thin body habitus are the risk factors of superior mesenteric syndrome.

3. CT/CTA abdomen. CTA can determine the aortomesenteric angle and shows the distance between aorta and SMA. Amount of fat loss around SMA, duodenal compression, and severity of duodenal distension can be directly visualized.

4. The aortomesentric angle of 22° is the critical angle below which superior mesenteric artery syndrome may occur.

5. Left lateral decubitus and prone positions cause widening of the aortomesenteric angle, so the duodenal obstruction may disappear.

Pearls

- This is a well-known complication of scoliosis surgery, trauma, and anorexia nervosa.
- In SMA syndrome, aortomesenteric angle: between 10° and 22° (normal= 45°-65°). Aorta SMA distance: <8 mm (normal = 10-20 mm).
- Aim of initial conservative treatment is to decompress the third part of duodenum and replenish the mesenteric fat. If this fails, then surgery may be necessary.
- It is important to make an early diagnosis to avoid complications, including death.
- Nutcracker syndrome is compression of the left renal vein between the SMA and the aorta (associated with flank pain and hematuria).

Suggested Readings

Mathenge N, Osiro S, Rodriguez II, Salib C, Tubbs RS, Loukas M. Superior mesenteric artery syndrome and its associated gastrointestinal implications. *Clin Anat.* 2014;27(8):1244-1252.

Yakan S, Calıskan C, Kaplan H, Deneclı AG, Coker A. Superior mesenteric artery syndrome: a rare cause of intestinal obstruction. Diagnosis and surgical management. *Indian J Surg.* 2013 Apr;75(2):106-110.

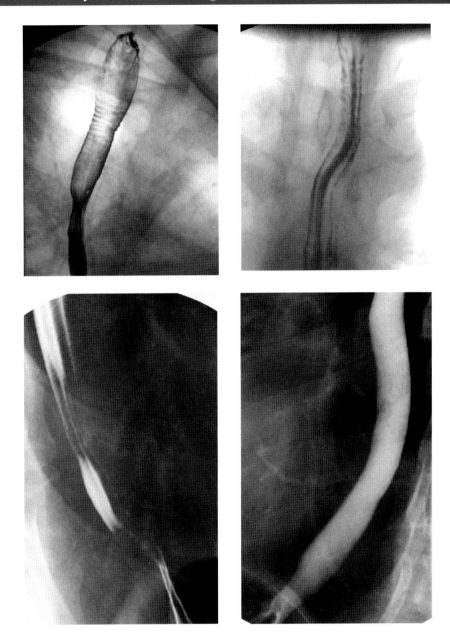

1. What is the diagnosis based on the two figures on top?

2. What is the diagnosis in a different patient based on the two figures on the bottom?

3. What is the expected finding on mucosal biopsy?

4. What is the fearful complication associated with this condition?

5. What is the possible etiology of this condition?

Eosinophilic esophagitis (ringed esophagus)   Case 63 (3538)

Case ranking/difficulty: **Category:** Esophagus

Answers

1. Since concentric rings persist on subsequent image, the diagnosis is eosinophilic esophagitis.

2. Since concentric rings disappeared on subsequent image, the diagnosis is feline esophagus.

3. Eosinophilic infiltration is the expected finding on mucosal biopsy.

4. Emesis or endoscopic-induced perforation is the frequent and fearful complication.

5. It is thought to be related to food allergens. More than half of the cases are associated with peripheral eosinophilia.

Pearls

- Child with gastroesophageal reflux symptoms, but negative PH monitoring and not responding to antireflux medication should raise the suspicion of eosinophilic esophagitis.
- Recurrent food impaction should also raise the possibility of eosinophilic esophagitis.
- Persistent multiple concentric rings on esophagram is a characteristic appearance of eosinophilic esophagitis (transient in feline esophagus).
- Risk of emesis or endoscopic-induced perforation is a frequent complication.

Suggested Readings

Assiri AM, Saeed A. Incidence and diagnostic features of eosinophilic esophagitis in a group of children with dysphagia and gastroesophageal reflux disease. *Saudi Med J.* 2014 Mar;35(3):292-297.

Levine JS, Pollard RE, Marks SL. Contrast videofluoroscopic assessment of dysphagic cats. *Vet Radiol Ultrasound.* 2014;55(5):465-471.

Pasha SF, DiBaise JK, Kim HJ, et al. Patient characteristics, clinical, endoscopic, and histologic findings in adult eosinophilic esophagitis: a case series and systematic review of the medical literature. *Dis Esophagus.* 2007 Oct;20(4):311-319.

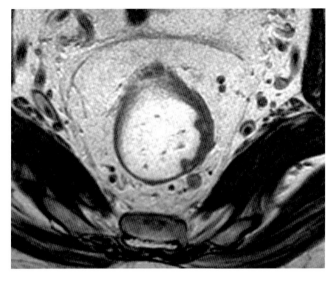
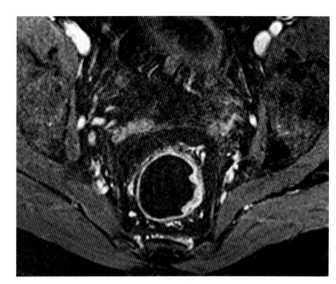
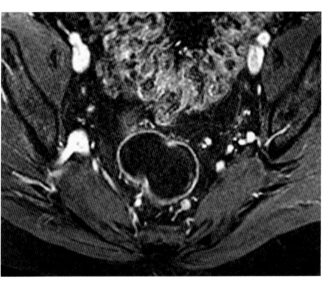
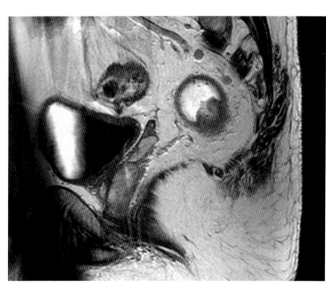

1. What is the most likely diagnosis?

2. What is the role of MR imaging in rectal cancer?

3. What is the role of dynamic contrast-enhanced T1W MRI sequence in locoregional staging?

4. What is the single most useful MR sequence for locoregional staging?

5. What is the role of CT in rectal cancer?

Case ranking/difficulty:

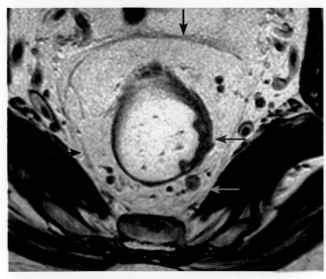

Axial MR T2W image shows irregular focal thickening of the left lateral rectal wall (*red arrow*) and enlarged lymph node (*green arrow*) in the 5-o'clock position. Rectum is filled with ultrasound gel. Mesorectal fascia is a thin low signal line surrounding the perirectal fat (*blue arrows*).

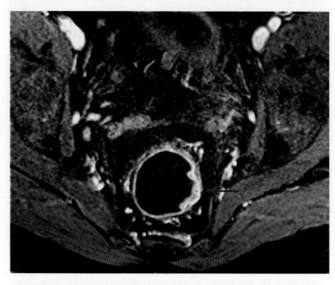

Contrast-enhanced T1W MR image shows enhancement of the irregular focal rectal wall thickening (*red arrow*). It does not give any additional value in locoregional staging.

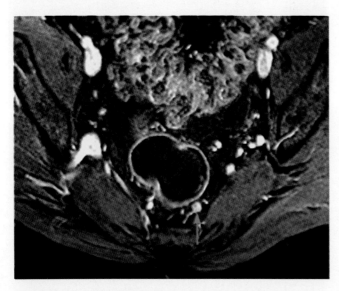

An enhancing perirectal lymph node in the 5-o'clock position (*green arrow*).

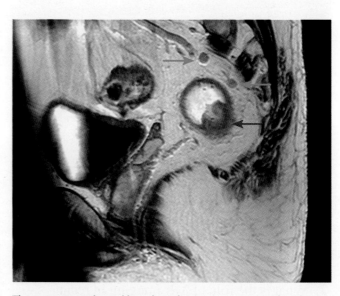

There are two enlarged lymph nodes (*green arrows*) within the perirectal fat and rectal mass (*red arrow*) is again seen.

Answers

1. Irregular mass lesion with enhancing perirectal lymph node is highly suggestive of rectal cancer.

2. MRI is a crucial investigation for making management decisions in cases of nonmetastatic locally invasive rectal cancer. Circumferential resection margin (CRM) positive cases need neoadjuvant chemoradiation followed by total mesorectal resection (TME) whereas CRM negative cases need only TME.

3. It will not give any additional value in locoregional staging.

Contrast-enhanced MR imaging shows enhancement of the irregular focal wall thickening.

4. T2-weighted sequence is the only sequence needed for assessment of local tumor invasion and detection of local lymph nodes. The essential images are T2-weighted images in at least two orthogonal planes to the long axis of rectal cancer. DWI is also useful to assess the response to treatment.

5. The role of CT in rectal cancer is to detect distal metastasis.

Pearls

- Both MRI and endorectal US are useful in locoregional staging.
- Contrast-enhanced MR image will not give any additional value in locoregional staging.
- In some cases, it is difficult to differentiate tumor infiltration from a desmoplastic reaction.
- While T stage is a strong predictor of overall prognosis, the CRM is an important predictor of local recurrence.
- CRM and extramural vessel invasion (EMVI) are not a part of TNM, but should be mentioned since they are independent predictors of prognosis and local recurrence.

Suggested Readings

Dewhurst CE, Mortele KJ. Magnetic resonance imaging of rectal cancer. *Radiol Clin North Am*. 2013 Jan;51(1):121-131.

Iannicelli E, Di Renzo S, Ferri M, et al. Accuracy of high-resolution MRI with lumen distention in rectal cancer staging and circumferential margin involvement prediction. *Korean J Radiol*. 2014;15(1):37-44.

Tong T, Yao Z, Xu L, et al. Extramural depth of tumor invasion at thin-section MR in rectal cancer: associating with prognostic factors and ADC value. *J Magn Reson Imaging*. 2014;40(3):738-744.

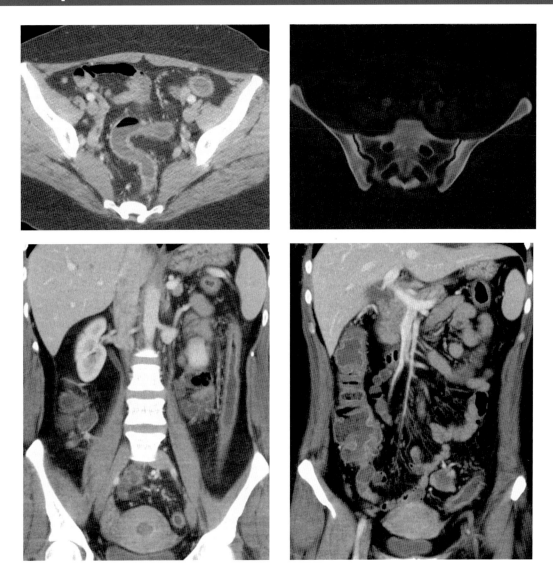

1. What is the differential diagnosis for these findings and what is the most likely diagnosis in a 36-year-old female?

2. What is the common biliary manifestation associated with ulcerative colitis?

3. What is the percentage of rectal involvement in this disease?

4. What is the best investigation for diagnosing ulcerative colitis?

5. What complication of ulcerative colitis is most likely to be fatal?

Case ranking/difficulty:

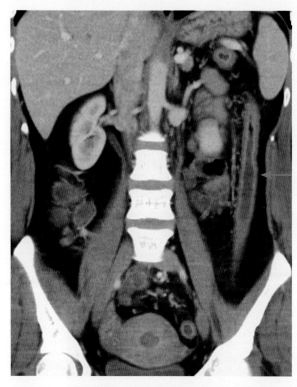

Coronal CT image in portal venous phase demonstrates the descending colonic involvement (*arrow*).

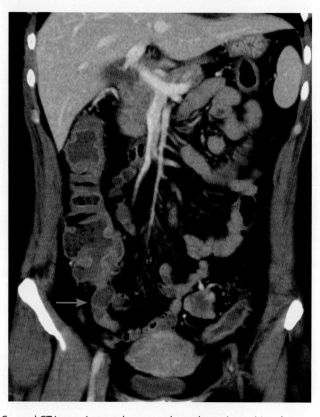

Coronal CT image in portal venous phase shows (*arrow*) involvement of descending colon, cecum, and terminal ileum (backwash ileitis).

Answers

1. Ulcerative colitis, Crohn disease, pseudomembranous colitis, infectious colitis, and ischemic colitis are in the differential diagnosis. The continuous involvement and backwash ileitis favor the correct diagnosis of UC over Crohn. Lack of exposure to antibiotics, lack of hospitalization, and lack of fever are against pseudomembranous and infectious colitis. Ischemic colitis would be most unusual in a 36-year-old woman.

2. Up to 5% of patients with ulcerative colitis develop primary sclerosing cholangitis. Interestingly, colectomy does not cure the biliary disease.

3. 95% cases of UC have rectal involvement. It is present in about 20% of patients with Crohn disease.

4. Colonoscopy with biopsy is the best test for diagnosis of ulcerative colitis. Mucosal biopsy shows cryptitis and crypt abscesses. Sometimes the pathology is inconclusive. Differentiation of ulcerative colitis from Crohn disease is important for management.

5. Toxic megacolon occurs in 5% to 10% of cases. Transverse colonic distension >6 cm in the setting of systemic toxicity is suggestive of toxic megacolon.

Pearls

- CT identification of colonic wall thickness greater than 5 mm is predictive of colonic pathology and requires further investigation.
- Halo (target) sign suggests a benign etiology of bowel disease.
- Rectum is almost always (95%) involved in UC but relatively spared in Crohn disease.
- Terminal ileal involvement is seen in about 90% of Crohn patients.
- In backwash ileitis (10%-25% of UC), the patulous ileocecal valve and absence of ulceration and peristalsis in the terminal ileum can distinguish the diagnosis of UC from Crohn.
- Toxic megacolon is a potentially fatal complication of UC in which the colon is dilated to more than 6 cm in diameter accompanied by systemic toxicity.
- Adenocarcinoma can develop in 3% to 5 % of cases of UC, risk starts after 10 years.

Suggested Readings

Horton KM, Corl FM, Fishman EK. CT evaluation of the colon: inflammatory disease. *Radiographics.* 2000;20(2):399-418.

Kawamoto S, Horton KM, Fishman EK. Pseudomembranous colitis: spectrum of imaging findings with clinical and pathologic correlation. *Radiographics.* 1999;19(4):887-897.

Patel B, Mottola J, Sahni VA, et al. MDCT assessment of ulcerative colitis: radiologic analysis with clinical, endoscopic, and pathologic correlation. *Abdom Imaging.* 2012 Feb;37(1):61-69.

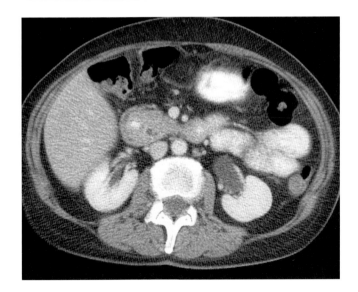 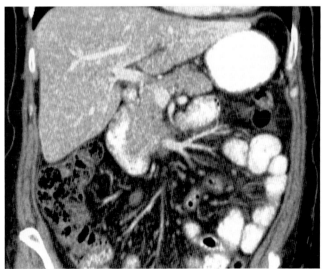

1. What is the most likely diagnosis?

2. What is the most common presentation of this condition in adults, if symptomatic?

3. What is the most common presentation of this condition in children?

4. What are the in utero ultrasonographic findings of this condition?

5. What is the treatment of annular pancreas if symptomatic in neonates?

Case ranking/difficulty:

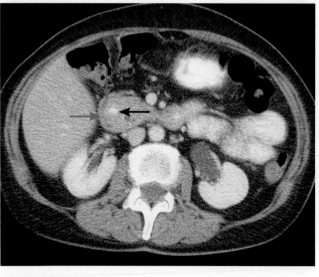

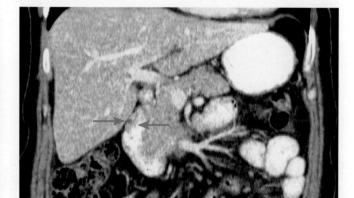

Axial CT image demonstrates a rind of pancreatic tissue with duct (*green arrows*) encircling the second part of the duodenum filled with oral contrast (*black arrow*).

Coronal CT image shows a thin rind of pancreatic tissue with duct (*arrows*) along the lateral wall of the second part of the duodenum.

Answers

1. Note the course of the pancreatic duct around the duodenum consistent with annular pancreas.

2. If symptomatic, it is usually present as a focal pancreatitis in the head and annulus. This condition is mostly asymptomatic and detected as an incidental finding during imaging.

3. During the neonatal period, features of gastric outlet obstruction is the usual presentation of annular pancreas.

4. Double bubble sign, polyhydramnios, and enlarged pancreatic head are the in utero ultrasonographic features of annular pancreas.

5. Gastrojejunostomy or duodenojejunostomy are the treatment options if annular pancreas is symptomatic during neonatal period.

Pearls

- In children, the most common clinical presentation is features of duodenal obstruction. In adults, it is mostly asymptomatic. If symptomatic, the presentations are acute pancreatitis, peptic ulcer disease or duodenal obstruction.

- Complete annular pancreas shows a rind of pancreatic tissue and duct around the 2nd part of duodenum. Incomplete annular pancreas shows a rim of pancreatic tissue incompletely around the duodenum, gives rise to 'Crocodile jaw appearance' of pancreatic head. The risk of duodenal obstruction is same as complete annular pancreas.

Suggested Readings

Sandrasegaran K, Patel A, Fogel EL, Zyromski NJ, Pitt HA. Annular pancreas in adults. *AJR Am J Roentgenol.* August 2009;193(2):455-460.

Türkvatan A, Erden A, Türkoğlu MA, Yener Ö. Congenital variants and anomalies of the pancreas and pancreatic duct: imaging by magnetic resonance cholangiopancreaticography and multidetector computed tomography. *Korean J Radiol.* January 2014;14(6):905-913.

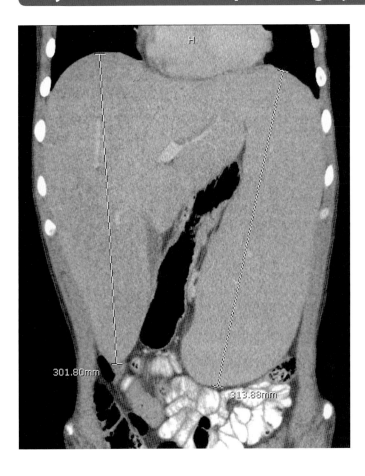 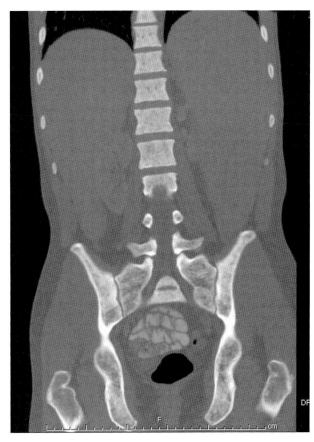

1. What is the diagnosis and what kind of
   neoplasm is it according to the World Health
   Organization?

2. What are the main radiographic manifestations
   of myelofibrosis?

3. Approximately 50% of patients with primary
   myelofibrosis have a defect in the gene for
   what enzyme?

4. What are the MRI characteristics of marrow in
   advanced myelofibrosis?

5. What tumor can myelofibrosis evolve into?

Case ranking/difficulty:

Answers

1. Based on the hepatosplenomegaly, bone sclerosis and extramedullary hematopoiesis the best diagnosis is myelofibrosis.

   In 2008, the World Health Organization reorganized its classification scheme for myeloid neoplasms. Primary myelofibrosis is classified as a myeloproliferative neoplasm, along with chronic myelogenous leukemia, polycythemia vera, essential thrombocythemia, and several other disorders.

2. The primary disorder is related to the marrow fibrosis that is the result of growth factors released by atypical megakaryocytes. This accounts for the skeletal findings. Hematopoiesis is displaced to extramedullary locations, including the spleen, liver, and multiple other locations.

3. Approximately 50% of patients with primary myelofibrosis have a defect in the gene encoding for Janus kinase 2. This has led to the development of newer drug therapies for primary myelofibrosis. Ruxolitinib and other newer agents are Janus kinase inhibitors that have shown some promise in treatment.

4. Due to the degree of fibrosis and sclerosis myelofibrosis has low signal characteristics on both T1W and T2W sequences. Similar findings can be noted in other marrow disorders such as mastocytosis or osteosclerosis.

5. Myelofibrosis can develop from essential thrombocytosis (ET) and polycythemia vera (PV), in which case it is secondary myelofibrosis. However, myelofibrosis can also evolve into acute myelogenous leukemia, as can ET and PV.

Pearls

- Marrow replacement disorder characterized by myelofibrosis and extramedullary hematopoiesis.
- Splenomegaly, hepatomegaly, extramedullary hematopoiesis, and osteosclerosis are common radiographic manifestations.
- Massive splenomegaly along with bone changes suggests the diagnosis.

Suggested Readings

Campbell PJ, Green AR. The myeloproliferative disorders. *N Engl J Med.* 2006;355(23):2452-2466. Epub 2006/12/08. doi: 10.056/NEJMra063728.

Guermazi A, de Kerviler E, Cazals-Hatem D, Zagdanski AM, Frija J. Imaging findings in patients with myelofibrosis. *Eur Radiol.* 1999;9(7):1366-1375. Epub 1999/08/25.

Kutti J, Ridell B. Epidemiology of the myeloproliferative disorders: essential thrombocythaemia, polycythaemia vera and idiopathic myelofibrosis. *Pathol Biol (Paris).* 2001;49(2):164-166. Epub 2001/04/25.

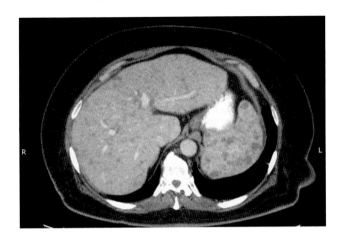 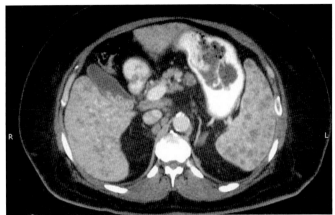

1. What is the most likely diagnosis, assuming that the patient appears better than the images suggest?

2. In what demographic is sarcoidosis more common?

3. Can abdominal sarcoidosis be hypermetabolic on PET/CT?

4. How does splenic nodular sarcoidosis appear on MRI?

5. Approximately what percentage of patients with sarcoidosis will have hepatosplenic findings on imaging studies?

Case ranking/difficulty:

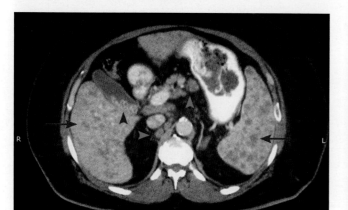

Axial portal venous phase CT at a lower level again shows numerous diffuse hypodensities throughout the liver and spleen (*red arrows*). Gallstones are incidentally noted (*red arrowhead*). Numerous small lymph nodes are noted (*green arrowheads*).

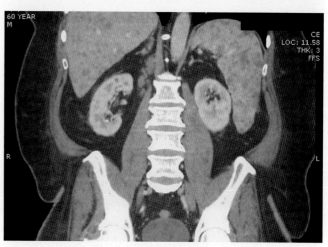

Coronal portal venous phase CT shows the multiple hypodensities in the liver and spleen, as well as the splenomegaly.

Answers

1. Hemangiomas are usually solitary lesions in the spleen, or at least few in number. Microabscesses would be a thought, but there is usually a history of immunosuppression, the lesions often have some peripheral enhancement, the lesions are not as solid as sarcoidosis, and the patient would likely be ill. Lymphoma is a thought also because it is a systemic illness and can involve the liver, spleen, and lymph nodes, as in this case. The lesions in lymphoma are more discrete than are the lesions in sarcoidosis, and there may be disease elsewhere. Metastatic disease is possible, although metastases to the spleen are unusual and are not so numerous, and there would likely be a history of malignancy elsewhere.

   Sarcoidosis is the best choice, especially given the additional history that the patient seems to be better than the images would suggest.

2. In the United States, the incidence is highest in African Americans and in women. The incidence in African Americans is at least three times that of the base rate.

3. Abdominal lymphadenopathy and abdominal organ involvement in sarcoidosis can be hypermetabolic on PET/CT, including diffuse splenic hypermetabolic activity. This can be confusing if considering lymphoma in the differential diagnosis.

4. Sarcoid nodules in the spleen are low signal on T1W, low signal on T2W, and they do not enhance early. They may become less conspicuous on delayed images after the administration of contrast.

5. On autopsy series, hepatosplenic disease is relatively common, but on imaging studies only about 5% to 15% of patients with sarcoidosis have findings. Symptomatic liver or splenic disease is unusual.

Pearls

- Characterized by noncaseating epithelioid granulomas involving primarily the liver, spleen, and lymph nodes. Other abdominal organs can be rarely affected.
- Rare for abdominal involvement to cause complications.
- Important to differentiate from malignancy such as metastatic disease or lymphoma.

Suggested Readings

Britt AR, Francis IR, Glazer GM, Ellis JH. Sarcoidosis: abdominal manifestations at CT. *Radiology*. 1991;178(1):91-94. Epub 1991/01/01. doi: 10.1148/radiology.178.1.1984330.

Prabhakar HB, Rabinowitz CB, Gibbons FK, O'Donnell WJ, Shepard JA, Aquino SL. Imaging features of sarcoidosis on MDCT, FDG PET, and PET/CT. *AJR Am J Roentgenol*. 2008;190(3 suppl):S1-S6. Epub 2008/03/08. doi: 10.2214/ajr.07.7001.

Warshauer DM, Lee JK. Imaging manifestations of abdominal sarcoidosis. *AJR Am Roentgenol*. 2004;182(1):15-28. Epub 2003/12/20. doi: 10.2214/ajr.182.1.1820015.

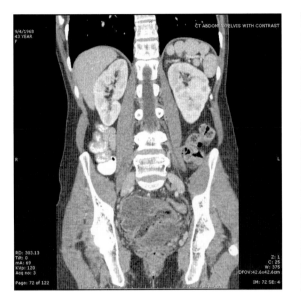
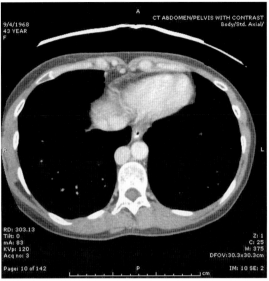
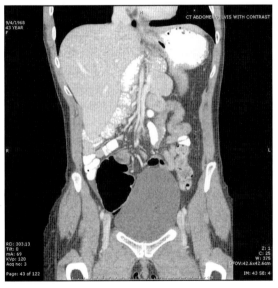
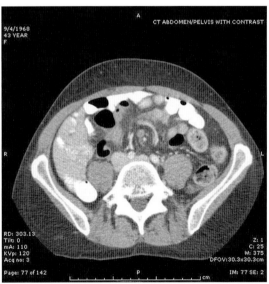

1. What is the diagnosis?

2. What is polysplenia also called?

3. Where is the SMA normally located relative to the SMV?

4. Describe the bronchial anatomy in asplenia.

5. What additional pulmonary disorder is sometimes associated with the heterotaxy syndromes?

Case ranking/difficulty:

Category: Spleen

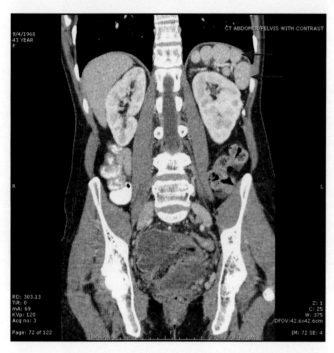

Coronal portal venous phase CT shows multiple spleens in the left upper quadrant (*red arrows*). Note that there is not a dominant spleen, as would be seen in the case of one or more splenules.

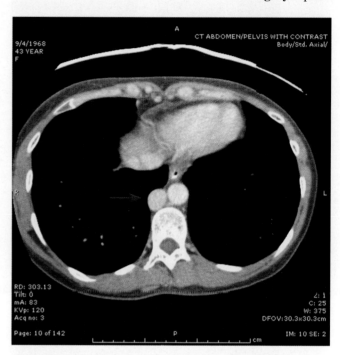

Axial contrast-enhanced CT shows enlarged azygous vein (*red arrow*) at a level slightly above the diaphragm, correlating with azygous continuation of the IVC.

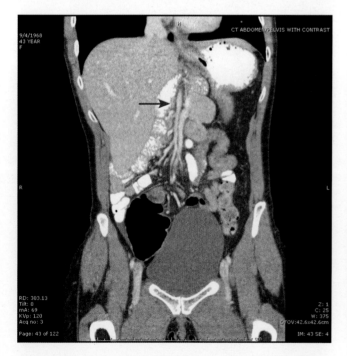

Coronal portal venous phase CT shows reversal of the SMA/SMV relationship (*red arrow*) with the SMA on the right and associated malrotation of bowel.

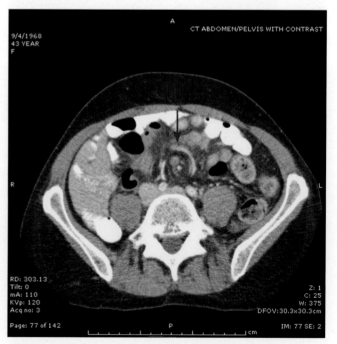

Axial portal venous phase CT shows a whirled appearance of the mesenteric vessels and surrounding fat corresponding to malrotation (*red arrow*).

Answers

1. The images show that there is azygous continuation of the IVC, multiple spleens of somewhat similar size in the left upper quadrant, and malrotation of bowel. Without ancillary findings one might consider multiple splenules or splenosis, although the spleens are somewhat similar in size, numerous, and there is no evidence of trauma. Given the other findings, this fits into a diagnosis of polysplenia.

2. Polysplenia and asplenia are both part of the heterotaxy syndromes, disorders in the normal development of asymmetry within the chest and abdomen. Bilateral left sidedness occurs when the left-sided structures are "duplicated" in a sense. In the lung, this means that the right lung has bronchial anatomy of the normal left side, a hyparterial main bronchus that is long. Left isomerism is the same thing as bilateral left sidedness. Right isomerism and bilateral right sidedness refer to asplenia.

3. Near its origin, the SMA is normally located to the left of the SMV. In malrotation, this relationship is usually different, with the SMA being located outside its normal position. In this case, it is located to the right of the SMV.

4. In asplenia, there is bilateral right sidedness, or right isomerism, so the normal bronchial anatomy on the right is duplicated in the left lung, so the left lung is trilobed with a short eparterial bronchus.

5. There is a diverse group of disorders termed "ciliopathies." Primary ciliary dyskinesia is included in that classification, and there is some evidence to suggest that the heterotaxy syndromes may be related to a disorder of cilia during development. There is an association, with some patients with heterotaxy syndromes also having primary ciliary dyskinesia.

Pearls

- Complex group of developmental anomalies involving abnormal development of normal asymmetry in the chest and abdomen.
- Also known as bilateral right sidedness (asplenia or right isomerism) and bilateral left sidedness (polysplenia or left isomerism).
- Patients with asplenia generally have more severe cardiac anomalies and have the additional complication of asplenia that makes them prone to infectious/immunologic complications.
- Abdominal manifestations of polysplenia including polysplenia, azygous continuation of the IVC, variable position of the stomach and liver, short pancreas, preduodenal portal vein, bowel malrotation/volvulus, biliary atresia, and bowel atresias and duplications.

Suggested Readings

Applegate KE, Goske MJ, Pierce G, Murphy D. Situs revisited: imaging of the heterotaxy syndrome. *Radiographics*. 1999;19(4):837-852; discussion 853-8544. Epub 1999/08/28. doi: 10.1148/radiographics.19.4.g99jl31837.

Dilli A, Gultekin SS, Ayaz UY, Kaplanoglu H, Hekimoglu B. A rare variation of the heterotaxy syndrome. *Case Rep Med*. 2012;2012:840453. Epub 2012/07/20. doi: 10.1155/2012/840453.

Kim SJ. Heterotaxy syndrome. *Korean Circ J*. 2011;41(5):227-232. Epub 2011/07/07. doi: 10.4070/kcj.2011.41.5.227.

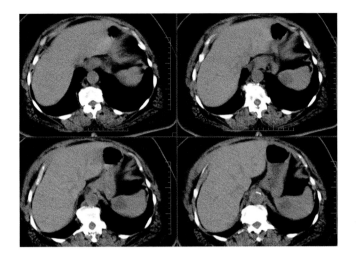
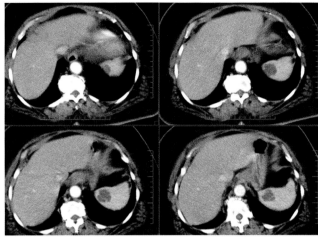
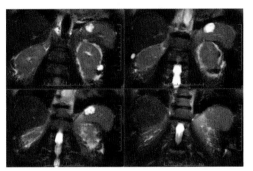
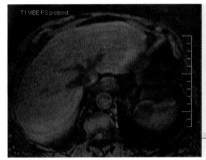
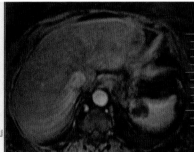

1. What is the most likely diagnosis?

2. What is the typical location for a solitary splenic lymphangioma?

3. When do the vast majority of lymphangiomas (anywhere) present?

4. What is the typical appearance of splenic lymphangiomas on MRI?

5. What are the different types of splenic lymphangiomas?

Case ranking/difficulty:

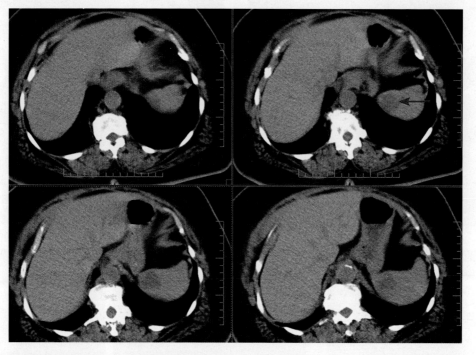

Noncontrast CT shows a hypodense subcapsular lesion with lobular contours (*red arrow*).

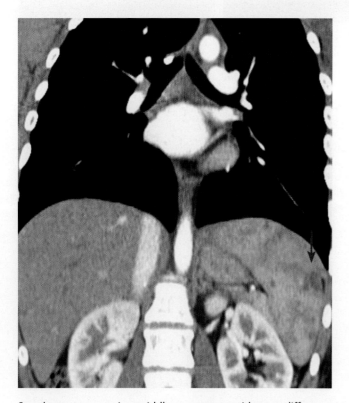

Supplementary case in a middle-age woman with more diffuse involvement of the spleen showing multiple irregular hypodense foci within the spleen (*red arrow*). Splenic lymphangiomatosis. The patient also had systemic involvement.

Answers

1. A solitary, subcapsular, multicystic lesion with lobular margins and slightly enhancing septae is most likely a lymphangioma.

   Abscess, lymphoma, cystic metastasis, primary or secondary cysts, and hemangioma could all be considered in the differential diagnosis. Ultrasound or MRI may be helpful in clarification, along with the clinical history.

   Lymphoma is hypodense on CT, but does not appear cystic on US or MRI, and it is unusual to have a solitary well-defined lesion. Cystic metastases are possible, but rare, and there would usually be a history of primary malignancy. Abscesses appear cystic, but they are often multiple, or there are satellite lesions, and the patients have signs and symptoms of infection. Primary or secondary cysts are a consideration but may not have as many septae or lobulations as the case here. Hemangioma is also a thought, but they are not cystic, and they often demonstrate a peripheral to central enhancement pattern.

2. Particularly when solitary, splenic hemangiomas have been described as most often having a subcapsular location, possibly related to the proximity of splenic lymphatics in this location.

3. Lymphangiomas, in general, present early in life, with 80% to 90% presenting prior to the second year of life. It is unusual for them to present after the age of 20. If a splenic lesion suggestive of a lymphangioma is seen in a child one should be aware that there may be extrasplenic lesions as part of a lymphangiomatosis syndrome.

4. Lymphangiomas are typically cystic lesions, so they are often low signal on T1W, high signal on T2W, and they may have septae (multilocular) that may or may not enhance. They are well defined and sharply marginated and may have lobular contours. Occasionally, they may have higher signal on T1W sequences owing to the presence of protein or hemorrhage within the cystic components.

5. Pathologically, splenic lymphangiomas are classified as capillary, cavernous, and cystic, based primarily on the size of the lymphatic spaces. The cystic variety is the most common. If the lymphatic spaces are small, they can have a more solid appearance on imaging studies.

Pearls

- Rare vascular neoplasm involving the spleen, either as an isolated finding or as part of lymphangiomatosis.
- Typically subcapsular location in the spleen. Well-marginated cystic or multicystic lesion with septae that may enhance.
- If seen in a pediatric patient, one should be alert to the possibility of extrasplenic disease.

Suggested Readings

Abbott RM, Levy AD, Aguilera NS, Gorospe L, Thompson WM. From the archives of the AFIP: primary vascular neoplasms of the spleen: radiologic-pathologic correlation. *Radiographics*. 2004;24(4):1137-1163. Epub 2004/07/17. doi: 10.1148/rg.244045006.

Caremani M, Occhini U, Caremani A, Tacconi D, Lapini L, Accorsi A, et al. Focal splenic lesions: US findings. *J Ultrasound*. 2013;16(2):65-74. Epub 2013/12/03. doi: 10.1007/s40477-013-0014-0.

Levy AD, Cantisani V, Miettinen M. Abdominal lymphangiomas: imaging features with pathologic correlation. *AJR Am Journal Roentgenol*. 2004;182(6):1485-1491. Epub 2004/05/20. doi: 10.2214/ajr.182.6.1821485.

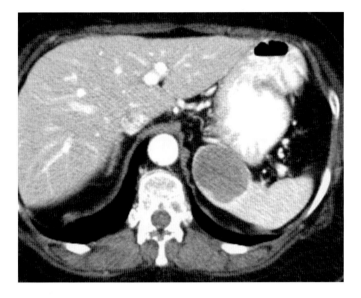
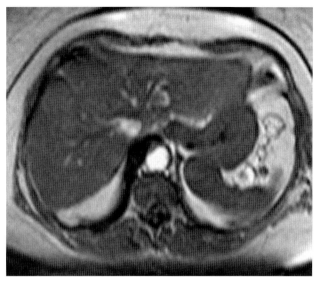

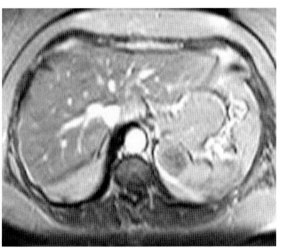
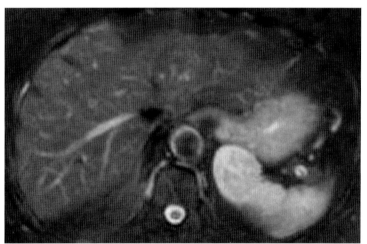

1. The diagnosis is the most common benign tumor in the spleen. What is that?

2. What are the different types of splenic hemangiomas, broadly speaking?

3. Which among hemorrhage/rupture, Kasabach-Merritt syndrome, infection, sepsis and neutropenia are possible complications.

4. Name some syndromes that are associated with splenic hemangiomas.

5. What are typical MRI features of splenic hemangioma?

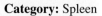
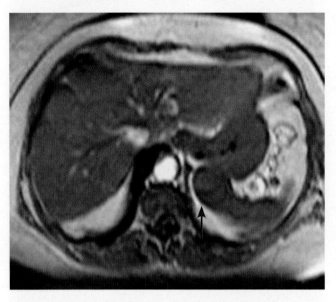

T1W axial MRI shows relatively isointense lesion (*red arrow*) within the medial aspect of the spleen.

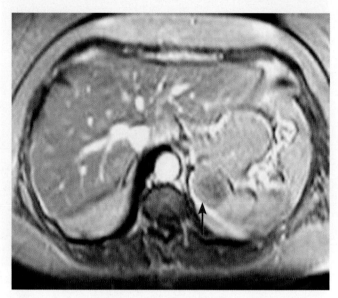

T1W postcontrast MRI shows slightly hypointense lesion (*red arrow*) within the medial aspect of the spleen.

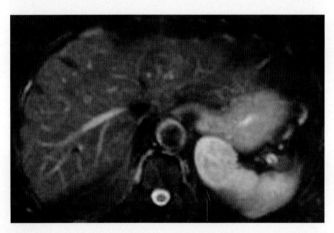

T2W fat saturated axial MRI shows the lesion (*red arrow*) in the medial aspect of the spleen. It is slightly hyperintense on T2W. They are typically somewhat more hyperintense than this.

Answers

1. Although relatively rare, hemangiomas are the most common benign tumor of the spleen, with a range of around 0.02% to 0.16% in some series. Congenital cysts, lymphangiomas, hamartomas, and littoral cell angioma are less common.

2. There are two pathologic types of splenic hemangiomas, capillary and cavernous. They can have different appearances on ultrasound examination with the capillary type more typically being hyperechoic and well defined, whereas the cavernous type is often more heterogeneous in appearance.

3. Spontaneous hemorrhage/rupture and Kasabach-Merritt syndrome are recognized complications. Kasabach-Merritt syndrome is also sometimes called hemangioma thrombocytopenia syndrome and is a consumptive thrombocytopenia related to the underlying tumor. In the older literature a significant number of cases of splenic hemangioma presented with spontaneous rupture.

4. Although rare, there are reported associations between splenic hemangioma and Klippel-Trenaunay-Weber, Gorham disease, Sturge-Weber, and von Hippel-Lindau. Klippel-Trenaunay-Weber is the association most commonly reported. There is no reported association with neurofibromatosis.

5. Typically, splenic hemangiomas are isointense to hypointense on T1W, hyperintense on T2W, and they have an enhancement pattern that proceeds from peripheral to central, although that is typically not as characteristic as the nodular and discontinuous pattern seen in hepatic hemangiomas.

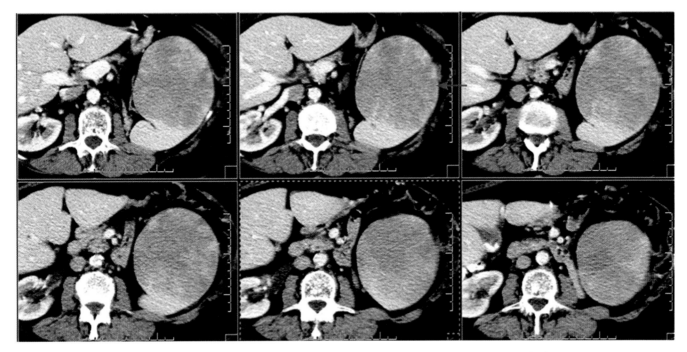

Supplementary case showing a much larger hypodense lesion within the spleen (*red arrow*) with peripheral inhomogeneous enhancement.

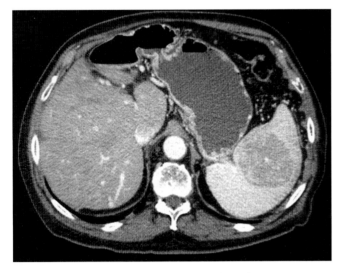

89-year-old male, incidental finding. Large hypodense splenic mass with inhomogeneous enhancement and central enhancement.

Pearls

- Most common primary benign tumor of the spleen.
- Usually solitary, well defined, and small (<2cm).
- Capillary variety usually hyperechoic and well defined on ultrasound. Cavernous types may be more complex on ultrasound.
- Imaging findings are typically not completely diagnostic. Differentiating from metastases or lymphoma can sometimes be problematic.

Suggested Readings

Abbott RM, Levy AD, Aguilera NS, Gorospe L, Thompson WM. From the archives of the AFIP: primary vascular neoplasms of the spleen: radiologic-pathologic correlation. *Radiographics*. 2004;24(4):1137-1163. Epub 2004/07/17. doi: 10.1148/rg.244045006.

Caremani M, Occhini U, Caremani A, Tacconi D, Lapini L, Accorsi A, et al. Focal splenic lesions: US findings. *J Ultrasound*. 2013;16(2):65-74. Epub 2013/12/03. doi: 10.1007/s40477-013-0014-0.

Levy AD, Cantisani V, Miettinen M. Abdominal lymphangiomas: imaging features with pathologic correlation. *AJR Am J Roentgenol*. 2004;182(6):1485-1491. Epub 2004/05/20. doi: 10.2214/ajr.182.6.1821485.

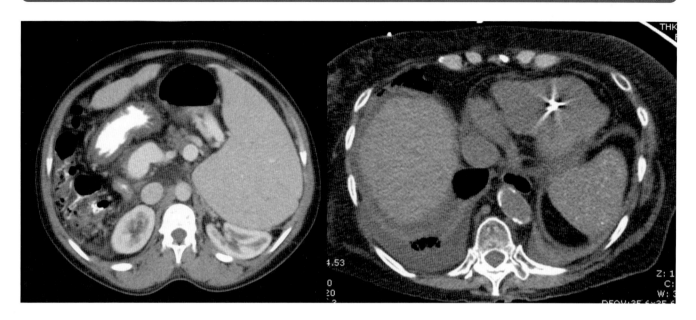

1. What are the splenic lesions and what are they called?

2. What is the most sensitive imaging modality in the detection of Gamna-Gandy bodies?

3. Approximately what percent of patients with portal hypertension have Gamna-Gandy bodies on MRI?

4. What is the treatment for Gamna-Gandy bodies?

5. On ultrasound, what other entities could be considered?

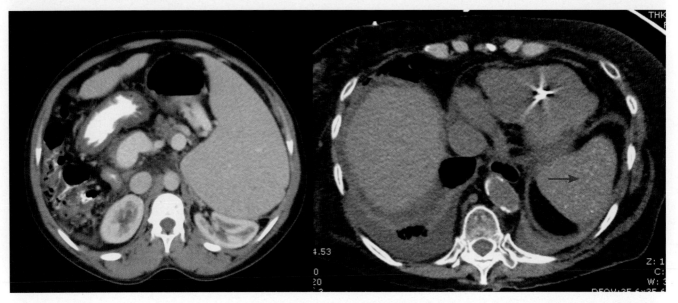

CT (*left panel*) shows splenomegaly with compression of the left kidney. Gamna-Gandy bodies are not particularly well seen on this CT, although they are seen on ultrasound examination. Unrelated case (*right panel*) does show multiple punctate calcifications within the spleen on CT (*red arrow*).

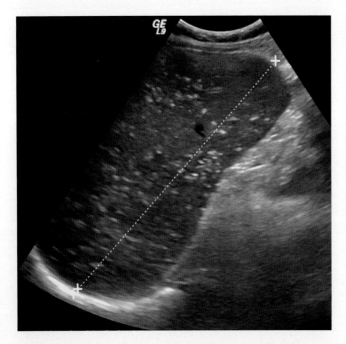

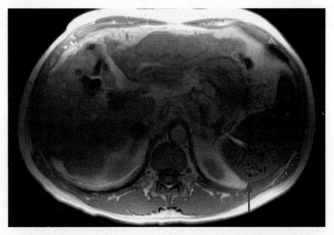

Supplementary case in 50-year-old male with cirrhosis. T1W gradient echo sequence with longer TE shows multiple small low signal foci within the spleen. The lesions are fairly well seen on most sequences, but because of their hemosiderin content, they are best seen on gradient echo sequences (*red arrow*).

US image through the spleen, the same patient as left panel of CT's above, shows splenomegaly as well as diffuse punctate hyperechoic foci throughout the spleen (*red arrow*).

Answers

1. The splenic lesions are known as splenic siderotic nodules or as Gamna-Gandy bodies. They are relatively common in patients with underlying liver disease and portal hypertension.

   The lesions do not resemble Gaucher lesions, hemangioma, lymphangioma, or littoral cell angioma.

2. Gamna-Gandy bodies contain hemosiderin and this makes them particularly conspicuous on gradient echo MRI images that have small flip angles and longer echo times because of the magnetic susceptibility effects. They have low signal on T1W, T2W, and T2* sequences. CT is relatively insensitive, depending on the size and calcium content of lesions. Ultrasound is relatively sensitive, and lesions appear as small, diffuse echogenic foci, with or without acoustic shadowing.

3. Approximately 10% of patients with portal hypertension have Gamna-Gandy bodies on MRI.

4. Gamna-Gandy bodies themselves do not require treatment. They may be a marker for the underlying disease such as portal hypertension or even schistosomiasis.

5. Granulomatous diseases (which includes sarcoidosis, tuberculosis, and histoplasmosis) can be included in the differential diagnosis, although the clinical history should help, and Gamna-Gandy bodies are small, echogenic (with or without shadowing), and fairly uniform, and there may be a history of portal hypertension or other risk factors.

Healed histoplasmosis is typically heavily calcified and has acoustic shadowing. Healed tuberculosis could have a similar appearance. Sarcoidosis can have various appearances including splenomegaly, diffuse infiltrative pattern, or other appearances. History would again be helpful.

Pearls

- Brightly echogenic small foci scattered through the spleen, primarily in patients with portal hypertension or hemolytic anemia.
- Low signal foci on T1W and T2W images on MRI with magnetic susceptibility effects related to the hemosiderin content.

Suggested Readings

Bhatt S, Simon R, Dogra VS. Gamna-Gandy bodies: sonographic features with histopathologic correlation. *J Ultrasound Med.* 2006;25(12):1625-1629. Epub 2006/11/24.

Selçuk D, Demirel K, Kantarci F, Mihmanli I, Oğüt G. Gamna-Gandy bodies: a sign of portal hypertension. *Turk J Gastroenterol.* 2005;16(3):150-152. Epub 2005/10/26.

Yilmaz S, Yekeler E, Rozanes I. Education and imaging. Hepatobiliary and pancreatic: Gamna-Gandy bodies of the spleen. *J Gastroenterol Hepatol.* 2007;22(5):758. Epub 2007/04/21. doi: 10.1111/j.1440-1746.2007.04965.x.

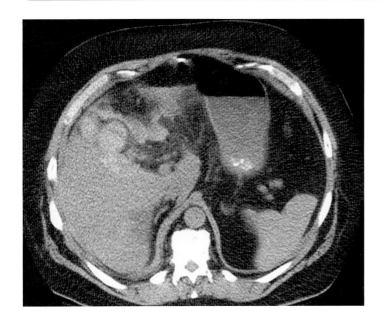 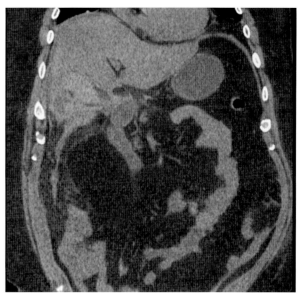

1. What is the diagnosis?

2. What is the classification system for gallbladder perforation?

3. What is the most common location in the gallbladder to perforate?

4. What is an estimate of mortality rates in gallbladder perforation?

5. Which imaging modality is superior in the evaluation of suspected gallbladder perforation?

Case ranking/difficulty:

Category: Gallbladder

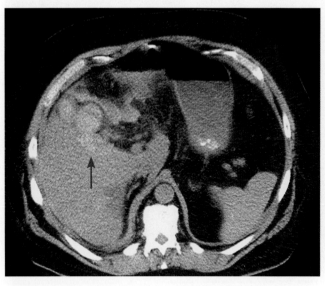

CT shows high-density material within the gallbladder fossa (*red arrow*) that is partially contained, corresponding to blood and pus.

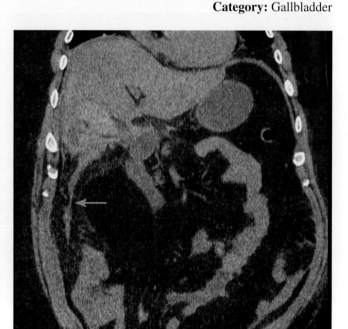

Coronal CT shows mixed density, but mostly blood (*red arrow*) within the gallbladder fossa with material tracking inferiorly into the abdomen (*green arrow*).

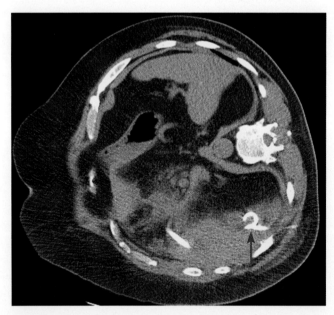

Postoperative CT showing percutaneous drain in place for treatment of abscess and hemorrhage (*red arrow*).

Answers

1. There is hemorrhage partially contained within the gallbladder fossa but tracking inferiorly into the abdomen. There is no free air, but this would not normally be expected with gallbladder perforation. An ultrasound might help, but even with the CT one should be concerned about gallbladder perforation given that the hemorrhage is epicentered over the gallbladder.

2. There is a quite old classification system for categorizing gallbladder perforations introduced by Niemeier back in 1934. This is still in use today:

   Type I—Acute free perforation into the peritoneal cavity

   Type II—Subacute perforation with pericholecystic abscess

   Type III—Chronic perforation with cholecystoenteric fistula

3. Perforation is thought to be related to ischemic changes within the gallbladder wall. Increased intraluminal pressure compromises venous and lymphatic drainage from the gallbladder. The fundus has an inferior blood supply and is therefore susceptible to ischemia.

   In some cases, the insult may be a focus of infection developing within a Rokitansky-Aschoff space.

4. Reported statistics vary, and they have improved over time, but a reasonable estimate is 12% to 16%.

5. Ultrasound is often the initial modality used for evaluation, but it is operator dependent and there may be technical factors that interfere with getting a good examination. It is superior to CT in detecting gallstones. CT is superior in detecting direct and indirect signs of perforation. The "hole" sign, a defect in the gallbladder wall, is a specific sign that can sometimes be seen on ultrasound, but CT is superior in the detection of a wall defect in the setting of gallbladder perforation.

Pearls

- Severe complication of gallbladder disease with mortality rate near 15%.
- Fundus is the most common site of perforation.
- Niemeier classification into acute, subacute, and chronic types.
- Look for defect or bulge in gallbladder wall, with CT somewhat superior to ultrasound for detection of that direct sign.

Suggested Readings

Chiapponi C, Wirth S, Siebeck M. Acute gallbladder perforation with gallstones spillage in a cirrhotic patient. *World J Emerg Surg*. 2010;5:11. Epub 2010/04/27. doi: 10.1186/1749-7922-5-11.

Coppolino F, Gatta G, Di Grezia G, Reginelli A, Iacobellis F, Vallone G, et al. Gastrointestinal perforation: ultrasonographic diagnosis. *Crit Ultrasound J*. 2013;5 suppl 1:S4. Epub 2013/08/02. doi: 10.1186/2036-7902-5-s1-s4.

Morris BS, Balpande PR, Morani AC, Chaudhary RK, Maheshwari M, Raut AA. The CT appearances of gallbladder perforation. *Br J Radiol*. 2007;80(959):898-901. Epub 2007/10/03. doi: 10.1259/bjr/28510614.

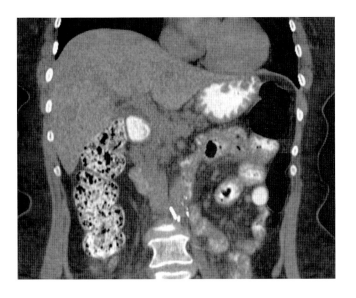
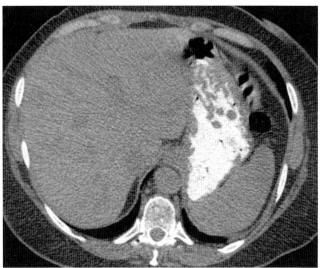

1. Where is the abnormality?

2. What is the most likely diagnosis of these stomach lesions?

3. What is the most common type of polyp in the stomach?

4. What is the most common presentation of gastric polyps?

5. What syndrome(s) are associated with gastric polyps?

Case ranking/difficulty:

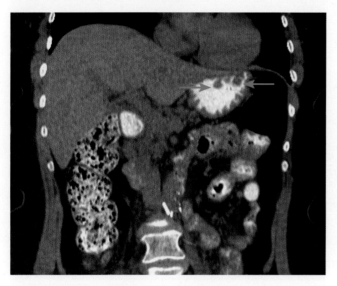

Coronal noncontrast CT shows pedunculated polyps (*green arrows*) from the stomach wall.

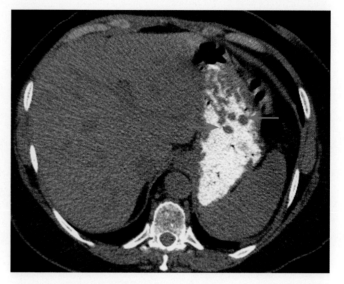

Axial noncontrast CT demonstrates multiple well-defined filling defects within the gastric lumen (*arrows*).

Answers

1. Multiple pedunculated filling defects arising from stomach fundal wall.

2. The small gastric filling defects attached to the wall are likely to be gastric polyps.

3. Hyperplastic polyps are the most common type of gastric polyps.

4. Gastric polyps most commonly present as incidental findings on upper GI endoscopy.

5. Peutz-Jeghers syndrome, Gardner syndrome, Cronkhite-Canada syndrome, and juvenile polyposis are all associated with gastric polyps. Adenomatous polyps develop in half of the cases of familial polyposis and Gardner syndrome.

- Surveillance endoscopy after 1 year is an acceptable method of follow-up after removal of gastric fundal polyp.
- There is no adenoma-carcinoma sequence in the stomach in contrast to the colon. However, patients with gastric adenomas have an increased risk of adenocarcinoma elsewhere in the stomach.

Suggested Readings

Boyd JT, Lee L. Portal hypertension-associated gastric polyps. *BMJ Case Rep*. 2014.

Jang HW, Jeong HY, Kim SH, et al. Adenocarcinoma occurring in a gastric hyperplastic polyp treated with endoscopic submucosal dissection. *J Gastric Cancer*. 2013 Jun;13(2):117-120.

Shaib YH, Rugge M, Graham DY, Genta RM. Management of gastric polyps: an endoscopy-based approach. *Clin Gastroenterol Hepatol*. 2013 Nov;11(11):1374-1384.

Pearls

- Fundic gland polyps are common where PPI are commonly used.
- Hyperplastic polyps are common where *H Pylori* infection is common.
- Adenoma and carcinoids are neoplastic polyps.
- Familial polyposis syndrome needs consideration whenever fundic gland polyp seen before the age of 40 years. Polyps >1cm, >20 polyps, fundic gland polyp in the antrum, and additional duodenal adenoma.

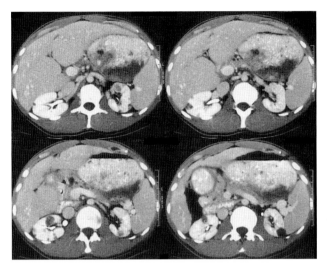
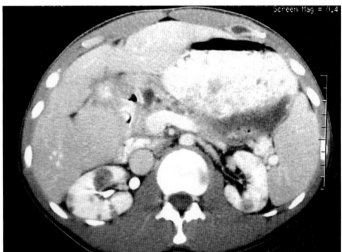

1. What is the best diagnosis?

2. What are the renal manifestations of von Hippel Lindau?

3. What are the pancreatic manifestations of von Hippel Lindau?

4. What criteria need to be met to make the diagnosis of VHL?

5. What are the features of neuroendocrine tumors of the pancreas in VHL?

Case ranking/difficulty:

Category: Pancreas

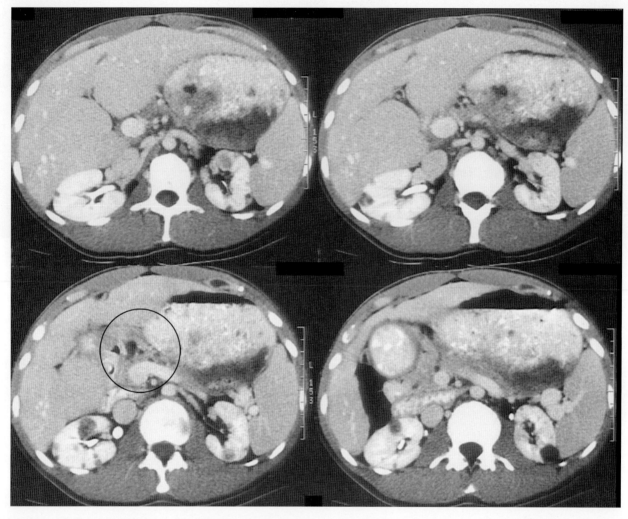

CT showing multiple small pancreatic cysts (*circle*) lower left and multiple renal masses, some cysts, some indeterminate, and some solid.

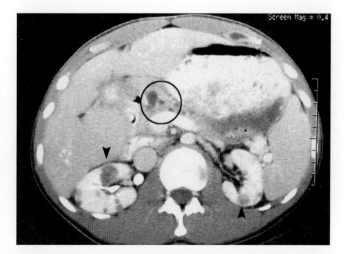

Annotated lower left image showing pancreatic cysts (*circle*) and the largest two renal masses looking solid (*arrowheads*).

Answers

1. The combination of multiple renal cell carcinomas and multiple renal cysts and pancreatic cysts is diagnostic of von Hippel Lindau (VHL) disease.

2. Hemangioblastome, renal cell adenoma, renal cell carcinoma (20-45%), renal hemangioma, and cortical renal cyst (75%) are the renal masses seen in VHL. RCC's often multicentric, bilateral when present.

3. Pancreatic masses in VHL are hemangioblastoma, cysts (50%-91% of patients), microcystic adenoma (12%), nonfunctioning islet cell tumors (5%-17% and associated with pheochromocytoma), and adenocarcinoma (rare).

4. Criteria for the diagnosis of von Hippel Lindau (VHL) include the following:

   (1) More than one hemangioblastoma in the CNS

   (2) One CNS hemangioblastoma and visceral manifestations of VHL

   (3) One manifestation and a known family history of VHL.

5. Neuroendocrine (islet cell) tumors occur in 5% to 17% of VHL patients and more frequently in VHL patients with pheochromocytomas. Most are nonhyperfunctioning, large, but slow growing, and usually picked up at screening. Malignancy and metastases in these tumors is much lower in VHL (~10%) than sporadic cases (60-90%). Because of the slow rate of growth and the low probability of metastases, VHL islet cell tumors may be observed rather than immediately removed.

Pearls

- Criteria for the diagnosis of von Hippel Lindau are:
  (1) More than one hemangioblastoma in the CNS
  (2) One CNS hemangioblastoma and visceral manifestations of VHL
  (3) One manifestation and a known family history of VHL
- Systemic manifestations of VHL are:
  - Retina: hemangioblastoma and retinal angiomatosis
  - Central nervous system: hemangioblastoma of cerebellum, cerebrum, medulla oblongata or spinal cord; syringomyelia, meningioma, AVM of the cervical cord, and posterior fossa epidermoid.
- Labyrinth: endolymphatic sac neoplasm
- Lung: cyst
- Heart: rhabdomyoma
- Kidney: hemangioblastoma, renal cell adenoma, renal cell carcinoma, renal hemangioma, cortical renal cyst
- Bladder: hemangioblastoma
- Epididymis/testis: cysts of the epididymis, clear cell papillary cystadenoma of the epididymis, hypernephroid tumor of the epididymis, and testicular germ cell tumor
- Broad ligament: papillary cystadenoma
- Adrenal gland: pheochromocytoma
- Pancreas: hemangioblastoma, cysts, microcystic adenoma, nonfunctioning islet cell tumors, adenocarcinoma
- Liver: cyst, adenoma, angioma, and carcinoid of the common bile duct
- Spleen: angioma and cyst
- Skin: nevus and café au lait spot
- Bone: cyst and hemangioma
- Miscellaneous: omental and mesenteric cysts and paraganglioma

Suggested Readings

Bhavsar AS, Verma S, Lamba R, Lall CG, Koenigsknecht V, Rajesh A. Abdominal manifestations of neurologic disorders. *Radiographics*. 2013;33(1):135-153, 10.148/rg.31125097.

Leung RS, Biswas SV, Duncan M, Rankin S. Imaging features of von Hippel-Lindau disease. *Radiographics*. October 2008;28(1):65-79; quiz 323.

Shinagare AB, Giardino AA, Jagannathan JP, Van den Abbeele AD, Ramaiya NH. Hereditary cancer syndromes: a radiologist's perspective. *AJR Am J Roentgenol*. December 2011;197(6):W1001-W1007.

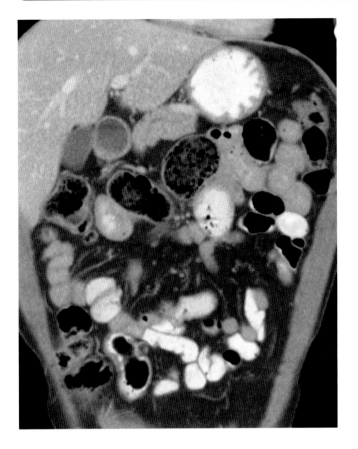 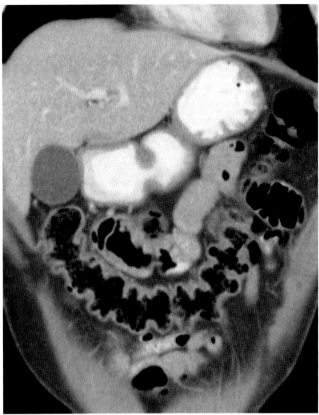

1. What is the correct diagnosis?

2. What are the CT findings of jejunal diverticulosis?

3. What are the possible complications of jejunal diverticulosis?

4. How is jejunal diverticulosis different from its colonic counterpart?

5. What is the best imaging modality for diagnosing jejunal diverticulosis?

Case ranking/difficulty:

Category: Small bowel

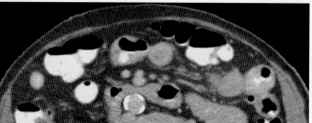

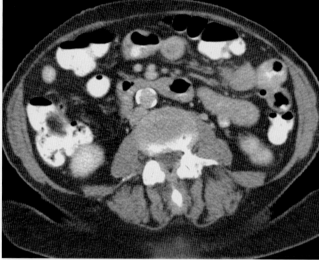

Axial CT shows the same outpouchings (*green arrows*) with food residue.

(Different patient: case 2) Multiple ovoid outpouchings with air fluid levels.

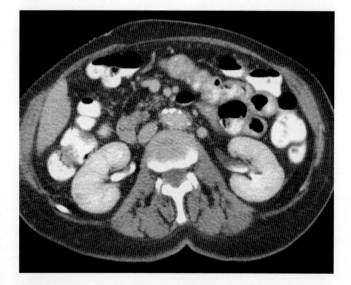

(Different patient: case 2) Barium follow-through demonstrates the diverticulosis, best diagnosed during scrolling through images.

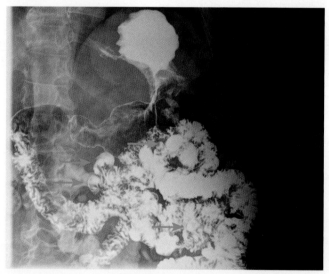

(Different patient: case 2) Barium follow-through confirms the presence of jejunal diverticulosis (*green arrows*). The findings are easy to miss.

Answers

1. Multiple outpouchings from the jejunum represent jejunal diverticulosis.

2. Round or ovoid outpouchings, filled with fluid, air or oral contrast, imperceptible thin wall, and absence of mucosal folds.

3. The possible complications are bacterial overgrowth due to stasis, diverticulitis (infection, perforation), bleeding,

diarrhea, malabsorption, and obstruction from enterolith formation or intussusception.

4. Infections are uncommon. Mostly multiple and more common in proximal jejunum. Incidence is less than colonic diverticula.

5. Even though both small bowel follow-through and enteroclysis are usually diagnostic, enteroclysis can better demonstrate the presence of jejunal diverticula.

Pearls

- Consider jejunal diverticulosis in an elderly patient presenting with unexplained diarrhea without previous history of malabsorption.
- One of the causes of pneumoperitoneum without peritonitis.
- Easy to detect while scrolling through images. Sagittal and coronal reconstructed images will be helpful.
- Difficult to detect when the bowel is dilated (associated with hypomotility).
- Contrary to colonic diverticula, diverticulitis is rare in jejunal diverticula.

Suggested Readings

Fintelmann F, Levine MS, Rubesin SE. Jejunal diverticulosis: findings on CT in 28 patients. *AJR Am J Roentgenol*. 2008 May;190(5):1286-1290.

Macari M, Faust M, Liang H, Pachter HL. CT of jejunal diverticulitis: imaging findings, differential diagnosis, and clinical management. *Clin Radiol*. 2007 Jan;62(1):73-77.

Mantas D, Kykalos S, Patsouras D, Kouraklis G. Small intestine diverticula: is there anything new? *World J Gastrointest Surg*. 2011 Apr;3(4):49-53.

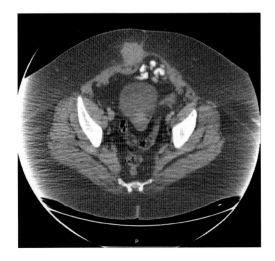

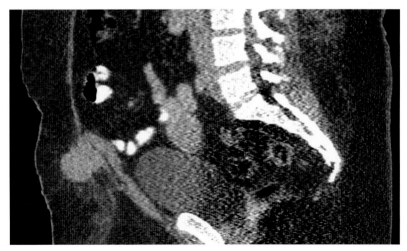

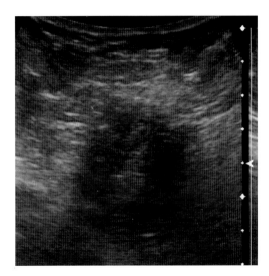

1. Given the history, what is your leading diagnosis?

2. What is the most common location for scar endometriosis?

3. What is the proposed mechanism for most cases of scar endometrioma?

4. What is the latency from a surgical procedure to the development of scar endometrioma?

5. What are the possible treatments for scar endometrioma?

Case ranking/difficulty:

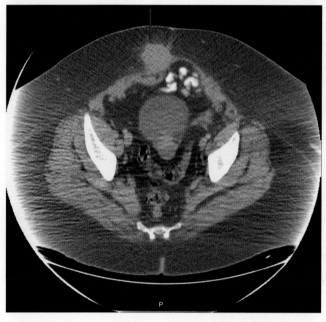

Axial portal venous phase CT shows a soft tissue density mass with irregular margins (*red arrow*) located in the subcutaneous fat anterior to the right rectus abdominis muscle. Clinically, this was located near a surgical scar from prior C-section.

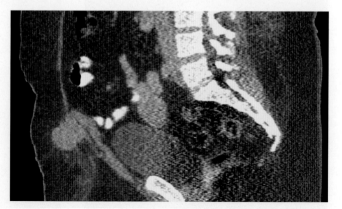

Reformatted sagittal portal venous phase CT again shows the soft tissue density mass largely situated within subcutaneous fat in the suprapubic region.

Answers

1. Desmoid tumor, hematoma, abscess, and metastatic disease can be considered but in a patient with a history of prior cesarian section, cyclical pain, and a mass scar endometrioma is the leading diagnosis.

2. Cesarian section scars are the most common location for scar endometriosis.

3. Most patients with scar endometriomas are thought to acquire them via transplantation of endometrial tissue into a surgical incision at the time of the procedure. One supporting piece of evidence for this is that many patients with scar endometriomas do not have pelvic endometriosis.

   Vascular or lymphatic spread, metaplasia, or transplantation from pelvic endometriomas could explain some cases, but these are in the minority.

4. The latency period from the initial surgical procedure (usually cesarian section) to the clinical presentation with symptoms can be highly variable, with ranges reported from 1 month to 20 years.

5. Wide surgical excision is the most common therapy. Surgical margins need to be generous to prevent the chance of recurrence. Patients and physicians sometimes opt for hormonal therapy. At the time of menopause the endometrioma may regress without other treatment.

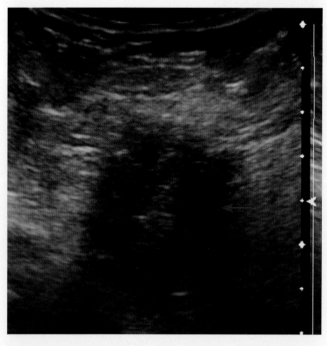

Sagittal ultrasound image from biopsy faintly shows the biopsy needle and the hypoechoic mass on ultrasound (*red arrow*).

Pseudomembranous colitis

Category: Colorectum

Case ranking/difficulty:

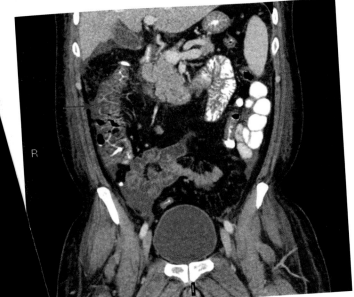

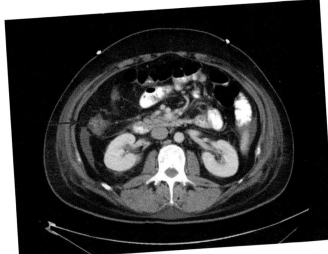

Axial portal venous phase CT shows bowel wall thickening and edema of the ascending colon (*red arrow*) and a small amount of ascites.

...nal portal venous phase CT shows bowel wall thickening and ...a with obliteration of the lumen of the ascending colon and ...cordion" appearance (*red arrow*). There is a small amount of

...findings are that of bowel wall thickening and
...na involving predominantly the right colon, although
...hole colon is not shown on the images. There is
...small amount of ascites. Typhlitis would be a
...eration, but it appears to involve a long segment
...ight colon, at least, and there is a small amount of
...The patient had in fact been on antibiotics for an
...d period of time within the hospital, and the test
...ficile was positive.

...er that we are looking for is the accordion sign.
...med by oral contrast material within the bowel
...g compressed by the surrounding edematous
...Although seen in pseudomembranous colitis,
...n sign can be present in other infectious
...schemic colitis.

...dies CT demonstrated a relatively low
...the detection of pseudomembranous
...sitive predictive value in one study was
...o one can suggest it when there are
...ings. Normally, the diagnosis is made or
...laboratory analysis of stool.

...ts have diarrhea and some degree of
...require fluid and electrolyte support.
...eatment is to eradicate the *C difficile*
...can be done with antibiotics, usually

vancomycin or metronidazole, and some people use probiotics. Fecal transplant is sometimes used for cases refractory to standard therapy.

5. *C difficile* is largely a nosocomial infection acquired in the hospital. It is easily spread by fomites. Outbreaks with particular strains in hospitals worldwide are not uncommon.

Pearls

- Hospitalized elderly population is particularly at risk, often a nosocomial disease.
- History of recent antibiotic therapy or chemotherapy.
- Bowel wall edema over a long segment of colon in conjunction with history is helpful in suggesting the diagnosis.

Suggested Readings

Ash L, Baker ME, O'Malley CM Jr, Gordon SM, Delaney CP, Obuchowski NA. Colonic abnormalities on CT in adult hospitalized patients with Clostridium difficile colitis: prevalence and significance of findings. *AJR Am J Roentgenol.* 2006;186(5):1393-1400. Epub 2006/04/25. doi: 10.214/ajr.4.697.

Bartlett JG. Narrative review: the new epidemic of Clostridium difficile-associated enteric disease. *Ann Intern Med.* 2006;145(10):758-764. Epub 2006/11/23.

Carter GP, Rood JI, Lyras D. The role of toxin A and toxin B in Clostridium difficile-associated disease: past and present perspectives. *Gut Microbes.* 2010;1(1):58-64. Epub 2010/07/29. doi: 10.161/gmic...0768.

Pearls

- Cyclically painful mass in a surgical scar (eg, C-section). Many patients will have constant pain. Some are asymptomatic.
- Consider the diagnosis in women who have had surgical procedures and who have pain close to a surgical scar, particularly if the uterus had been opened.
- There have been cases reported in relation to other abdominal and pelvic procedures, including amniocentesis (along the tract).
- Rare cases of malignant transformation into endometrial cancer.

Suggested Readings

Al-Jabri K. Endometriosis at caesarian section scar. *Oman Med J.* 2009;24(4):294-295. Epub 2009/10/01. doi: 10.5001/omj.2009.59.

Anand M, Deshmukh SD. Massive abdominal wall endometriosis masquerading as desmoid tumour. *J Cutan Aesthet Surg.* 2011;4(2):141-143. Epub 2011/10/07. doi: 10.4103/0974-2077.85043.

Hensen JH, Van Breda Vriesman AC, Puylaert JB. Abdominal wall endometriosis: clinical presentation and imaging features with emphasis on sonography. *AJR Am J Roentgenol.* 2006;186(3):616-620. Epub 2006/02/25. doi: 10.2214/ajr.04.1619.

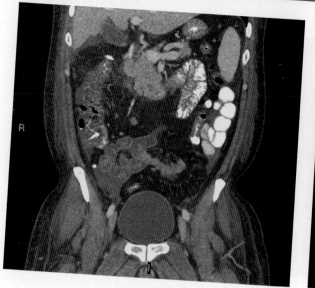 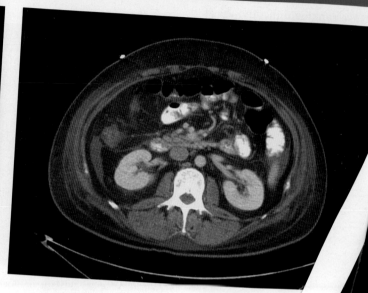

1. What is the most likely diagnosis?

2. What radiologic sign is seen here?

3. How sensitive is CT for the detection of pseudomembranous colitis?

4. What is the usual treatment for *C difficile* infection?

5. Where are most *C difficile* infections acquired?

Cor
eder
an "a
ascite

Answe

1. The
eder
the
also
consi
of the
ascites
extende
for *C di*

2. The answ
This is fo
lumen bei
bowel wal
the accordi
colitides or

3. In several stu
sensitivity fo
colitis. The po
around 88%, s
compatible fin
confirmed with

4. Since most patie
dehydration they
Another aim of tr
from the gut. This

270

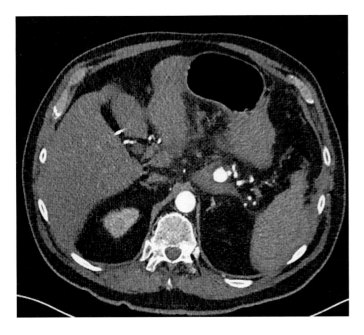 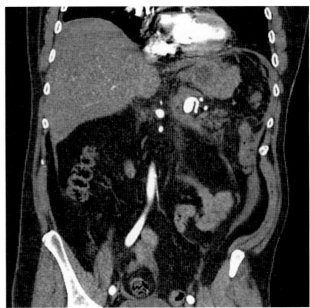

1. What is the most likely diagnosis?

2. How many times more common are splenic artery aneurysms relative to splenic artery pseudoaneurysms?

3. What size cutoff is frequently used as a threshold for the treatment of asymptomatic splenic artery aneurysms?

4. It is recommended that splenic artery pseudoaneurysms be treated regardless of size. True or false.

5. Which more often has mural thrombus and mural calcification, splenic artery aneurysm, or pseudoaneurysm?

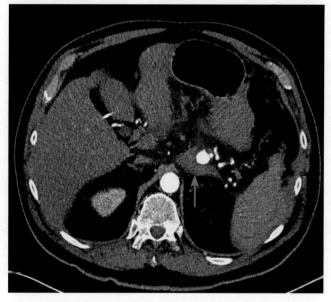

Axial arterial phase CT shows an enhancing round structure contiguous with the splenic artery (*red arrow*). There is soft tissue density posterior to this related to hemorrhage (*green arrow*). There is a crescent of soft tissue density surrounding the spleen related to perisplenic hemorrhage (*blue arrow*). No active bleeding.

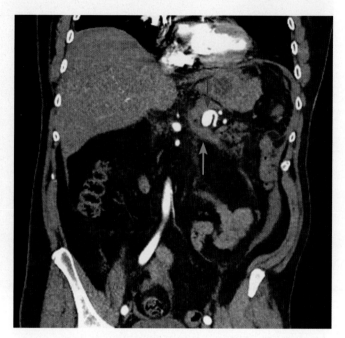

Coronal arterial phase CT again shows the well-defined enhancing structure contiguous with the splenic artery (*red arrow*), and there is soft tissue density surrounding this inferiorly (not pancreas) corresponding to hemorrhage (*green arrow*).

Answers

1. There is a small aneurysm involving the splenic artery with surrounding local and perisplenic hemorrhage. The spleen itself is intact, and no history of trauma is given. There is no collection to suggest a pseudocyst, and there is no evidence for pancreatitis.

   A pseudoaneurysm can be suggested by a history that includes a risk factor for a pseudoaneurysm or by a symptomatic patient since aneurysms are usually not symptomatic until they rupture. On imaging, they may be more irregular (ie, not as round and smooth) than an aneurysm with surrounding thrombus and hemorrhage.

   Aneurysms more commonly have mural calcification and mural thrombus, and they have a more regular appearance than pseudoaneurysms. They are usually asymptomatic until they rupture (as in this case).

2. Splenic artery aneurysms are much more common than splenic artery pseudoaneurysms. Estimates vary, but they may be approximately 20 times more common.

3. Opinions slightly vary, but 2 cm is frequently cited as the threshold size for treatment of asymptomatic splenic artery aneurysms. The risk of rupture is increased in patients with portal hypertension, pregnant patients, and in patients undergoing liver transplantation.

4. Because pseudoaneurysms are more often symptomatic and because of a significant mortality rate when ruptured it is recommended that all splenic artery pseudoaneurysms be treated, either endovascularly or surgically.

5. Splenic artery aneurysms and pseudoaneurysms have somewhat different etiologies with some overlap. Pseudoaneurysms are more often related to pancreatitis, trauma, surgical instrumentation, or peptic ulcer disease (ie, there is an insult or injury to the vessel), whereas aneurysms develop spontaneously in relation to certain other risk factors. Like in other atherosclerotic vessels, mural thrombus or mural calcification is not uncommon in splenic artery aneurysms.

Pearls

- Splenic aneurysm is much more common than a pseudoaneurysm.
- 2.0-cm threshold for consideration of elective repair of asymptomatic splenic artery aneurysm.
- Splenic pseudoaneurysms should be repaired. Patients with recent trauma or pancreatitis are particularly at risk.

Suggested Readings

Agrawal GA, Johnson PT, Fishman EK. Splenic artery aneurysms and pseudoaneurysms: clinical distinctions and CT appearances. *AJR Am J Roentgenol*. 2007;188(4): 992-999. Epub 2007/03/23. doi: 10.214/ajr.6.794.

Lakin RO, Bena JF, Sarac TP, et al. The contemporary management of splenic artery aneurysms. *J Vasc Surg*. 2011;53(4):958-964; discussion 65. Epub 2011/01/11. doi: 10.016/j.vs.010.0.55.

Saad NE, Saad WE, Davies MG, Waldman DL, Fultz PJ, Rubens DJ. Pseudoaneurysms and the role of minimally invasive techniques in their management. *Radiographics*. 2005;25 suppl 1:S173-S189. Epub 2005/10/18. doi: 10.148/rg.5si055503.

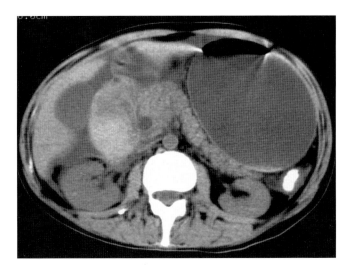 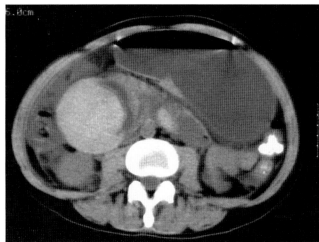

1. What is the most likely diagnosis?

2. In what time frame do uncomplicated duodenal hematomas generally resolve with conservative measures?

3. What specific CT findings suggest perforation?

4. What is the concentric ring sign in MR imaging of large hematomas in the abdomen?

5. Name three causes of spontaneous small bowel intramural hematomas?

Case ranking/difficulty:

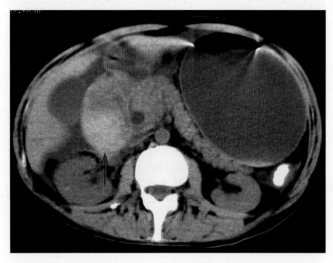

Axial noncontrast CT shows marked distention of the stomach and large hyperdense mass (*red arrow*) interposed between the head of the pancreas and the gallbladder. There is a small amount of free intraperitoneal fluid.

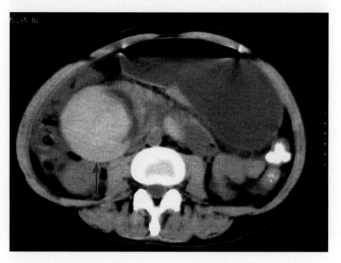

Axial noncontrast CT shows gastric distention and a somewhat better defined hyperdense mass (*red arrow*) involving the duodenum. The density of the mass is consistent with acute hemorrhage.

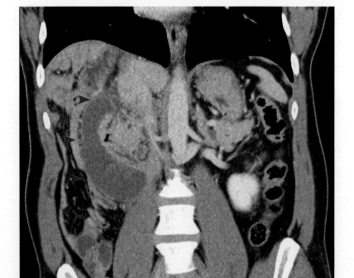

Companion case. Coronal portal venous phase CT shows a near fluid density collection conforming to the course of the duodenum (*red arrowheads*). It is not clear from the image whether it is intraluminal or mural, although other images (see stack) demonstrate areas of higher density within the collection and demonstrate that it is intramural.

Answers

1. The high-density material within the intramural portion of the duodenum is most consistent with hemorrhage, or duodenal hematoma.

   There is no sign of perforation on this examination. There is no mass in the duodenum to suggest a gangliocytic paraganglioma, and an ulcer or duodenitis would not produce a large high-density mass-like structure in the duodenum.

2. In general, uncomplicated duodenal hematomas will resolve in approximately 10 to 15 days with conservative treatment, that being nasogastric suction and dietary support or parenteral nutrition. There are reports of hematomas being drained percutaneously as well. Surgery is reserved for cases that do not respond to conservative measures.

3. It can be difficult to diagnose duodenal injury with CT sensitivity being near 80%. In cases where a patient will not otherwise undergo laparotomy it is important to distinguish isolated duodenal hematoma or edema from duodenal perforation. In a well-performed study two signs that indicate perforation are air in the right anterior pararenal space and extravasated contrast in the right anterior pararenal space. The other findings (thickening of the duodenal wall, intraperitoneal fluid, and pneumoperitoneum) can be seen without duodenal perforation, although you might want to explain pneumoperitoneum.

4. As a hematoma evolves in the abdomen it goes through a stage after a couple of weeks where there is central intermediate signal on T1W corresponding to clot. This is surrounded around the periphery by a band of high signal on T1W and another outer band of low signal on T1W. Although this is an interesting finding, it does not appear until later in the evolution of the hematoma and is not that useful in the acute setting. These findings can also be seen in hematomas involving other parts of the abdomen.

5. Although rare, spontaneous intramural hemorrhage does occur in the small bowel, not just the duodenum. Risk factors include, but are not limited to, anticoagulation therapy, bleeding disorders, and vasculitides.

Pearls

- Possible complication of nonaccidental trauma in children.
- Handlebar injuries, all-terrain vehicle accidents, sports trauma, other etiologies in children.
- Distinguish between perforation and simple hematoma. Air or contrast in right anterior pararenal space is specific finding.

Suggested Readings

Abbas MA, Collins JM, Olden KW. Spontaneous intramural small-bowel hematoma: imaging findings and outcome. *AJR Am J Roentgenol.* 2002;179(6):1389-1394. Epub 2002/11/20.doi:10.2214/ajr.179.6.1791389.

Jayaraman MV, Mayo-Smith WW, Movson JS, Dupuy DE, Wallach MT. CT of the duodenum: an overlooked segment gets its due. *Radiographics.* 2001;21 Spec No:S147-160. Epub 2001/10/13. doi: 10.1148/radiographics.21.suppl_1.g01oc01s147.

Velmahos GC, Tabbara M, Gross R, Willette P, Hirsch E, Burke P, et al. Blunt pancreatoduodenal injury: a multicenter study of the Research Consortium of New England Centers for Trauma (ReCONECT). *Arch Surg.* 2009;144(5):413-419; discussion 419-420. Epub 2009/05/20. doi: 10.1001/archsurg.2009.52.

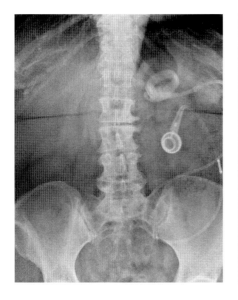 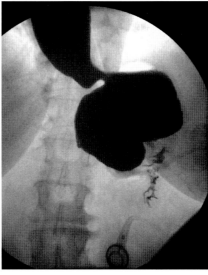 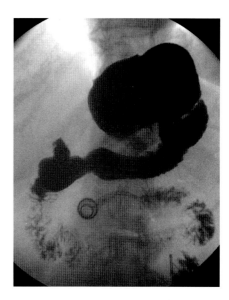

1. What is the complication in this patient with bariatric surgery?

2. What are the radiographic manifestations of gastric band slippage?

3. What are the names of other common types of bariatric surgery in USA?

4. What is the best modality to evaluate gastric band slippage?

5. What is the best view for upper GI contrast evaluation after gastric banding surgery?

Case ranking/difficulty: **Category:** Stomach

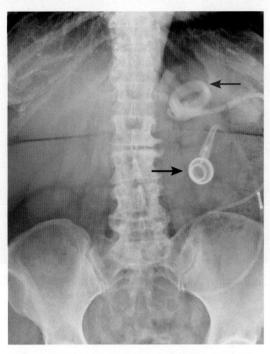

Plain radiography in frontal projection shows open ring appearance of the band ("O" sign) and phi angle >58°. Subcutaneous port (*black arrow*), connecting tube (*green arrow*) and band (*red arrow*).

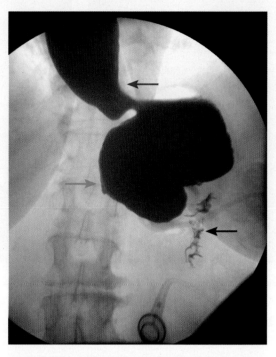

Upper GI study shows large dilated gastric pouch (*green arrow*) and esophagus (*red arrow*) with collapsed stomach (*black arrow*) distal to gastric band.

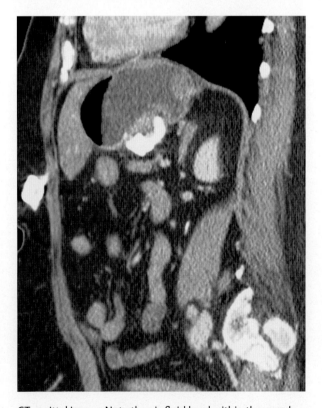

CT sagittal image: Note the air-fluid level within the pouch.

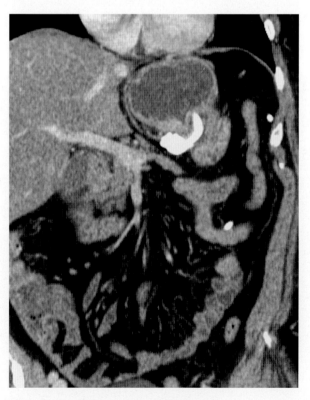

CT coronal view: Distended gastric pouch.

Answers

1. Gastric band slippage. On plain radiography, rectangular appearance of superimposed band about 5 cm below the left diaphragm suggestive of appropriately positioned band. On fluoroscopic barium study, there is small pouch, narrow stoma, and opacification of the remainder of stomach. Pouch dilatation occurs in up to 25% of patients as a long-term sequela. In gastric band erosion, the band appears as a filling defect.

2. Phi angle >58°, "O" sign and lateral eccentric pouch dilatation are the radiographic manifestations of gastric band slippage. Phi angle is the superior angle between long axis of band and long axis of the vertebral column.

3. Roux-en-Y gastric bypass, vertical sleeve gastrectomy, jejunoileal bypass, vertical-banded gastroplasty, and biliopancreatic diversion are the other common types of bariatric surgery in USA.

4. UGI barium study is the modality of choice to evaluate gastric band slippage.

5. Profile view of band allows best visualization of pouch and stoma. The supine left posterior oblique is the best position for evaluation of patients after Roux-en-Y gastric bypass surgery. Supine position helps distend the pouch adequately for demonstration of leak.

Pearls

- Identification of 'O' signs and Phi angle >58° are the most helpful plain radiographic findings for early diagnosis of gastric band slippage and useful for triage the patient as severe band slippage may be an acute surgical emergency.
- Further confirmation can be made by upper GI barium series under fluoroscopy.
- CT may be helpful in doubtful cases and also useful when abscess or bowel obstruction suspected.

Suggested Readings

Chandler RC, Srinivas G, Chintapalli KN, Schwesinger WH, Prasad SR. Imaging in bariatric surgery: a guide to postsurgical anatomy and common complications. *AJR Am J Roentgenol.* January 2008;190(1):122-135.

Prosch H, Tscherney R, Kriwanek S, Tscholakoff D. Radiographical imaging of the normal anatomy and complications after gastric banding. *Br J Radiol.* September 2008;81(969):753-757.

Sonavane SK, Menias CO, Kantawala KP, et al. Laparoscopic adjustable gastric banding: what radiologists need to know. *Radiographics.* 2012;32(4):1161-1178.

Incidental masses discovered on ultrasound exam performed for fatty food intolerance

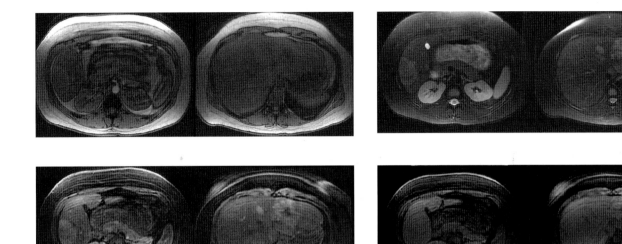

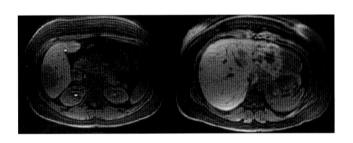

1. What is the most likely diagnosis?

2. What type of examination is most helpful in distinguishing a hepatic adenoma from focal nodular hyperplasia?

3. Hepatic adenomas have no malignant potential. True or false.

4. What are the main complicating features of hepatic adenomas?

5. What is the atoll sign?

Case ranking/difficulty:

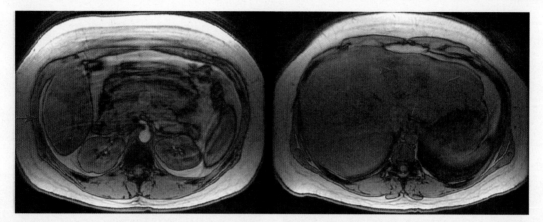

Axial T1W MRI prior to contrast, out of phase. There are two separate lesions. One is in the right hepatic lobe inferiorly and has an elliptical shape (*red arrow*). It is slightly hyperintense on T1W. The other lesion is in the left hepatic lobe and is somewhat less conspicuous (*red arrowheads*). It is nearly isointense to adjacent liver and has a mildly hypointense irregular center region.

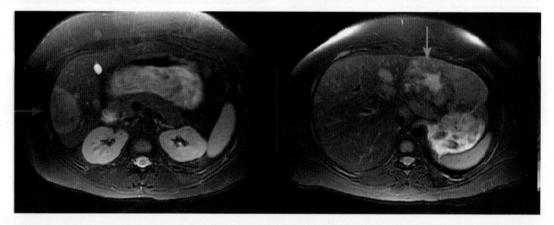

T2W axial MRI prior to contrast. The lesion in the right hepatic lobe is mildly hyperintense to liver on T2W and has an elliptical shape with sharp margins (*red arrow*). The lesion in the left hepatic lobe is more conspicuous on T2W (*green arrow*). The peripheral portion is only mildly hyperintense to liver (less so than the other lesion), and the central irregular area and fairly hyperintense.

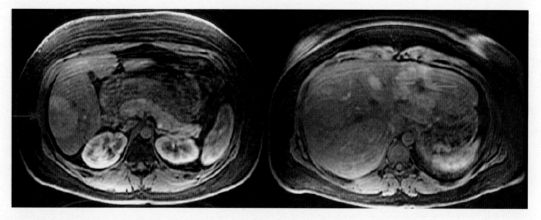

T1W gradient echo fat saturated images after contrast in the arterial phase show both lesions are fairly conspicuous and enhance. The lesion in the right hepatic lobe (*red arrow*) is fairly homogeneous. The central scar for the lesion in the left hepatic lobe is low signal intensity on T1W (*green arrow*).

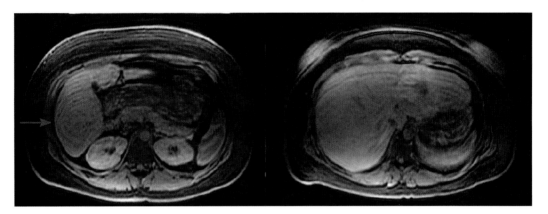

T1W gradient echo fat saturated images after contrast in the portal venous phase show that the lesion in the right hepatic lobe is nearly isointense to liver (*red arrow*). The lesion in the left hepatic lobe shows some persistent hyperintensity with the low-intensity central scar.

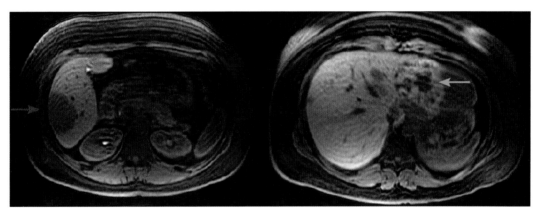

T1W gradient echo fat saturated images 20 minutes after contrast (Eovist, a hepatobiliary agent) administration show that the lesion in the right hepatic lobe is hypointense to liver (*red arrow*). The lesion in the left hepatic lobe is iso- to slightly hyperintense with the hypointense central scar (*green arrow*).

Answers

1. The most likely diagnosis is a hepatic adenoma. It is slightly hyperintense on T2W, enhances in the arterial phase on T1W GRE sequences, is nearly isointense on portal venous phase, and is hypointense in the late hepatobiliary phase.

   Focal nodular hyperplasia is usually relatively inconspicuous on noncontrast MRI, except for the scar, when present, which is high signal on T2W, enhances intensely in the arterial phase and then is nearly isointense on portal venous phase, and then iso- to hyperintense on delayed phase with hepatobiliary agents like Eovist. The second lesion in this case is focal nodular hyperplasia.

   The enhancement pattern here is not consistent with cavernous hemangioma, and cavernous hemangiomas are very high signal on T2W sequences.

   Hepatocellular carcinoma is a thought, but except for the two lesions the liver is otherwise normal.

   Fibrolamellar hepatocellular carcinoma usually occurs in younger patients, often has a scar, may have calcifications, and has more heterogeneous enhancement.

2. Distinguishing between focal nodular hyperplasia and hepatic adenoma can be sometimes difficult. One useful difference histologically is that adenomas contain few Kupffer cells and when present they may be reduced in function. In addition, there are no bile ductules in adenomas and the hepatocytes in an adenoma may not function normally. A Tc99m sulfur colloid examination depends on Kupffer cell uptake of the radiopharmaceutical. Consequently, a scan should and often does show a photopenic region in the area of the adenoma, but scans are occasionally "warm" in the region of the adenoma.

An MRI scan with a hepatobiliary agent measures a different parameter, namely uptake and excretion of the contrast agent, but delayed scans usually do show hypointensity in the region of a hepatic adenoma while focal nodular hyperplasia is usually iso- to hyperintense.

A CT with contrast, US, and a tagged red cell study are not as helpful as is an MRI study.

3. Hepatic adenomas do have malignant potential. An estimate is that approximately 5% are/become malignant. If observation is the chosen management strategy one should be concerned if there is continued growth after an offending agent (if there is one) is discontinued.

4. Many hepatic adenomas are asymptomatic, or patients may have vague symptoms of right upper quadrant fullness or pain. Rarely, there is a palpable abnormality. Unfortunately, a not uncommon presentation is related to spontaneous hemorrhage and patients then present with acute abdominal pain.

Also, the nonsteatotic subtypes of hepatic adenomas have some malignant potential.

Biliary obstruction, liver failure, and portal vein thrombosis are not recognized common complications.

5. There are a number of subtypes of hepatic adenoma, and some of these can be suggested on the basis of imaging. The HNF-1 alpha inactivated/steatotic subtypes (also called L-FABP–negative tumors) have increased intracellular lipid and can be detected with opposed phase imaging. An atoll sign can be seen in the inflammatory/telangiectatic subtype of hepatic adenoma, and beta-catenin positive tumors can have a central scar and poorly demarcated areas of increased T2W signal. The distinction is important because beta-catenin positive tumors and inflammatory/telangiectatic subtypes can have an increased risk of malignancy.

Pearls

- Clonal population of cells.
- Multiple subtypes now recognized. HNF-1 alpha inactivated (steatotic type) is characterized by intracellular lipid and does not carry risk of transformation to hepatocellular carcinoma.
- Beta-catenin and inflammatory (includes telangiectatic variant) carry some risk of malignant transformation. For the inflammatory type this is by virtue of a small percentage that also have the beta-catenin mutation.
- Increasing frequency or detection related to "metabolic syndrome."
- Typically occur in women of childbearing on oral contraceptive pills.
- Propensity for spontaneous hemorrhage.

Suggested Readings

Chang CY, Hernandez-Prera JC, Roayaie S, Schwartz M, Thung SN. Changing epidemiology of hepatocellular adenoma in the United States: review of the literature. *Int J Hepatol.* 2013;2013:604860. Epub 2013/03/20. doi: 10.1155/2013/604860.

Grazioli L, Bondioni MP, Haradome H, Motosugi U, Tinti R, Frittoli B, et al. Hepatocellular adenoma and focal nodular hyperplasia: value of gadoxetic acid-enhanced MR imaging in differential diagnosis. *Radiology.* 2012;262(2):520-529. Epub 2012/01/28. doi: 10.1148/radiol.11101742.

van Aalten SM, Thomeer MG, Terkivatan T, Dwarkasing RS, Verheij J, de Man RA, et al. Hepatocellular adenomas: correlation of MR imaging findings with pathologic subtype classification. *Radiology.* 2011;261(1):172-181. Epub 2011/08/31. doi: 10.1148/radiol.11110023.

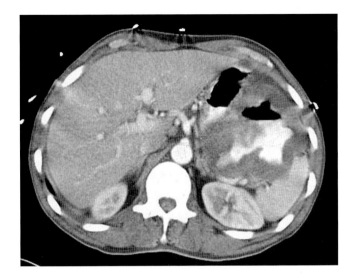
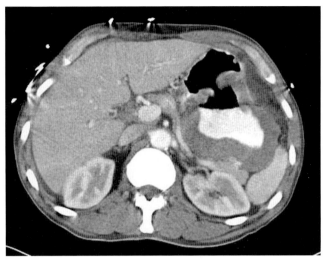
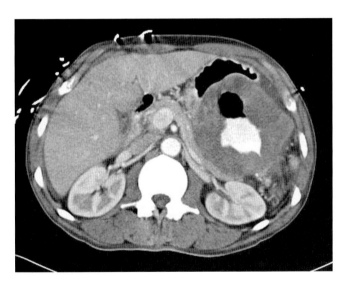
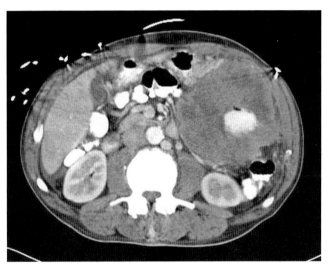

1. What is the most likely diagnosis?

2. What two syndromes have an association with gastrointestinal stromal tumors?

3. What medications are specifically effective in treating most gastrointestinal stromal tumors?

4. What is the immunohistochemical stain commonly used to diagnose gastrointestinal stromal tumors?

5. Which imaging modality is most helpful in assessing therapeutic response to Kit-selective tyrosine kinase inhibitors?

Case ranking/difficulty:

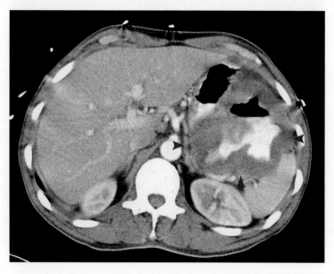

Contrast-enhanced CT shows soft tissue density rind (*red arrowheads*) involving the wall of the stomach and encroaching upon the lumen.

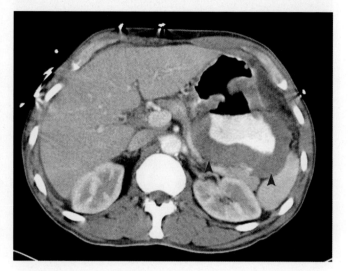

Contrast-enhanced CT at a slightly lower level shows the ulcerated exophytic soft tissue density tumor with a thick wall (*red arrowheads*).

Answers

1. Given the exophytic nature of the mass with a thick wall and ulceration, a GIST and leiomyosarcoma are the most likely diagnoses.

   Prior to the 1990s the distinction between gastrointestinal stromal tumors and leiomyosarcoma was not well elucidated, so many tumors previously diagnosed as leiomyosarcoma were probably actually gastrointestinal stromal tumors. Gastrointestinal stromal tumors are the most common mesenchymal neoplasm of the GI tract with leiomyosarcomas being much less common.

   Neural tumors of the stomach do occur, although they are rare, usually submucosal and not as exophytic as GISTs.

   Lipomas would have fat density on CT.

   Desmoid tumors usually occur in the setting of trauma, surgery, or in familial polyposis syndrome, and intra-abdominal desmoid tumors usually involve the mesentery or retroperitoneum. The abdominal wall is a common location.

2. Gastrointestinal stromal tumors (GISTs) do have an association with Carney triad (GISTs, pulmonary chondroma, and extra-adrenal paraganglioma) and with neurofibromatosis type I.

3. Many gastrointestinal stromal tumors (GISTs) are sensitive to treatment with a Kit-selective tyrosine kinase inhibitor (eg, imatinib). Newer agents are also available. Treatment for a GIST initially involves surgery, particularly when the tumor can be completely resected. However, imatinib and other agents can be used to control locally advanced or metastatic disease. They are also being used in neoadjuvant and adjuvant settings.

4. Positive CD117 (c-Kit) staining is useful in identifying gastrointestinal stromal tumors. CD3 is useful in identifying T-cell lymphomas. CD45 is useful in non-Hodgkin lymphoma and leukemias. CEA is useful in detecting adenocarcinomas, whereas AFP is useful in detecting liver and germ cell tumors.

5. PET/CT provides the best information regarding a therapeutic response as the metabolic activity of the tumor may decrease substantially before a significant anatomic change is noted. In addition, some patients' tumors develop resistance to a Kit-selective tyrosine kinase inhibitor, necessitating a change to another agent. PET/CT can be used to assess the therapeutic response in such cases as well and may help guide selection of an appropriate agent.

Pearls

- c-Kit (CD117) immunoreactivity for GIST.
- Response to imatinib and other Kit-selective tyrosine kinase inhibitors for GIST.
- Many GISTs were previously identified as leiomyomas or leiomyosarcomas.
- Association with Carney triad and neurofibromatosis type I with GIST.

Suggested Readings

Abraham SC. Distinguishing gastrointestinal stromal tumors from their mimics: an update. *Adv Anat Pathol.* 2007;14(3):178-188. Epub 2007/04/25. doi: 10.1097/PAP.0b013e318050aa66.

Aggarwal G, Sharma S, Zheng M, Reid MD, Crosby JH, Chamberlain SM, et al. Primary leiomyosarcomas of the gastrointestinal tract in the post-gastrointestinal stromal tumor era. *Ann Diagn Pathol.* 2012;16(6):532-540. Epub 2012/08/25. doi: 10.1016/j.anndiagpath.2012.07.005.

Sandrasegaran K, Rajesh A, Rydberg J, Rushing DA, Akisik FM, Henley JD. Gastrointestinal stromal tumors: clinical, radiologic, and pathologic features. *AJR Am J Roentgenol.* 2005;184(3):803-811. Epub 2005/02/25. doi: 10.2214/ajr.184.3.01840803.

29-year-old male with fever, weight loss, and acquired immunodeficiency syndrome

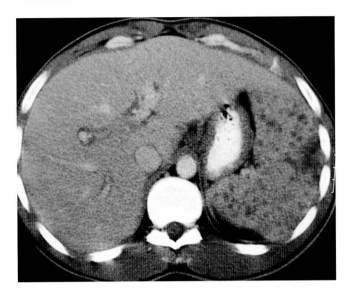 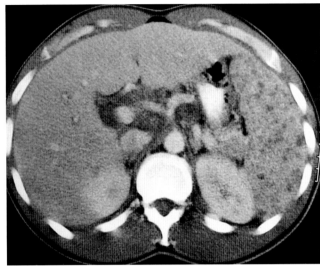

1. What is the most likely diagnosis?

2. Ultrasound is not useful in the evaluation of abdominal tuberculosis. True or false?

3. What are the three categories of peritoneal involvement in abdominal tuberculosis?

4. What appearance does acute adrenal involvement have on CT?

5. What percentage of all cases of tuberculosis in the US are extrapulmonary?

Case ranking/difficulty:

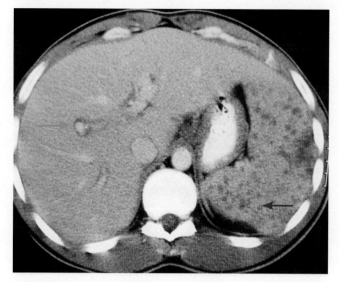

Axial portal venous phase CT shows multiple small low-density foci (*red arrow*) with some areas of confluence within the spleen. Also noted is circumferential low density around the portal vein (*green arrow*) corresponding to edema.

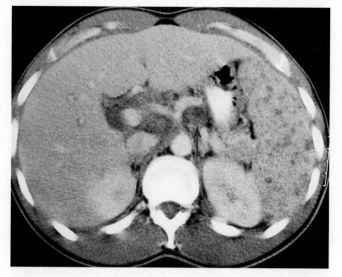

Axial portal venous phase CT shows periaortic adenopathy with multiple lymph nodes demonstrating low-density centers (*red arrow*). Also noted are the multiple low-density splenic lesions.

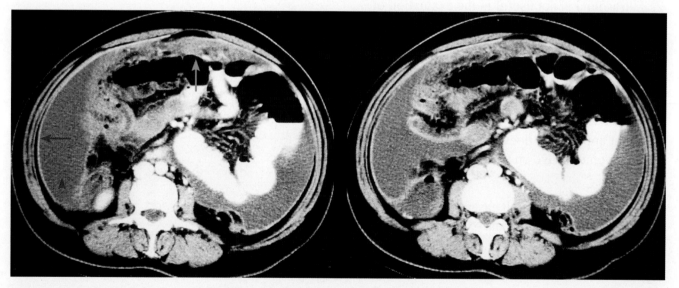

Supplementary case, 38-year-old female with HIV, increasing abdominal girth, and fever. CT shows ascites (*red arrowhead*), thickened and enhancing peritoneum (*red arrow*), and mesenteric thickening (*green arrow*).

Answers

1. The combination of multiple splenic lesions, abdominal lymphadenopathy with low-density centers, and immunodeficiency favors a diagnosis of disseminated tuberculosis. The lymph nodes in abdominal tuberculosis sometimes have peripheral enhancement with a low-density center.

Primary splenic lymphoma is rare, and the splenic involvement is usually larger in size and nonuniform.

Splenic abscesses due to bacteria are usually larger in size when compared to disseminated tuberculosis, and there are often daughter abscesses adjacent to the primary abscess.

Splenic hamartomas are usually solitary, larger, and have variable enhancement characteristics.

Whipple disease and celiac sprue are two diseases that primarily affect bowel but which can cause low-density lymphadenopathy within the abdomen, so-called cavitating mesenteric lymph node syndrome in celiac sprue. Lymphangioleiomyomatosis is another condition that can cause abdominal lymphadenopathy with low-density centers.

2. Although not the preferred modality, ultrasound can be useful in the evaluation of suspected abdominal tuberculosis. It can detect and characterize ascites, and it can detect lymphadenopathy or solid organ involvement. Hepatosplenic involvement usually manifests as hypoechoic lesions varying from less than 1 mm to as large as 10 mm.

3. Peritoneal involvement in abdominal tuberculosis is categorized into three main types. The wet type is the most common and has free or loculated ascites, frequently with hyperdense fluid. The fibrotic type is characterized by omental caking and matting of bowel loops. The dry type is characterized by mesenteric thickening, fibrous adhesions, and caseous nodules. There may be some overlap between types.

4. Acute adrenal gland involvement most often presents as bilateral involvement and enlargement, sometimes with hypodense areas related to caseous necrosis. This evolves to bilateral small glands, sometimes with speckled calcification.

One should be aware that adrenal involvement with tuberculosis can cause adrenal insufficiency.

5. In the United States approximately 20% of cases of tuberculosis are extrapulmonary. This includes lymphatic, pleural, bone and joint, genitourinary, meningeal, peritoneal, and other, so abdominal cases account for only a small percentage of the total number of cases. Tuberculosis in the United States peaked in the early 1990s, and the incidence has been declining since.

Pearls

- Adenopathy with low-density center is suggestive of TB in the right clinical setting.
- Whipple disease and Sprue are other diseases that can show lymph nodes with low-density centers. In Sprue this is called cavitating mesenteric lymph node syndrome.
- Approximately 20% of cases of tuberculosis in the United States are extrapulmonary.

Suggested Readings

Burrill J, Williams CJ, Bain G, Conder G, Hine AL, Misra RR. Tuberculosis: a radiologic review. *Radiographics*. 2007;27(5):1255-1273. doi: 10.148/rg.75065176.

Dong P, Wang B, Sun QY, Cui H. Tuberculosis versus non-Hodgkin's lymphomas involving small bowel mesentery: evaluation with contrast-enhanced computed tomography. *World J Gastroenterol*. 2008;14(24):3914-3918. Epub 2008/07/09.

Engin G, Acunaş B, Acunaş G, Tunaci M. Imaging of extrapulmonary tuberculosis. *Radiographics*. 2000;20(2):471-488. doi: 10.148/radiographics.0..00mc07471.

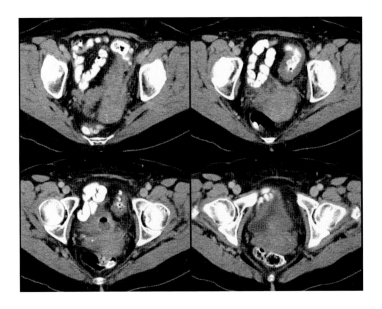
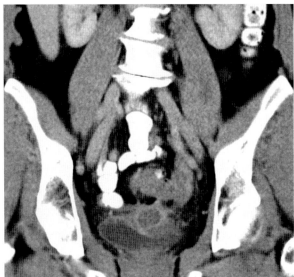

1. Based on the above images what is the most likely diagnosis?

2. What are the various causes of herald lesions of the bladder?

3. What are the imaging features of herald lesions?

4. What are the MR findings of early invasion of the bladder due to cervical carcinoma?

5. What are the potential complications of herald lesions?

Case ranking/difficulty:

Category: Colorectum

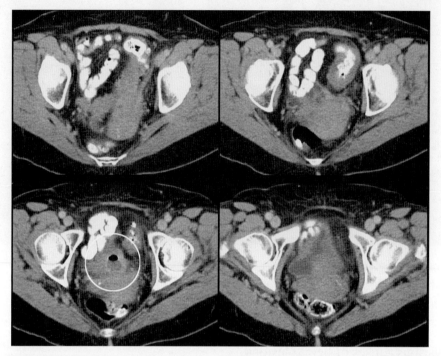

Nephrographic phase of CT urogram shows sigmoid wall thickening and diverticula. There is a small mass with an air-fluid level (*circle*) between the colon and the bladder burrowing into the bladder and thickening its wall. There is mild pericolic fat infiltration.

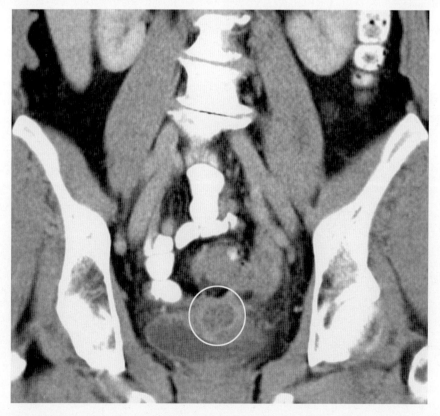

Coronal nephrographic phase of CT urogram shows the small mass (*circle*) in the bladder dome. Stranding extends from it to the colon.

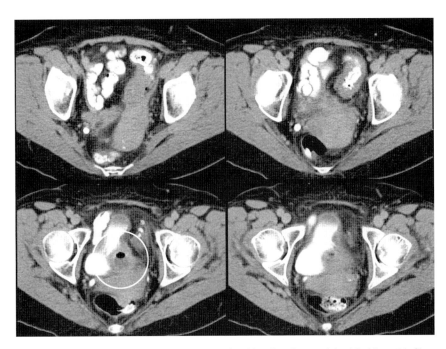

Excretory phase of CT urogram shows the small mass (*circle*) with air-fluid level in dome of the bladder with fibrous stranding between it and the sigmoid.

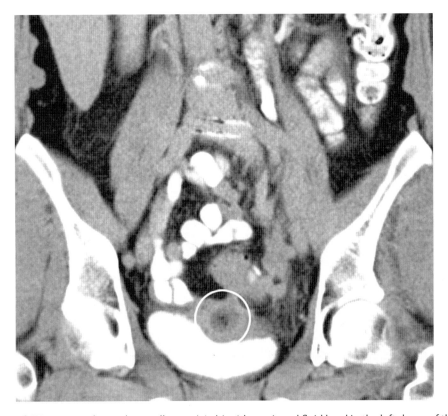

Coronal excretory phase of CT urogram shows the small mass (*circle*) with an air and fluid level in the left dome of the bladder, causing bladder wall thickening.

Answers

1. Bladder carcinoma is possible but air-fluid level is unlikely and colon wall thickening is hard to explain. Urachal carcinoma is more anterior. Crohn disease with impending colovesical fistula is possible but less likely than diverticulitis. The long segment colon wall thickening is more likely diverticulitis than colon carcinoma.

2. Cystoscopic focal mucosal lesions of the urinary bladder caused by extrinsic inflammatory and neoplastic processes seen at cystoscopy herald encroachment or invasion of the bladder and are called herald lesions. Diverticulitis is the most common cause. Other causes are Crohn disease, colonic carcinoma, endometriosis, and gynecologic malignancy.

3. Imaging features depend on the stage and type of pelvic disease, amount of bladder contact, and depth of invasion. The affected area may appear as a small bladder filling defect or as a focal contour abnormality or focal wall thickening. Margin may be spiculated, lobulated, or smooth. When the cause is diverticulitis, there is usually a small gas-containing mass between the bladder and the sigmoid colon invading the bladder dome, causing wall thickening. Signs of sigmoid diverticulitis are usually present and are often mild/chronic.

4. MR of cervical carcinoma invading the bladder has been reported to show nodularity and irregularity of the posterior bladder wall mass(es) protruding into the bladder lumen, high signal intensity of the anterior aspect of the posterior wall of the bladder, and abnormal soft-tissue strands in the uterovesical space.

5. Without treatment the extrinsic disease causing a herald lesion will progress, leading to fistula development. Colovesical fistulas are difficult to demonstrate by cystography. CT or a contrast study of the colon is more likely to be diagnostic. Gas but usually not feces is transmitted through a colovesical fistula. Involvement of the ureterovesical junction by the extrinsic process can lead to ipsilateral hydronephrosis. Fecaluria is less common than pneumaturia but can occur.

Pearls

- A cystoscopic herald lesion is a focal mucosal lesion of the urinary bladder caused by an extrinsic inflammatory or neoplastic process.
- Its radiologic counterpart is a disease process extrinsic to the bladder that produces a focal bladder wall abnormality at imaging (originally excretory urography or cystography, now most often CT). Identification of the imaging abnormality can precede the diagnosis of the primary disease.
- Excretory urography or cystography: Small bladder filling defect or focal contour abnormality or focal wall thickening. Spiculated, lobulated, or smooth margin.
- CT: Small gas-containing mass between the bladder and the sigmoid colon invading the bladder dome, causing wall thickening. Signs of sigmoid diverticulitis are usually present and are often mild/chronic.

Suggested Readings

Flisak ME, Kalbhen CL, Predey TA, Demos TC. Radiographic herald lesion of the urinary bladder: pictorial essay. *Australas Radiol*. August 2000;44(3):261-265.

Goldman SM, Fishman EK, Gatewood OM, Jones B, Siegelman SS. CT in the diagnosis of enterovesical fistulae. *AJR Am J Roentgenol*. June 1985;144(6):1229-1233.

Kitamura M, Namiki M, Nonomura N, Monden T, Okuda H, Sonoda T. A pseudotumor of the urinary bladder secondary to diverticulitis of the sigmoid colon with colo-vesical fistula: a case report. *Urol Int*. April 1987;42(3):234-236.

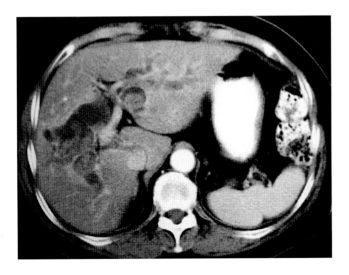 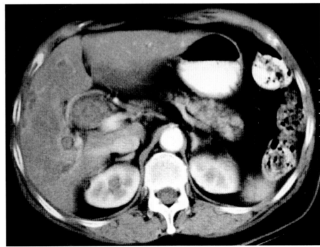

1. What is the most likely diagnosis?

2. What type of intrahepatic stones is formed in recurrent pyogenic cholangitis?

3. What is the approximate risk of developing cholangiocarcinoma with recurrent pyogenic cholangitis?

4. Which population has the highest incidence of recurrent pyogenic cholangitis?

5. What are the potential complications?

Case ranking/difficulty:

Category: Biliary tract

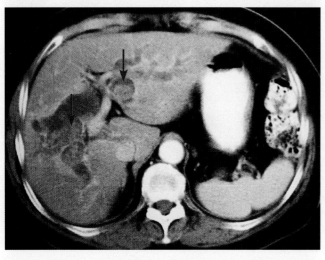

Axial portal venous phase CT shows intrahepatic biliary dilatation involving the right and left lobes with some periductal enhancement (*green arrows*) and intraductal stones and "mud" (*red arrows*).

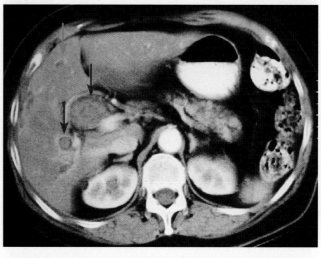

Axial CT at a lower level shows more intrahepatic pigmented stones (*red arrows*), intrahepatic ductal dilatation, and periductal enhancement (*green arrows*).

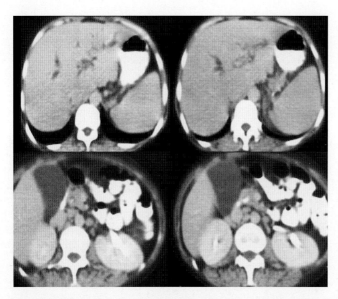

Second companion case in a 58-year-old male with right upper quadrant pain and elevated LFTs showing intrahepatic ductal dilatation and intrahepatic stones within the left biliary tree (seen well on the following cholangiogram).

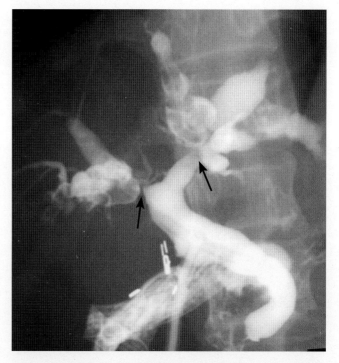

Companion case from a 58-year-old male. Cholangiogram with T tube in place showing biliary strictures (*black arrows*), ductal dilatation, and intraductal filling defects corresponding to pigment stones.

Answers

1. The presence of biliary ductal stone disease and cholangitis suggests a diagnosis of recurrent pyogenic cholangitis.

   Bacterial cholangitis without stone disease occurring in the United States is usually due to obstruction or instrumentation. Primary sclerosing cholangitis usually has multiple strictures with pruning of the intrahepatic biliary tree. Caroli disease has saccular dilatation of the biliary tree with variable degrees of involvement of the intrahepatic ducts and sometimes shows a central dot sign. Biliary hamartomas (von Meyenburg complexes) are multiple small nodules that are hypodense on CT and hyperintense on T2W MRI.

2. The stones formed in recurrent pyogenic cholangitis are bilirubin stones. Some hypothesize that *Escherichia coli* production of a beta-glucuronidase deconjugates bilirubin and contributes to the production of bilirubin stones.

3. As with many other diseases affecting the biliary tree and causing bile stasis and inflammation (eg, primary sclerosing cholangitis), there is a small risk of developing cholangiocarcinoma when there is underlying recurrent pyogenic cholangitis. The risk is estimated to be in the range of 5%.

4. For reasons that may be as much related to diet and socioeconomic status as it is to genetics, the highest incidence of recurrent pyogenic cholangitis is in patients living in Southeast Asia. The incidence is also higher in Southeast Asians who immigrate to the United States.

   The fact that the worldwide distribution of liver parasites is similar to the distribution of recurrent pyogenic cholangitis does suggest some causal relationship there as well.

5. Ductal strictures can result in intrahepatic bilomas, and hepatic abscess is a complication that may require intervention and drainage. As already mentioned, the risk of developing cholangiocarcinoma is approximately 5%. Portal vein thrombosis and biliary cirrhosis are also complications in long-standing disease.

Pearls

- Intra- and extrahepatic duct dilatation with pigment stones in Southeast Asians.
- Associated with parasitic infection (*Clonorchis sinensis*, *Ascaris lumbricoides*, *Fasciola hepaticum*), although stone formation may be related to *E coli* infection.

Suggested Readings

Catalano OA, Sahani DV, Forcione DG, et al. Biliary infections: spectrum of imaging findings and management. *Radiographics*. 2009;29(7):2059-2080. doi: 10.148/rg.97095051.

Chan FL, Man SW, Leong LL, Fan ST. Evaluation of recurrent pyogenic cholangitis with CT: analysis of 50 patients. *Radiology*. 1989;170(1 pt 1):165-169. Epub 1989/01/01. doi: 10.148/radiology.70..909092.

Federle MP, Jeffrey RB, Woodward PJ, Borhani AA. *Diagnostic Imaging: Abdomen*. Salt Lake City, UT: Amirsys; 2010, III(2):18-21. ISBN: 9781931884716.

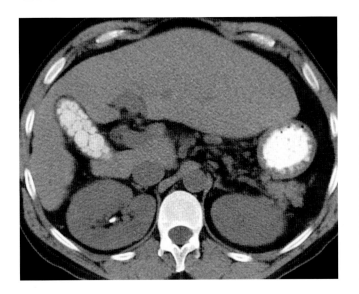 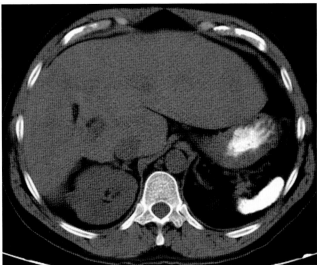

1. What are the radiological findings?

2. What are the causes of splenic calcifications? What is the best diagnosis in this patient?

3. What disease does sickle cell trait protect against?

4. What are the abdominal imaging findings of sickle cell disease?

5. What is the renal malignancy associated with sickle cell trait?

Sickle cell disease with autosplenectomy

Case 87 (3208)

Case ranking/difficulty:

Answers

1. Calcified spleen, gallstones, right renal stone, and features of liver cirrhosis are the radiological findings in this case.

2. Sickle cell disease, tuberculosis, histoplasmosis, and SLE cause splenic calcifications. Tuberculosis and histoplasmosis usually have nodular calcifications in other organs such as liver, adrenals, and mesenteric lymph nodes. There are reports that SLE can cause asplenia and a small, calcified spleen on occasion. Sickle cell disease is the best diagnosis with the findings enumerated above.

3. Sickle cell trait protects against malaria explaining the genes persistence in areas affected by malaria.

4. Common abdominal findings include gallstones, small calcified spleen, and hemosiderosis. Renal papillary necrosis is seen in sickle trait.

5. Renal medullary carcinoma is a rare epithelial malignant tumor arising from collecting duct epithelium. The tumor is almost exclusively seen in young African Americans with the sickle cell hemoglobinopathies, mainly sickle cell trait (SCT), rarely sickle cell disease. Most patients present with metastatic disease and have a poor prognosis. At imaging it is a central infiltrative renal mass.

Pearls

- Vaso-occlusive phenomena and hemolysis are the two major causes of increased morbidity and mortality.
- Asplenia is a feature of >90% of cases of homozygous sickle cell disease at 5 years of age and susceptible to infection.
- Gallbladder sludge is seen in almost all patients. Gallstones are seen in about 50% of adult and 20% of children.
- Lifelong blood transfusions make these patients more vulnerable to hepatitis and leads to liver parenchymal disease.
- Sickle cell trait patients are at risk for papillary necrosis and medullary carcinoma of the kidney.

Suggested Readings

Hung HH, Chen TS, Su CW. Pancreatic duct disruption with autosplenectomy. *Gastroenterology*. 2009 Dec;137(6):e7-e8.

Lonergan GJ, Cline DB, Abbondanzo SL. Sickle cell anemia. *Radiographics*. 2001;21(4):971-994.

Marsh A, Golden C, Hoppe C, Quirolo K, Vichinsky E. Renal medullary carcinoma in an adolescent with sickle cell anemia. *Pediatr Blood Cancer*. 2014 Mar;61(3):567.

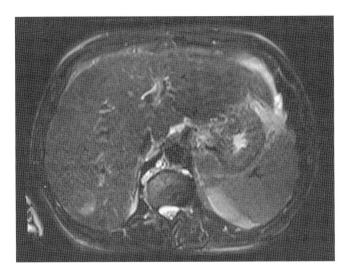
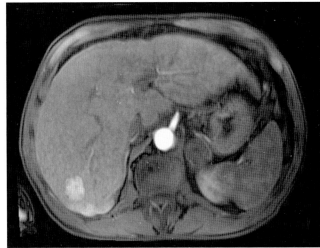

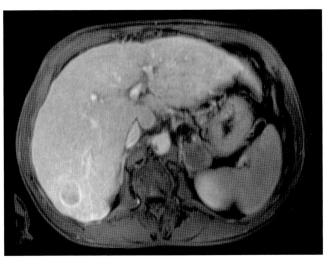
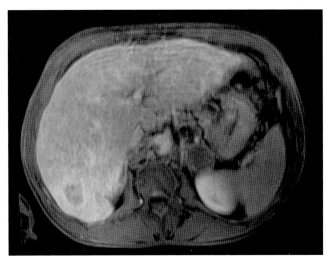

1. What is the most likely diagnosis?

2. What arterial enhancing masses can be confused with HCC?

3. What is the size limit for a single HCC lesion in the Milan eligibility criteria for liver transplant?

4. What are the nonsurgical treatment options for HCC patients?

5. What is the preferred imaging screening modality for the patients at risk of HCC?

Case ranking/difficulty: 🌑🌑

Answers

1. Arterial enhancement, contrast washout, and capsular enhancement in a patient with known hepatitis C infection are the most consistent with hepatocellular carcinoma.

2. Fibronodular hyperplasia, hepatocellular adenoma, arterioportal shunt, hypervascular metastasis, and hemangioma can have arterial enhancement and be confused with HCC. Venous phase washout and capsular enhancement are characteristics of HCC useful in differential diagnosis.

3. Single mass <5 cm, up to 3 masses each smaller than 3 cm, no vascular invasion, and no extrahepatic lesions are the Milan liver transplant eligibility criteria.

4. Radiofrequency ablation, transcatheter arterial chemoembolization, chemotherapy, yttrium therapy, cryotherapy, and percutaneous ethanol injection are nonsurgical treatment options.

5. The available screening tools are serum alpha-fetoprotein and ultrasonography. Alpha-fetoprotein has high false-positive rates and low sensitivity. US is the preferred imaging screening modality with a preferred time interval of 6 months. It has sensitivity of 60% to 80% and specificity of 45% to 95%.

Pearls

- Annual incidence of HCC in cirrhotic patients is 3% to 5%.
- All hepatitis carriers need surveillance by US at 6 month intervals. Serum AFP is controversial due to low sensitivity and false positives.
- TACE is useful both for controlling the tumor burden while the patient waits for liver transplantation and as palliative treatment for larger tumors.
- When the diagnosis of HCC tumor is not achieved by imaging, percutaneous biopsy may be indicated.

Suggested Readings

Ayuso C, Rimola J, García-Criado A. Imaging of HCC. *Abdom Imaging*. 2012 Apr;37(2):215-230.

Parente DB, Perez RM, Eiras-Araujo A, et al. MR imaging of hypervascular lesions in the cirrhotic liver: a diagnostic dilemma. *Radiographics*. 2012;32(3):767-787.

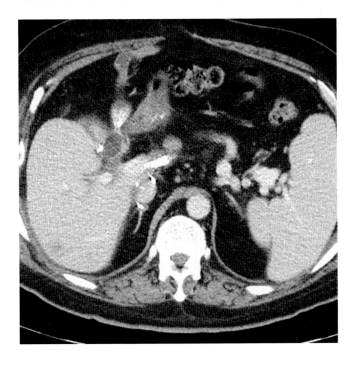
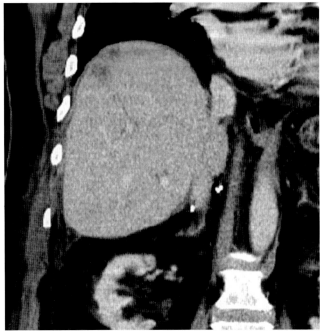

1. What are the findings?

2. What is the next investigation?

3. What is the best diagnosis?

4. What is the initial treatment of bilioenteric anastomotic stricture?

5. What is the diagnostic test for delayed liver transplant rejection?

Case ranking/difficulty:

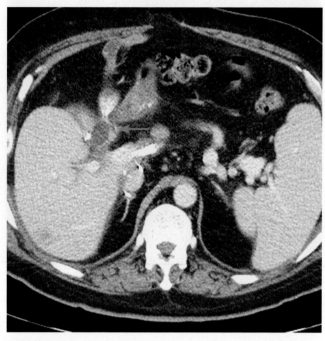

Axial portal venous CT shows extrahepatic biliary duct dilatation above the bilioenteric anastomosis (*green arrow*), but without significant intrahepatic biliary duct dilatation.

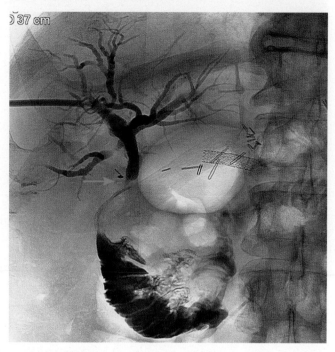

Cholangiography shows definite stricture at the anastomotic site (*green arrow*).

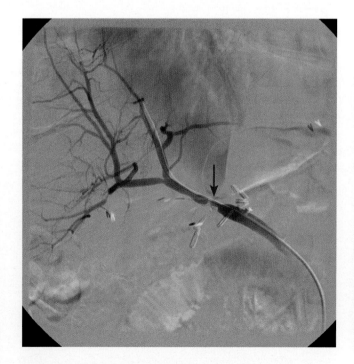

The patient had a short segmental hepatic artery stenosis (*red arrow*) at anastomotic site earlier.

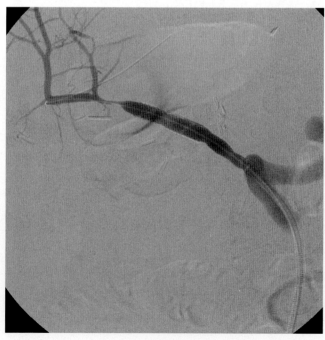

The hepatic artery stenosis was successfully treated by balloon dilatation and stenting.

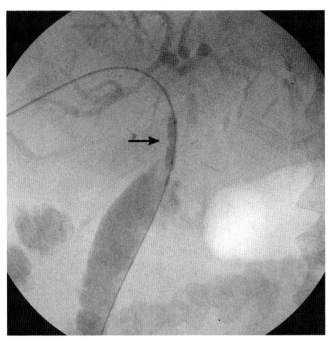

Balloon waist (a definite sign of stricture) at the anastomotic site (*black arrow*).

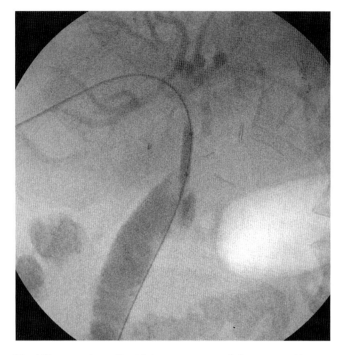

The biliary anastomotic stricture was successfully managed by serial balloon dilatations.

Answers

1. There is extrahepatic biliary duct dilatation without significant dilatation of intrahepatic biliary ducts. Multiple peripheral liver lesions are likely areas of biliary necrosis as a consequence of hepatic artery stenosis.

2. MRCP is the investigation of choice in cases of suspected biliary obstruction. Even if negative strongly suspected biliary obstruction is not excluded. PTC in cases of suspected bilioenteric anastomosis stricture or ERCP in cases of suspected duct-to-duct biliary anastomosis stricture should be performed. Biliary scintigraphy is a useful test for biliary leak. The sensitivity of US is very low since more than 60% of bilioenteric anastomotic strictures are without intrahepatic biliary duct dilatation.

3. The best diagnosis is bilioenteric anastomosis stricture with multiple intrahepatic abscesses. Infarcts extend up to the capsule, and so less likely. IVC is widely patent and normal enhancement. Pseudoaneurysm should enhance similar to artery.

4. Serial balloon dilatation and placement of larger stent/ drainage tubes at 3-month intervals up to 1 year is often successful. This can be done by ERCP (duct-to-duct anastomosis) or by PTC (bilioenteric anastomosis). Surgery is the next option. Nonanastomotic strictures are very difficult to treat. Treatment depends on location, number, and severity of strictures. Surgery should be tried before the development of liver fibrosis. Retransplantation may be needed.

5. Liver biopsy is the only test which can diagnose delayed liver transplant rejection. Ductopenic (vanishing bile duct) syndrome is loss of small intrahepatic biliary ducts due to any cause. The most common reason is acute or chronic rejection.

Pearls

- Significant intrahepatic dilatation is absent in more than 60% cases of bilioenteric anastomotic stricture.
- In case of biliary stricture or leak, a Doppler study of the hepatic artery should be performed to confirm patency.
- Even though MRCP is a sensitive test for diagnosis of biliary stricture direct cholangiography should be performed despite negative MRCP if the

clinical picture is strongly suspicious for biliary obstruction.

- PTC is the best choice for bilioenteric anastomosis with ERCP best for duct-to-duct anastomosis.
- Nonanastomotic strictures (ischemic strictures) are less common, mostly hilar or multiple, intrahepatic, and difficult to treat. Frequently retransplantation is needed.
- US and color Doppler imaging has an important role in posttransplant liver to confirm the vascular patency and postoperative fluid collection.

Suggested Readings

Crossin JD, Muradali D, Wilson SR. US of liver transplants: normal and abnormal. *Radiographics*. 2010 Mar;23(5):1093-1114.

Kochhar G, Parungao JM, Hanouneh IA, Parsi MA. Biliary complications following liver transplantation. *World J Gastroenterol*. 2013 May;19(19):2841-2846.

Seehofer D, Eurich D, Veltzke-Schlieker W, Neuhaus P. Biliary complications after liver transplantation: old problems and new challenges. *Am J Transplant*. 2013 Feb;13(2):253-265.

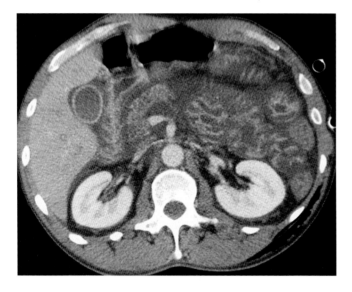
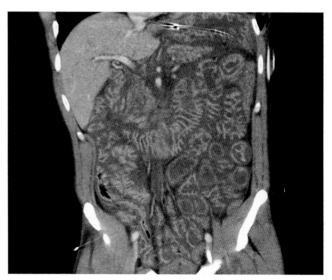
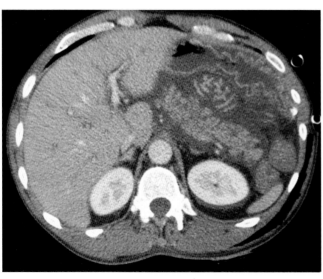
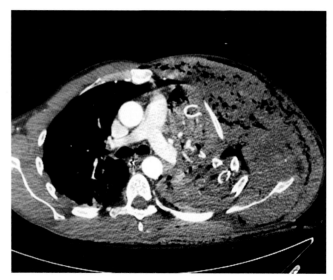

1. What is the diagnosis?

2. What is the expected finding in adrenals in shock bowel?

3. What are the pathophysiological changes in shock bowel?

4. What are the possible liver findings in shock bowel?

5. What is the treatment for this shock bowel?

Case ranking/difficulty:

Category: Small bowel

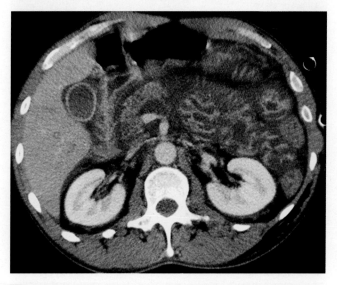

Portal venous phase CT show intense diffuse small bowel mucosal enhancement and thin caliber of IVC (*green arrow*).

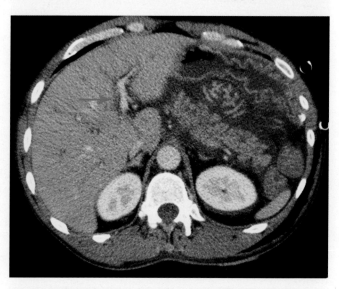

CT shows bulky pancreas with peripancreatic edema, periportal edema (*green arrow*), and relatively normal enhancement of adrenals, liver, and spleen. Slit-like IVC is noticed.

Answers

1. CT hypotensive complex. The mesenteric inflammatory changes tend to be more in the peripancreatic region in acute pancreatitis.

2. Intense contrast enhancement of both adrenals is a finding in shock bowel. It does not have to be present; if two or more signs of shock bowel are present, the diagnosis is suggested.

3. Slow perfusion, altered capillary permeability, interstitial leakage of contrast, and loss of bowel fluid resorption are the pathophysiologic changes in shock bowel.

4. Intense arterial enhancement, heterogenous, hypoenhancing liver, and perivascular edema are all potential findings in shock bowel.

5. Urgent fluid resuscitation is the treatment for shock bowel.

Pearls

- CT hypotension complex is an indicator of impending hemodynamic instability and reversible if prompt fluid resuscitation performed.
- Traumatic bowel injury and bowel ischemia are the two mimickers that need to be excluded as these conditions need urgent surgical attention.
- Hypoperfusion to spleen or pancreas may mimic splenic vascular pedicle injury or pancreatic injury.
- Mortality of these patients with shock bowel is high up to 70%, due to other injuries.

Suggested Readings

Lubner M, Demertzis J, Lee JY, Appleton CM, Bhalla S, Menias CO. CT evaluation of shock viscera: a pictorial review. *Emerg Radiol.* 2008 Jan;15(1):1-11.

Prasad KR, Kumar A, Gamanagatti S, Chandrashekhara SH. CT in post-traumatic hypoperfusion complex—a pictorial review. *Emerg Radiol.* 2011 Apr;18(2):139-143.

Tarrant AM, Ryan MF, Hamilton PA, Benjaminov O. A pictorial review of hypovolaemic shock in adults. *Br J Radiol.* 2008 Mar;81(963):252-257.

35-year-old female presenting with hepatomegaly and anemia

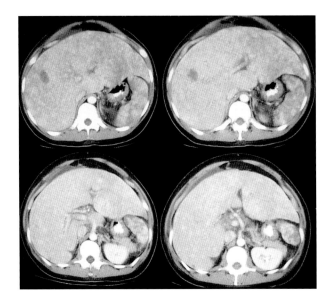

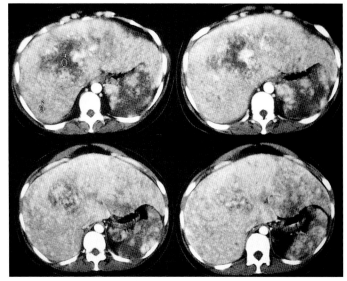

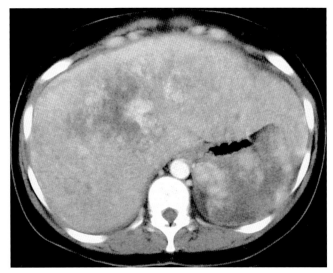

1. What is the most likely diagnosis?

2. Which two diseases have been associated with the development of hepatic angiosarcoma.

3. AFP is positive in hepatic angiosarcoma. True or false.

4. What are complications of hepatic angiosarcoma?

5. Which environmental exposures have been implicated in the development of hepatic angiosarcoma?

Case ranking/difficulty:

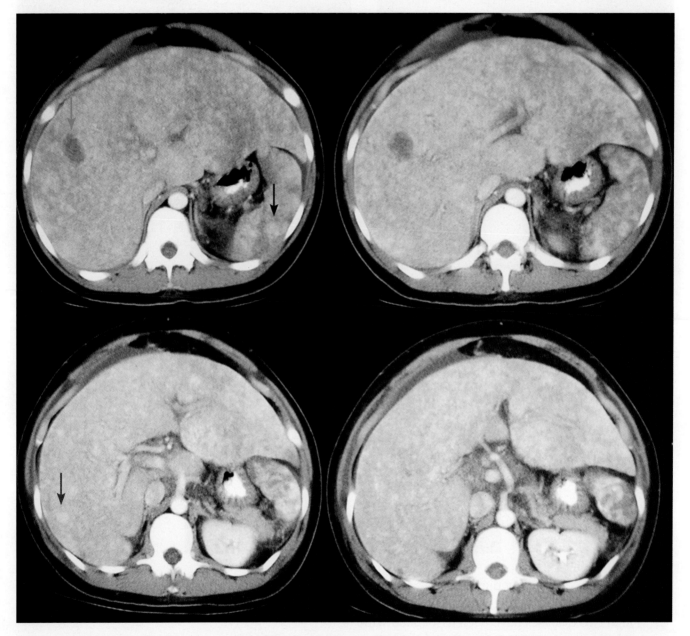

Composite portal venous phase CT shows multiple diffuse small enhancing nodular lesions through the liver (*red arrow*) with other nonenhancing foci of decreased density (*green arrow*), and enhancing nodular lesions with the spleen (*blue arrow*). There is also hepatomegaly and adenopathy.

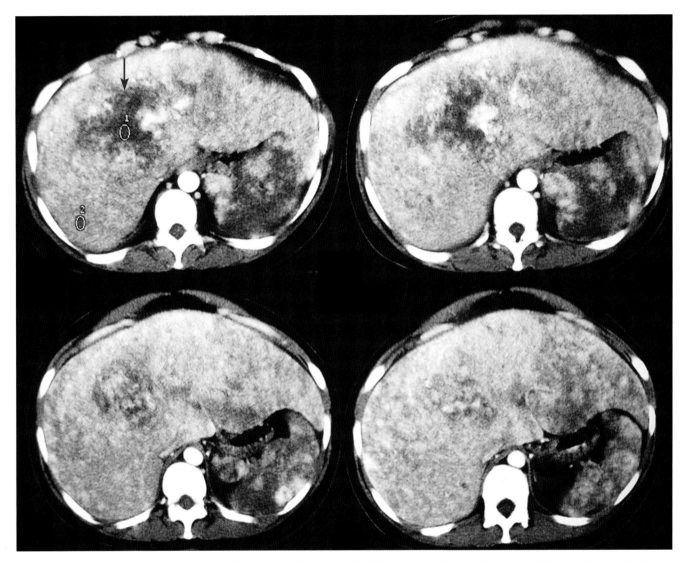

Composite portal venous phase CT (liver windows) again shows multiple diffuse enhancing nodular masses within the liver and spleen with scattered areas of lower attenuation (*red arrow*) within the liver.

Answers

1. Angiosarcoma involving the liver and spleen can have a variety of appearances, depending on the multiplicity of lesions, the presence of hemorrhage, necrosis, and enhancement characteristics. Lesions are frequently multiple, and the spleen can be involved along with the liver. Some cases have been described as having characteristics similar to cavernous hemangioma, but the appearance is usually not classic for cavernous hemangioma and there may be other features (multiplicity, atypical enhancement, hemorrhage, necrosis, history) that suggest the correct diagnosis.

Hepatocellular carcinoma usually occurs in diseased livers, and variably demonstrates a capsule, washout, and arterial phase enhancement. The LI-RADS system was recently introduced to classify lesions, and it may incorporate hepatobiliary agents in the future.

Focal nodular hyperplasia is usually relatively inconspicuous without contrast and is most conspicuous in the arterial phase. It may have a central scar. They usually are iso- to hyperintense on delayed images with hepatobiliary agents.

Hepatic adenomas usually occur in specific populations and can have variable appearances. They are often solitary, but can be multiple.

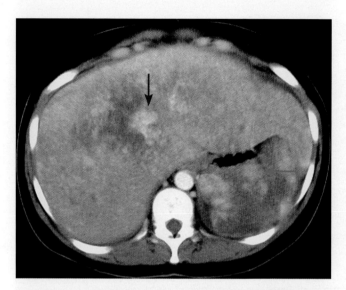

Axial portal venous phase CT shows enlarged and irregular vessels/vascularity within the liver (*red arrow*) and enhancing nodular lesions within the spleen (*green arrow*).

Pearls

- Related to environmental exposures. Thorotrast, vinyl chloride, arsenicals.
- Reported association with neurofibromatosis type I and hemochromatosis.

Suggested Readings

Bruegel M, Muenzel D, Waldt S, Specht K, Rummeny EJ. Hepatic angiosarcoma: cross-sectional imaging findings in seven patients with emphasis on dynamic contrast-enhanced and diffusion-weighted MRI. *Abdom Imaging*. 2013;38(4):745-754. Epub 2012/12/12. doi: 10.1007/s00261-012-9967-2.

Buetow PC, Buck JL, Ros PR, Goodman ZD. Malignant vascular tumors of the liver: radiologic-pathologic correlation. *Radiographics*. 1994;14(1):153-166. doi: doi:10.1148/radiographics.14.1.8128048.

Peterson MS, Baron RL, Rankin SC. Hepatic angiosarcoma: findings on multiphasic contrast-enhanced helical CT do not mimic hepatic hemangioma. *AJR Am J Roentgenol*. 2000;175(1):165-170. Epub 2000/07/06. doi: 10.2214/ajr.175.1.1750165.

2. Neurofibromatosis type 1 and hemochromatosis have been associated with the development of hepatic angiosarcoma.

3. AFP is not elevated in hepatic angiosarcoma. This can help differentiate it from hepatocellular carcinoma.

4. Hemoperitoneum is a potential complication and may occur spontaneously secondary to peripheral tumor rupture into the peritoneal cavity. There are frequently early and distant metastases, including the spleen in approximately 16% of cases.

5. Thorotrast (no longer used) exposure has been implicated in the development of hepatic angiosarcoma, as have vinyl chloride and arsenicals. Mercury and cadmium have not been implicated in the development of angiosarcoma, although they are otherwise toxic.

Abdominal pain and vomiting

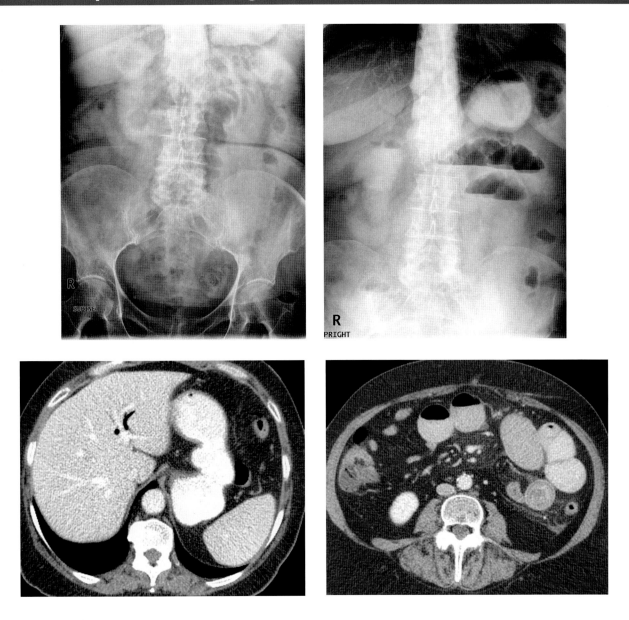

1. What are the radiological findings?

2. What is the diagnosis?

3. What is the most common cause of small bowel obstruction?

4. What is the commonest location of impaction of stone in gallstone ileus?

5. What is the commonest type of fistula in gallstone ileus?

Case ranking/difficulty:

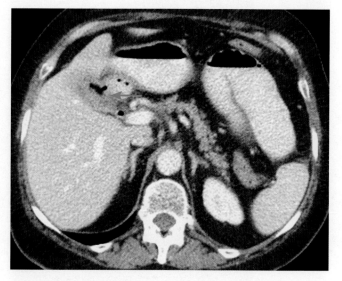

Axial CT image in portal venous phase shows air within the gallbladder and also in the cholecystoenteric fistula (*green arrow*).

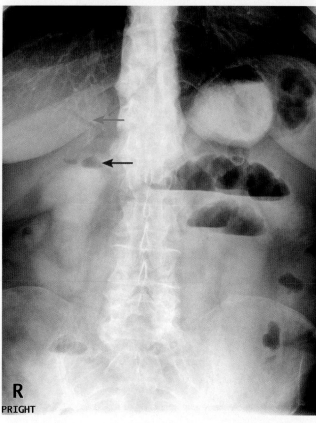

R
PRIGHT

Frontal abdominal radiograph in erect view show few air fluid levels in the left upper quadrant. Note the linear branching air lucency within the left intrahepatic biliary ducts (*green arrow*) and air within the gallbladder (*red arrow*).

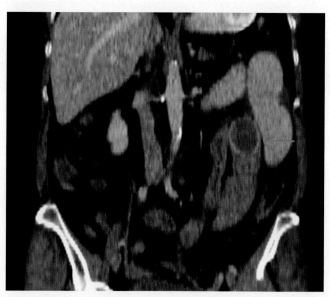

CT coronal image reveals the impacted gallstone (*green arrow*) within the jejunum with collapsed loop distally.

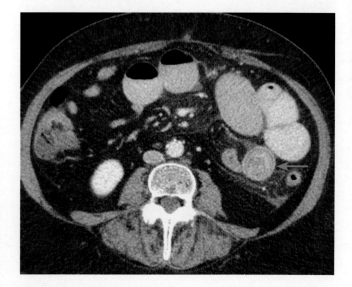

Impacted gallstone (*green arrow*).

Answers

1. Air within the biliary tract and air fluid levels within in the jejunal loops.

2. Impacted gallstone within the small bowel causes small bowel obstruction and air within the biliary duct due to fistulous connection between the biliary tract and bowel. These radiographic findings are highly suggestive of gallstone ileus. CT scan can demonstrate the cholesterol stone with or without rim of calcifications at the transition zone.

   Paraduodenal hernia shows dilated small bowel loops between pancreas and stomach due to herniation through the congenital or acquired mesenteric defect. Sentinel loops may be seen in this location in cases of acute pancreatitis.

3. Adhesion is the most common cause of small bowel obstruction, usually secondary to surgical manipulation.

4. It is the narrowest portion of small bowel. Next common site of impactions are jejunum and stomach.

5. The commonest type of fistula in gallstone ileus is cholecystoduodenal fistula (65% of cases).

Pearls

- The high mortality (5%-25%) and morbidity are mainly due to associated comorbidities in this elderly population.
- Rapid diagnosis reduces the mortality.
- Radiologist should note the presence of any stones within the dilated bowel proximal to the obstructing stone since removal of such stones may prevent recurrent obstruction (5%-10% of cases usually within 1-6 months).

Suggested Readings

Collins A, Coughlin D, Mullen M. Gallstone ileus. *J Emerg Med*. 2013 Feb;44(2):e277-e278.

Lassandro F, Romano S, Ragozzino A, et al. Role of helical CT in diagnosis of gallstone ileus and related conditions. *AJR Am J Roentgenol*. 2005 Nov;185(5):1159-1165.

Yu CY, Lin CC, Shyu RY, et al. Value of CT in the diagnosis and management of gallstone ileus. *World J Gastroenterol*. 2005 Apr;11(14):2142-2147.

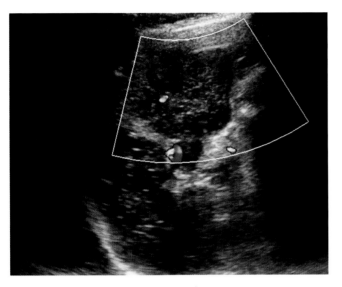
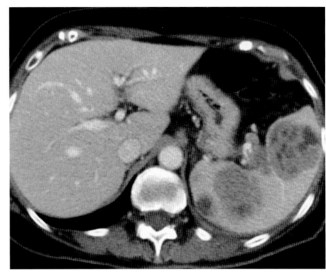
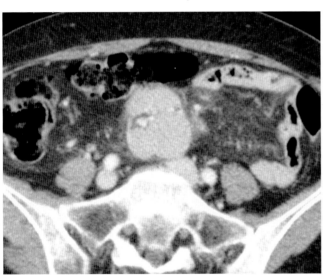
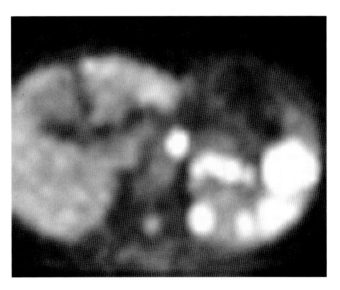

1. What is the most likely diagnosis for the masses in the spleen?

2. What is the most common subtype NHL?

3. What are the causes of mesenteric mass lesions?

4. What are the causes of high FDG avidity in lymph nodes?

5. What is the sensitivity of PET-CT for the detection of splenic lymphoma?

Case ranking/difficulty: **Category:** Spleen

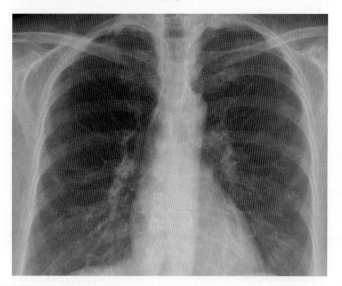

Plain radiography of chest in frontal projection demonstrates no lung opacity especially in the apices or no mediastinal widening.

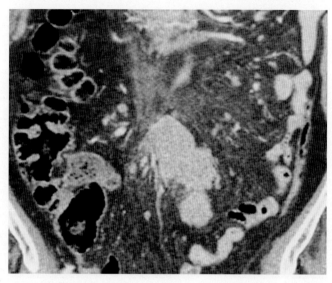

Coronal CECT shows bulky mesenteric lymph nodes with adjacent soft tissue mesenteric strands.

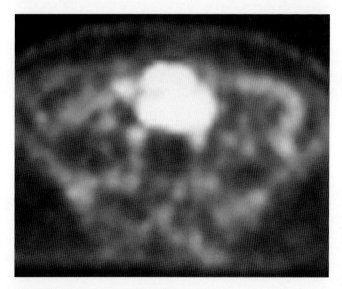

Axial PET image shows FDG avid mesenteric lymph nodes. Complete resolution after chemotherapy.

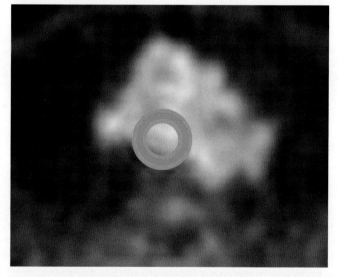

Axial PET image shows FDG avid subcarinal lymph node (*circle*). Involvement of both sides of diaphragm (stage III).

Answers

1. Findings are typical of splenic lymphoma. Multiple splenic abscesses are most commonly seen in patients with endocarditis, immunocompromise (AIDS), and s/p transplant. It shows typical fluid density with marginal enhancement. Fungal abscesses are usually multiple microabscesses, much smaller than the masses depicted, and usually without lymphadenopathy.

   Splenic metastasis is less common than lymphoma. The most common primaries to metastasize to spleen

   are melanoma, breast, lung, and ovary. Splenic infarcts are wedge shaped, peripheral, without mass effect, and nonenhancing except may be a rim enhancement. Tuberculous involvement of spleen causing large masses is rare, especially in the absence of disease elsewhere.

2. Diffuse large B-cell lymphoma (about 30%) followed by follicular lymphoma.

3. Lymphoma, peritoneal carcinomatosis, carcinoid tumor, desmoid, and sclerosing mesenteritis cause mesenteric masses. Ovarian and GI cancers are the most common

causes of peritoneal carcinomatosis usually manifest as multiple nodules in the mesentery and omentum.

4. Lymphoma, reactive hyperplasia, granulomatous disease, metastasis, and infection are all causes of increased metabolic activity in lymph nodes.

5. PET-CT is almost 100% sensitive (and 95% specific in the right clinical context) for splenic lymphoma. Splenic lymphomatous infiltration is isointense to normal splenic tissue on both T1- and T2-weighted images. So unenhanced MR is insensitive. However, MR is very sensitive for lymphomatous bone marrow infiltration.

Pearls

- NHL is the most common malignant tumor of the spleen.
- Lymphoma is the most common cause of mesenteric mass and lymphadenopathy.
- Calcifications of lymphomatous lesions are rare without treatment.
- New appearance of high FDG avid splenic lesion in a known low-grade lymphoma patient should raise the possibility of malignant transformation.
- Splenomegaly with hilar lymphadenopathy is suggestive of splenic lymphoma.
- Diminution of splenic size during treatment may be a reactive process and does not indicate splenic involvement.

Suggested Readings

Anis M, Irshad A. Imaging of abdominal lymphoma. *Radiol Clin North Am*. 2008 Mar;46(2):265-285, viii-ix.

Karlo CA, Stolzmann P, Do RK, Alkadhi H. Computed tomography of the spleen: how to interpret the hypodense lesion. *Insights Imaging*. 2013 Feb;4(1):65-76.

Tomita N, Takasaki H, Fujisawa S, et al. Standard R-CHOP therapy in follicular lymphoma and diffuse large B-cell lymphoma. *J Clin Exp Hematop*. 2013 Feb;53(2):121-125.

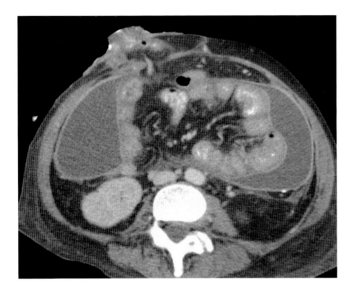 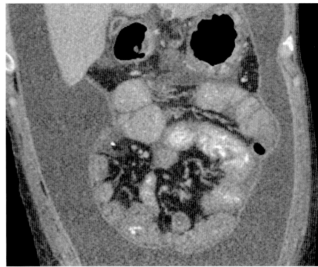

1. What is the most likely diagnosis?

2. What are the possible causes of sclerosing encapsulating peritonitis?

3. How does one differentiate simple peritonitis from sclerosing encapsulating peritonitis?

4. What are the radiological features of peritoneal carcinomatosis?

5. What is the treatment?

Case ranking/difficulty:

Category: Peritoneum

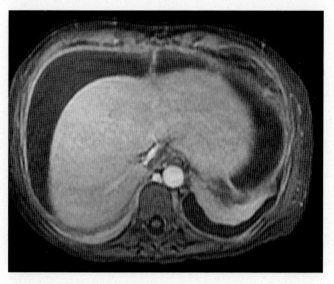

Axial CE MRI shows the thick enhancing peritoneum.

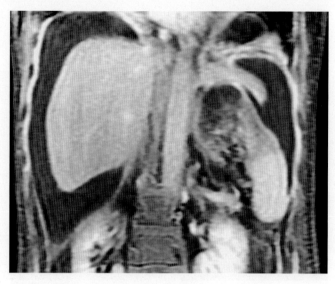

Coronal CE MRI shows a thick enhancing peritoneum.

Answers

1. The encapsulating membrane around the bowel loops in the center of the abdomen is a typical finding of sclerosing encapsulating peritonitis. There are no nodular deposits in the peritoneal cavity to suggest peritoneal carcinomatosis. Tuberculosis peritonitis is usually associated with necrotic enhancing retroperitoneal or mesenteric lymph nodes. The CT density of hemoperitoneum is higher (>30HU) than simple ascites.

2. The cause is unknown. It is postulated that excessive circulation of peritoneal fluid causes deposition of fibrin, which initiates the membrane formation.

3. In cases of simple peritonitis, the bowel loops are separated, there is no encasing membrane around the bowel loops and clinical features point to infection rather than bowel obstruction. Peritoneal calcifications or nodules are neither a feature of simple peritonitis nor sclerosing encapsulating peritonitis.

4. Omental caking, ascites, nodular peritoneal thickening, and peritoneal implants are all features of peritoneal carcinomatosis.

5. Membrane dissection with adhesiolysis is the surgical treatment of sclerosing encapsulating peritonitis.

Pearls

- Awareness of this entity is the key to the diagnosis.
- Direct visualization of the membrane on CT leads to an accurate diagnosis.
- Membrane dissection is the simple and effective treatment.

Suggested Readings

Gupta S, Shirahatti RG, Anand J. CT findings of an abdominal cocoon. *AJR Am J Roentgenol.* 2004 Dec;183(6):1658-1660.

Solak A, Solak İ. Abdominal cocoon syndrome: preoperative diagnostic criteria, good clinical outcome with medical treatment and review of the literature. *Turk J Gastroenterol.* 2012 Oct;23(6):776-779.

Térébus Loock M, Lubrano J, Courivaud C, et al. CT in predicting abdominal cocoon in patients on peritoneal dialysis. *Clin Radiol.* 2010 Nov;65(11):924-929.

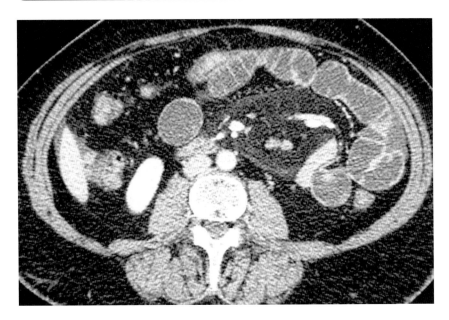 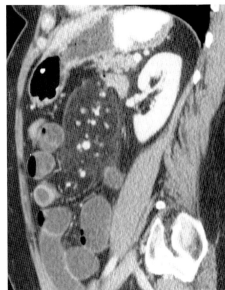

1. What is the most likely diagnosis?

2. What is the most common symptom of this condition?

3. What is the investigation useful to differentiate carcinoid from retractile mesenteritis?

4. What are the rare, but possible, complications of sclerosing mesenteritis?

5. What are the differentiating features of lymphoma from sclerosing mesenteritis?

Case ranking/difficulty:

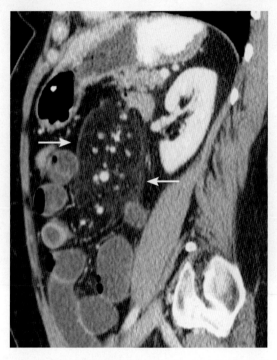

Sagittal CECT shows subtle ill-defined increased density in the root of mesentery with a thin pseudocapsule (*white arrows*).

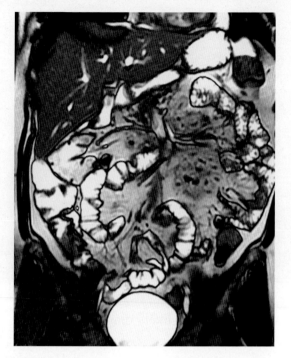

MRI FIESTA coronal image from the same patient shows ill-defined low signal intensity in the root of mesentery in relation to surrounding fat.

Answers

1. Small bowel obstruction is the primary finding. Sclerosing mesenteritis is an incidental finding. There is no bulky lymphadenopathy to suggest lymphoma. Secondary deposits to mesentery are usually from ovary or GI malignancy and associated with ascites and deposits in the other typical locations like liver or splenic surfaces, paracolic gutters, and pelvis. Carcinoid tumor has stellate appearance and usually associated with desmoplastic reaction and calcifications. It mimics the late stage of sclerosing mesenteritis (retractile mesenteritis).

2. Sclerosing mesenteritis is mostly identified as an incidental finding during imaging. However, it may cause nonspecific symptoms like abdominal pain. Rarely, it encases the mesenteric vessels and causes bowel ischemia.

3. Octreotide scan is positive in 80% of carcinoid tumors, but negative in retractile mesenteritis.

4. Complications of sclerosing mesenteritis are very rare. However, encasement of mesenteric vessels can cause bowel ischemia and warrant the surgery. Ureteric obstruction is also a reported complication.

5. Lymphoma never shows calcification unless treated. Presence of bowel mass favors the diagnosis of lymphoma.

Pearls

- Most common site is in the root of mesentery.
- In about 90% cases, it is an incidental finding on imaging.
- Search for any underlying malignancy such as lymphoma and GI malignancy.
- Fat ring sign may be helpful to differentiate it from other malignant process.

Suggested Reading

Horton KM, Lawler LP, Fishman EK. CT findings in sclerosing mesenteritis (panniculitis): spectrum of disease. *Radiographics*. 2003;23(6):1561-1567.

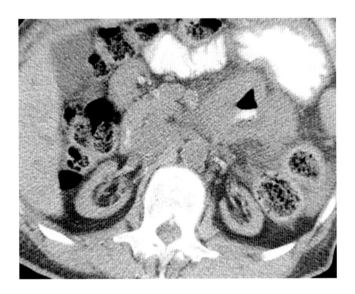 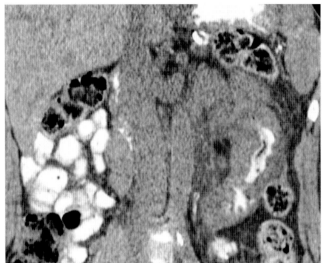

1. What is the most likely diagnosis?

2. What are the features of NHL in immunocompromised individuals that differ from those in immunocompetent patients?

3. What are the risk factors for development of secondary bowel lymphoma?

4. What are the radiological findings in favor of bowel lymphoma?

5. What is the imaging modality of choice for staging of PTLD?

Case ranking/difficulty: **Category:** Duodenum

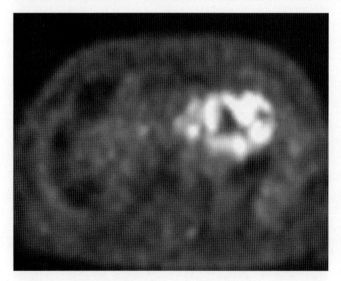

Axial PET reveals the high FDG avidity in the bowel wall thickening

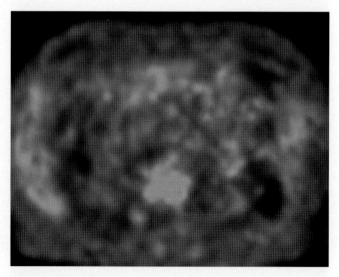

Resolution of PET avidity 4 months after treatment.

Answers

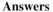

1. Posttransplantation lymphoproliferative disorder (PTLD). Note the absent bowel obstruction in spite of the gross bowel wall thickening in a patient with renal transplant. Although duodenum and jejunum are common locations for adenocarcinoma of small bowel, it usually presents with bowel obstruction and abdominal pain.

   GIST is an intramural well-circumscribed, exophytic focal mass. It may show aneurysmal dilatation like lymphoma if it cavitates into the lumen. Crohn disease is relatively uncommon in the jejunum and shows homogenous, uniform wall thickening with adjacent inflammatory stranding, and mesenteric fibrofatty proliferation.

   Carcinoid tumor is less common in jejunum than ileum. It usually shows calcification and mesenteric desmoplastic reaction.

2. NHL in immunocompromised individuals is higher grade, has a worse prognosis, is more prone to ulceration/perforation, and has higher frequency of extranodal disease. NHL in immunocompromised patients can affect any body part but are most common in the GI tract, lung, and brain.

3. *Helicobacter pylori* infection, celiac disease, HIV infection, and inflammatory bowel disease can cause secondary lymphoma of bowel.

4. 1. Bulky mass in the bowel wall

   2. Heterogeneously enhancing mass with luminal narrowing

   3. Relative preservation of adjacent fat planes

   4. Aneurysmal bowel dilatation without obstruction

   5. Bulky lymphadenopathy

   All are features of bowel lymphoma. Encasement of mesenteric vessels by lymph nodal masses and preservation of fat planes around the vessels (sandwich sign) are also typical findings of bowel lymphoma. Adenocarcinoma of bowel is more invasive with infiltrative margins and luminal narrowing. Bowel obstruction is likely.

5. High FDG avidity is the metabolic indicator of tumor viability. PET CT is most helpful in staging of the disease and in monitoring the response to treatment.

Pearls

- Always think about the possibility of PTLD in patients after organ transplantation who present with any mass lesion in the bowel or solid organ.
- Extranodal presentation is three to four times more common than nodal.
- Prognosis worse than NHL.
- Flow cytometry is used for immunophenotyping.
- Treatment is different for each subtype of PTLD and a core biopsy is needed for typing.

Suggested Readings

Borhani AA, Hosseinzadeh K, Almusa O, Furlan A, Nalesnik M. Imaging of posttransplantation lymphoproliferative disorder after solid organ transplantation. *Radiographics*. 2010 Jan;29(4):981-1000; discussion 1000-2.

Dhillon MS, Rai JK, Gunson BK, Olliff S, Olliff J. Post-transplant lymphoproliferative disease in liver transplantation. *Br J Radiol*. 2007 May;80(953):337-346.

Leite NP, Kased N, Hanna RF, et al. Cross-sectional imaging of extranodal involvement in abdominopelvic lymphoproliferative malignancies. *Radiographics*. 2007;27(6):1613-1634.

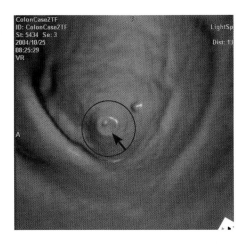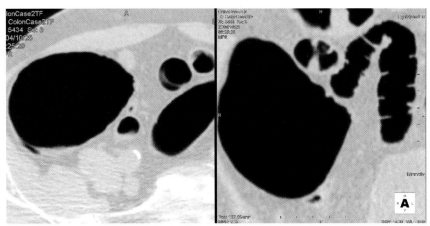

1. What is your differential diagnosis for the umbilicated abnormality in the above images? (I'll give you the small cecal polyp).

2. What is the best diagnosis after seeing additional images next two pages?

3. What is the danger of incorrect diagnosis of appendiceal intussusception?

4. What are the clinical manifestations of appendiceal intussusception?

5. What are the imaging manifestations of appendiceal intussusception?

Case ranking/difficulty:

Category: Colorectum

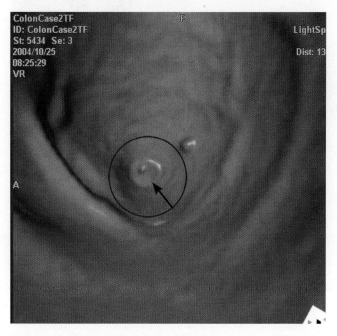

Endoluminal flythrough supine: Small umbilicated mass (*circle*) in the cecal tip adjacent to a small polyp (*arrow*).

Answers

1. Intussusception of the appendix and appendiceal carcinoid are good choices in view of the small mass and the nonvisualization of the appendix. An enlarged lymphoid follicle is possible. Umbilication is not likely in an inverted appendiceal stump. Flat lesions can have central depression so that is a good choice.

2. The filling of the appendix and disappearance of the mass with some residual swelling around the appendiceal orifice are diagnostic of transient appendiceal intussusception.

3. Correct diagnosis is vital in avoiding unnecessary and potentially catastrophic interventions like endoscopic excision or even more radical surgery in cases of suspected malignancy. Routine biopsy or attempted endoscopic "polypectomy" may result in perforation or bleeding requiring urgent surgical exploration.

4. Four presentation patterns of appendiceal intussusception are:

   1. Nonspecific symptoms including recurrent cramping abdominal pain, rectal bleeding, melena and mucous in stools, and change in bowel habits.

   2. RLQ pain mimicking appendicitis.

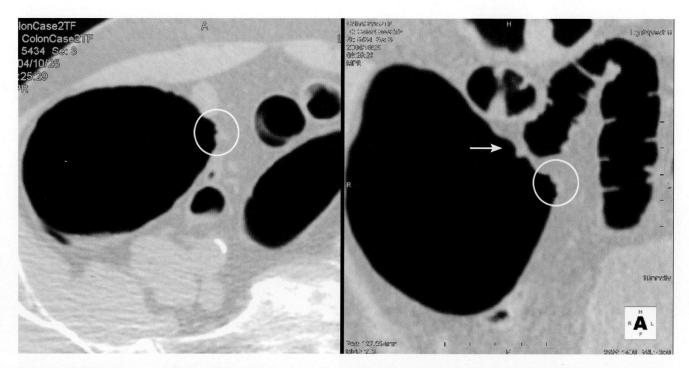

Supine axial (*left*) and coronal (*right*) 2D MPR confirming the small umbilicated mass (*circles*) and the small polyp (*arrow*). No visualization of the appendix.

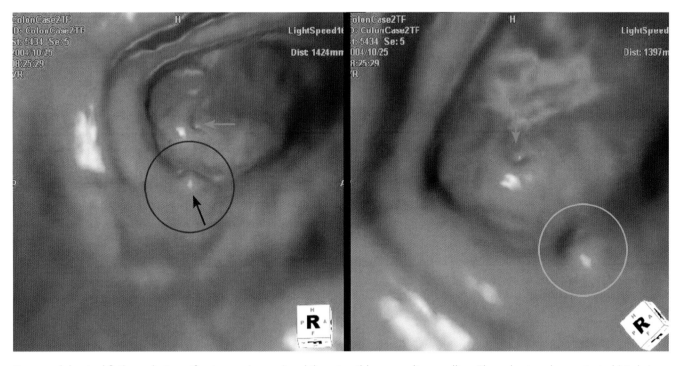

Prone endoluminal flythrough: An orifice is seen (*arrows*) and there is mild surrounding swelling. The polyp is redemonstrated (*circles*).

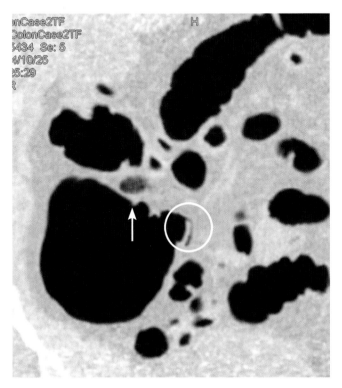

Coronal prone MPR shows a tiny appendix (*circle*) at the site of the orifice in the image. The polyp is redemonstrated (*arrow*) lateral to a bifid fold.

3. Days to months of abdominal pain and vomiting with or without diarrhea and melena suggesting intussusception.

4. Asymptomatic and incidentally diagnosed.

5. A cecal filling defect in the expected position of the appendix on single-contrast BE and a coiled spring appearance in the same area of the cecum on double-contrast BE and absent filling of the appendix have been described.

US: "Target-like" appearance and the "concentric ring sign" on axial US and an inverted appendix intruding into the cecum on longitudinal US have been reported.

CTC: Its appearance is polypoid. Intussusceptions may reduce during gas insufflation, resulting in a halo-like erythematous region (mild swelling on CTC) surrounding the appendiceal orifice.

Pearls

- BE: Cecal tip filling defect and/or coiled spring appearance, failure of appendiceal filling. Subsequent reduction implies no significant appendiceal pathology.
- US: "Target-like" appearance and the "concentric ring sign" and an inverted appendix intruding into the cecum.
- Optical colonoscopy or CT colonography: Appearance is commonly referred to as polypoid; intussusceptions may reduce during insufflation of gas (implying again no significant pathology), resulting in a halo-like erythematous region (round swelling on CTC) surrounding the appendiceal lumen. Appendiceal intussusception has been misdiagnosed endoscopically or on CTC as cecal polyp or carcinoma.
- In symptomatic patients, laparoscopic appendectomy is recommended. Surgery is unnecessary in asymptomatic patients.

Suggested Readings

Gollub MJ. Letter to the Editor. Inverted appendiceal orifice masquerading as a cecal polyp on virtual colonoscopy. *Gastrointest Endosc*. 2006;63:358.

Koff JM, Choi JR, Hwang I. Inverted appendiceal orifice masquerading as a cecal polyp on virtual colonoscopy. *Gastrointest Endosc*. 2005;62:308.

Salehzadeh A, Scala A, Simson JN. Appendiceal intussusception mistaken for a polyp at colonoscopy: case report and review of literature. *Ann R Coll Surg Engl*. September 2010;92(6):W46-W48.

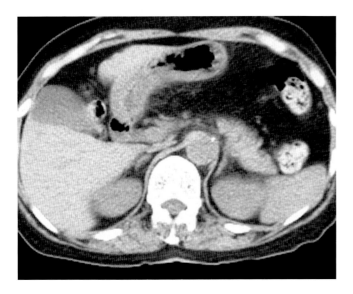
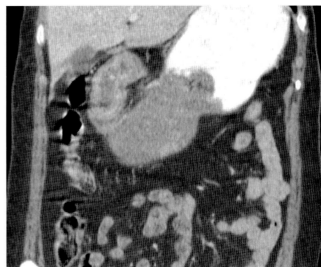

1. What is the differential diagnosis of this antral abnormality?

2. What are the characteristic features of mucinous adenocarcinoma of the stomach?

3. Which histological subtype of gastric carcinoma commonly causes bilateral ovarian metastatic deposits (Krukenberg tumor)?

4. What are the radiological findings that favor lymphoma over carcinoma?

5. What is the most common primary to metastasize to the stomach?

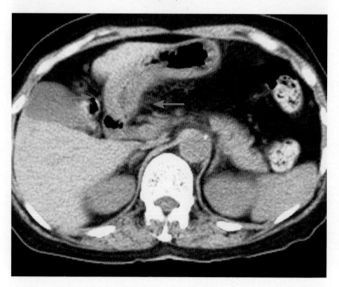

Noncontrast-enhanced CT (as a part of PET/CT) axial image shows circumferential antral wall thickening (*green arrows*).

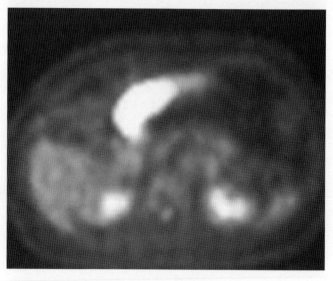

PET image demonstrates high FDG avidity at the site corresponding to the antral wall thickening.

Answers

1. The differential diagnosis of antral circumferential wall thickening includes gastritis, carcinoma, lymphoma, metastatic disease, and Crohn disease. Gastritis can affect any portion of the stomach, but is most common in the antral region. The common etiologies are alcohol, drug (NSAIDs), infections like *H pylori*. The primary imaging finding is fold thickening and ulcerations. Sometime, it appears as polypoidal mass.

   Varices are usually located around GE junction or gastric fundus. The commonest etiology is portal hypertension. Isolated fundal varices are due to splenic vein occlusion (pancreatitis or pancreatic cancer). The final diagnosis of this case is a low-grade adenocarcinoma, intestinal type.

2. Low CT density and calcifications are the characteristic features of mucinous adenocarcinoma of the stomach.

3. Signet ring cell carcinoma. Colorectal carcinoma is the next most common cause of Krukenberg tumor.

4. Findings in favor of stomach lymphoma are

   1. Transpyloric spread
   2. Relative preservation of overlying mucosal folds
   3. Marked thickening of the wall (>1 cm) and extensive involvement
   4. Presence of multiple bulky mesenteric lymph nodes

5. Breast and lung carcinoma are the two most common primaries metastasize to the stomach.

Pearls

- Gastric cancer has high geographical variation, with high prevalence in Japan and low in the USA.
- Double-contrast barium is more sensitive (90%-95%) than single contrast (75%) in detection of gastric cancer in reference to endoscopy.
- The primary role of CT is to evaluate for liver metastasis or local invasion.
- Endoscopic ultrasonography (EUS) plays a significant role in local staging by assessing depth of wall invasion and perigastric lymph nodes within 3 cm from gastric wall.

Suggested Readings

Ba-Ssalamah A, Prokop M, Uffmann M, Pokieser P, Teleky B, Lechner G. Dedicated multidetector CT of the stomach: spectrum of diseases. *Radiographics*. 2003;23(3):625-644.

Lim JS, Yun MJ, Kim MJ, et al. CT and PET in stomach cancer: preoperative staging and monitoring of response to therapy. *Radiographics*. 2006;26(1):143-156.

Shen Y, Kang HK, Jeong YY, et al. Evaluation of early gastric cancer at multidetector CT with multiplanar reformation and virtual endoscopy. *Radiographics*. 2011;31(1):189-99.

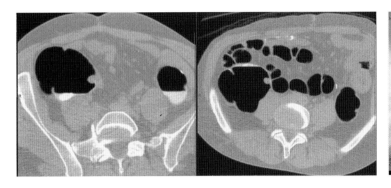
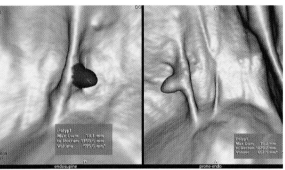

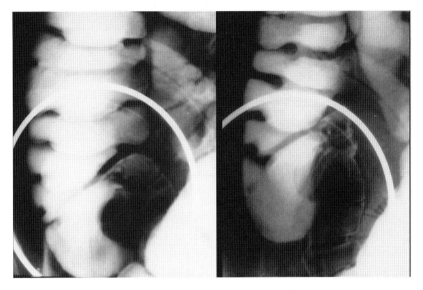

1. What is the best diagnosis on all images? Hint: Would I travel all the way from the Bronx to show you a polyp? (What my chairman would say when he was a visiting professor?)

2. What imaging features are shared by polyps and inverted appendiceal stumps?

3. How can intussusception of a normal appendix be differentiated from an inverted appendiceal stump?

4. What diseases have been reported in inverted appendiceal stumps?

5. What procedures may be needed if an inverted appendiceal stump is suspected on CTC?

Case ranking/difficulty: **Category:** Colorectum

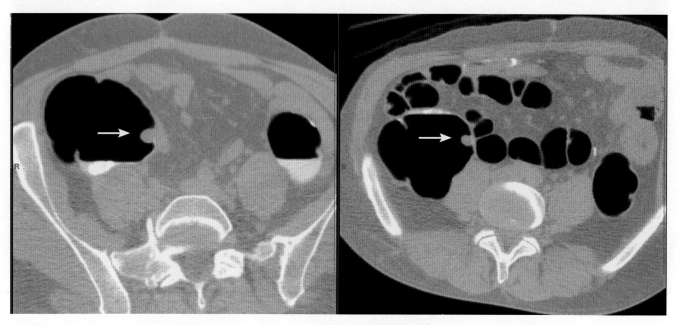

Supine (*left*) and prone (*right*) axial images from a CTC showing a sessile soft tissue attenuation polyp (*arrows*) attached to the medial cecal wall. It stays in the same location in both positions. The appendix is not seen.

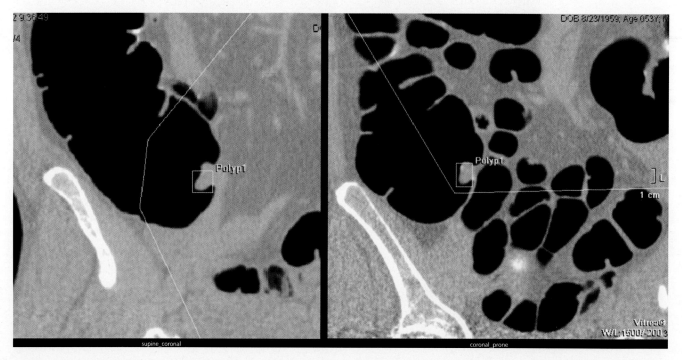

Supine (*left*) and prone (*right*) coronal images from a CTC showing a sessile polyp attached to the medial cecal wall in the expected location of the appendix. It stays in the same location in both positions. The appendix is not seen.

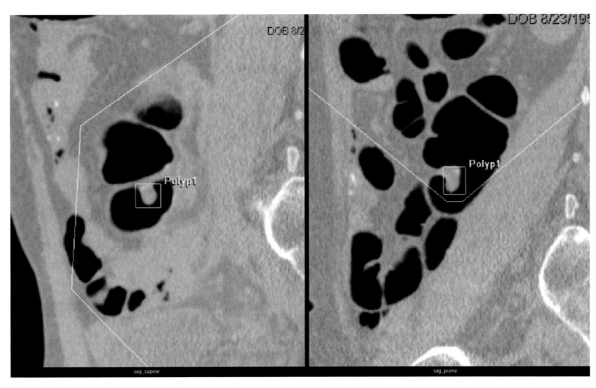

Supine (*left*) and prone (*right*) sagittal images from a CTC showing a sessile polyp that stays in the same location in both positions.

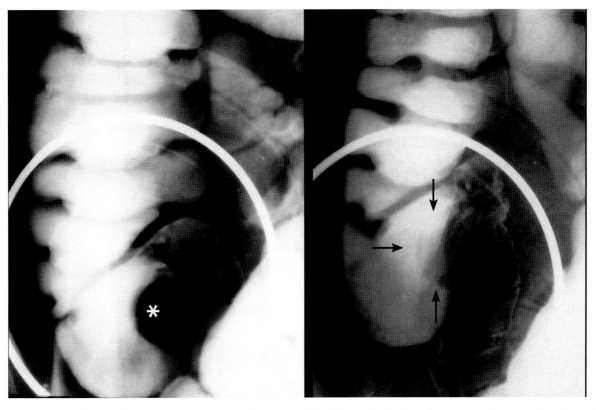

World's largest inverted appendiceal stump in a 25-year-old woman with abdominal pain 3 weeks s/p appendectomy. Spot films of cecum from barium enema show a large filling defect (*asterisk right, arrows left*) at the expected location of the appendix due to an inverted appendiceal stump.

Answers

1. Absence of the appendiceal orifice on endoluminal images and nonvisualization of the appendix on 2D images suggests appendectomy and an inverted stump. Querying the electronic medical record confirmed these suspicions and the best diagnosis is inverted appendiceal stump.

2. Both polyps and inverted appendiceal stumps have homogeneous soft-tissue attenuation, do not change location between supine and prone series, and will enhance with intravenous contrast.

3. Reduction of an appendiceal intussusception during the course of the examination may permit differentiation of it from inverted appendiceal stump. A history of appendectomy makes appendiceal intussusception very unlikely. The patient is very unlikely to know whether or not his or her stump was inverted.

4. Mucoceles and stump appendicitis have been reported in an inverted appendiceal stump. Other abnormalities that can affect a normal appendix are possible.

5. Endoscopic biopsy of an inverted appendiceal stump will show normal mucosa. This may be indicated when history is unclear. Deep biopsy is ill-advised due to risk of perforation.

Pearls

- Inverted appendiceal stump is not an easy diagnosis at CTC or optical colonoscopy without a history of appendectomy and operative report of stump inversion because there is often no imaging characteristic other than absence of the appendix to differentiate inverted appendiceal stump from polyp. An appendiceal stump might have mesenteric fat in its middle supporting the correct diagnosis.
- Even with clinical history of appendectomy you could get a polyp right at the old orifice.
- Appendiceal orifice almost always visible at good-quality endoluminal CTC unless submerged in fluid. Its absence suggests appendectomy. On 2D images absence of the appendix is a strong indicator of prior surgery.
- Endoscopy and biopsy may be required at times.

Suggested Readings

Gollub MJ. Letter to the Editor. Inverted appendiceal orifice masquerading as a cecal polyp on virtual colonoscopy. *Gastrointest Endosc*. 2006;63:358.

Mang T, Maier A, Plank C, Mueller-Mang C, Herold C, Schima W. Pitfalls in multi-detector row CT colonography: a systematic approach. *Radiographics*. July 2007;27(2):431-454.

Prout TM, Taylor AJ, Pickhardt PJ. Inverted appendiceal stumps simulating large pedunculated polyps on screening CT colonography. *AJR*. 2006;186(2):535-538.

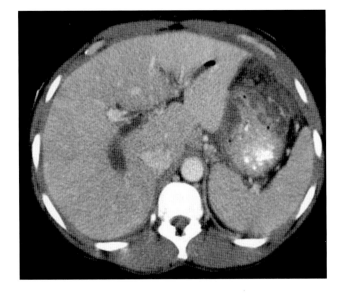 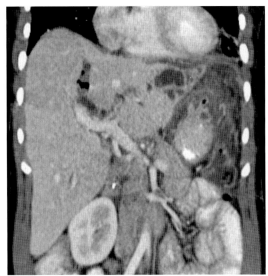

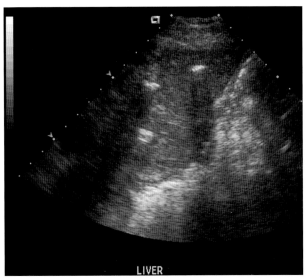

LIVER

1. What other feature does Caroli syndrome include when compared to Caroli disease?

2. Which specific feature on CT is helpful in making the diagnosis?

3. What genetic disorder is Caroli syndrome most strongly associated with?

4. What bile duct cyst classification is assigned to Caroli disease according to the Todani classification?

5. What is the another name for Caroli disease?

Case ranking/difficulty:

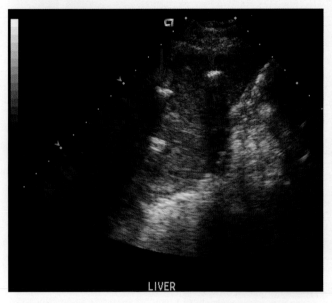

Grayscale ultrasound images demonstrates linear echogenic shadowing foci (*red arrows*) corresponding to air seen within the biliary tree on CT.

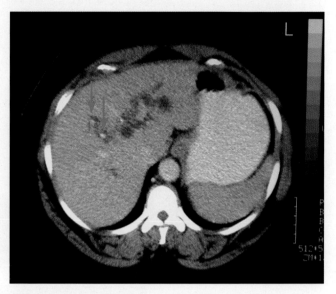

Companion case from a 38-year-old female with fever and elevated liver functions tests. Axial portal venous phase CT demonstrates dilatation of the biliary tree along with central enhancing foci, portal vein radicals, or "central dot sign" (*green arrows*), within dilated portion of the biliary tree, a finding suggestive of Caroli disease or Caroli syndrome.

Answers

1. Caroli syndrome includes the additional feature of congenital hepatic fibrosis and is thus a more severe form of the disease. Caroli disease affects only the larger intrahepatic and extrahepatic ducts and is not associated with congenital hepatic fibrosis.

2. Although cystic spaces, intraductal stones, and intrahepatic abscesses may all be seen, the "central dot sign" is perhaps the most specific finding, although it is not present in all cases. The dot is related to a portal vein radical situated in the midst of a dilated cystic space. The second case shown here shows an example. The other thing to note is that the cystic spaces communicate with the biliary tree.

3. The strongest association is with autosomal recessive polycystic kidney disease, although there have been cases thought to be related to autosomal dominant polycystic kidney disease.

4. Caroli disease is assigned the type V classification within the Todani classification of bile duct cysts, although some would argue that Caroli disease and syndrome should be classified separately since there is a genetic component and it is associated with renal disease.

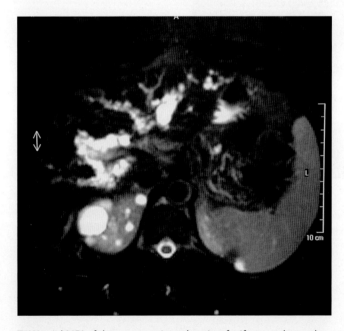

T2W axial MRI of the same patient showing fusiform and saccular dilatation of the biliary tree along with renal cystic disease noted within the right kidney.

5. The term "communicating cavernous biliary ectasia" is more descriptive and is sometimes used to refer to Caroli disease, although one should remember that the syndrome includes the additional feature of hepatic fibrosis.

Pearls

- Caroli syndrome includes congenital hepatic fibrosis.
- Caroli disease is cystic disease without fibrosis.
- Rare disorder.
- Todani type V choledochal cyst.
- Communication of cystic spaces with the biliary tree helps differentiate from other hepatic cystic diseases.

Suggested Readings

Lefere M, Thijs M, De Hertogh G, Verslype C, Laleman W, Vanbeckevoort D, Van Steenbergen W, Claus F. Caroli disease: review of eight cases with emphasis on magnetic resonance imaging features. *Eur J Gastroenterol Hepatol.* 2011 Jul;23(7):578-585.

Levy AD, Rohrmann CA, Jr., Murakata LA, Lonergan GJ. Caroli's disease: radiologic spectrum with pathologic correlation. *AJR Am J Roentgenol.* 2002;179(4):1053-1057. Epub 2002/09/20. doi: 10.2214/ajr.179.4.1791053.

Yonem O, Bayraktar Y. Clinical characteristics of Caroli's syndrome. *World J Gastroenterol.* 2007;13(13):1934-1937. Epub 2007/04/28.

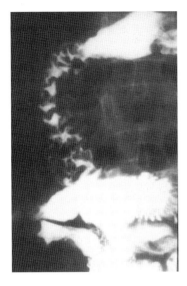 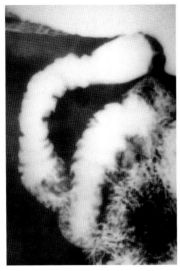 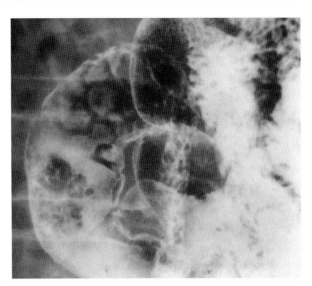

1. What is the best diagnosis for images on the left and in the center (on the same patient)? The image on the right is same diagnosis, different patient.

2. Villous adenomas are most frequent in what part of the bowel?

3. What conditions predispose to villous tumors of the duodenum?

4. What are the possible features of villous tumors on UGI?

5. What is the treatment of duodenal villous tumor?

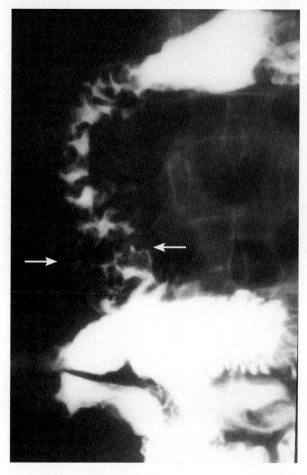

There is subtle widening at the junction of the second and third portions of the duodenum with a lacy mucosal pattern (*arrows*).

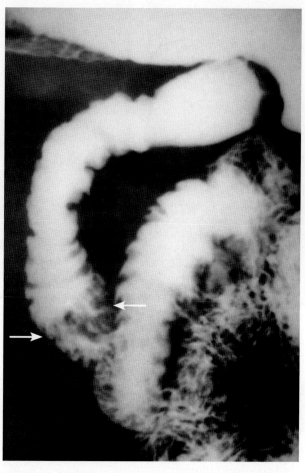

RAO with better filling shows a microlobulated polypoid filling defect (*arrows*) with some barium in interstices.

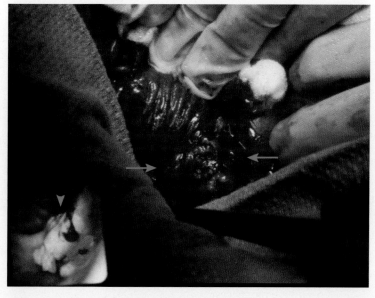

Lower left-hand corner is an endophoto (*arrowhead*) showing a small cauliflower-like mass. The red is bleeding from the biopsy site. Remainder of the image is an intraoperative photo of the small cauliflower-like mass (*arrows*).

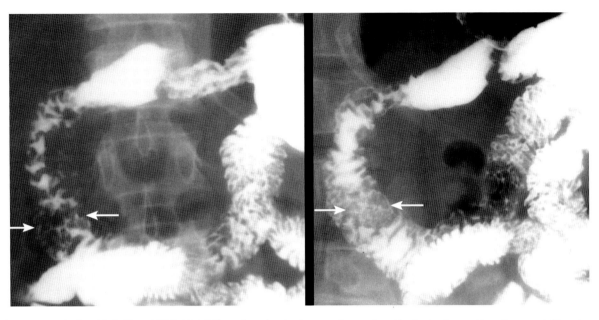

Second case, very similar. AP (*left*) and RAO (*right*) films show luminal expansion and a reticular barium pattern (*arrows, left*) and a small periampullary mass with reticular barium filling fine interstices (*arrows, right*).

Answers

1. The microlobulation and reticular barium filling interstices and the cauliflower appearance are consistent with villous tumor. The radiologist should not call it a villous adenoma; that diagnosis can only be made by the pathologist after adenocarcinoma is excluded. Duodenal lipomas are smooth submucosal masses. Brunner gland adenomas are usually in the duodenal bulb. Duodenal carcinomas are usually stenotic and distal to the ampulla, although foci of adenocarcinoma can be present in villous tumors.

2. Villous adenomas are rare in the small intestine as opposed to the colon and are most common (85%) in the duodenum and less common in the jejunum (10%) and they account for only 1% of duodenal tumors.

3. Although most duodenal villous tumors are sporadic they do occur in association with familial polyposis or Gardner syndrome.

4. Small duodenal villous tumors may appear as nonspecific smooth polypoid filling defects. Larger masses may have a soap bubble or cauliflower-like appearance. The frond-like projections often seen at gross inspection are visible radiographically because barium fills the interstices between the fingerlike projections.

5. Benign villous tumors may be treated with submucosal resection. Because of the risk of malignant transformation (or missed malignancy) serial endoscopic follow-up examinations are mandatory.

Malignant villous tumors in second portion of the duodenum require pancreatoduodenectomy. When the tumor location is more distal duodenal resection suffices.

Pearls

- The radiologist can only suggest a diagnosis of villous tumor. Differentiation between villous adenoma and carcinoma is by histology.
- Small duodenal villous tumors: Nonspecific smooth polypoid filling defects.
- Larger duodenal villous tumors: Soap bubble or cauliflower-like appearance. Barium fills the interstices between the fingerlike projections.
- CT: Variegated attenuation and variable enhancement patterns. Large tumors may have a characteristic surface gyral pattern.

Suggested Readings

Izgur V, Dass C, Solomides CC. Best cases from the AFIP: villous duodenal adenoma. *Radiographics*. January 2010;30(1):295-299.

Rueda O, Alvarez C, Vicente JM, Martel J, Escribano J. Quiz case of the month. Villous tumor of the duodenum. *Eur Radiol*. May 1997;7(6):951-952.

Vinnicombe S, Grundy A. Case report: obstructive jaundice secondary to an intussuscepting duodenal villous adenoma. *Clin Radiol*. July 1992;46(1):63-65.

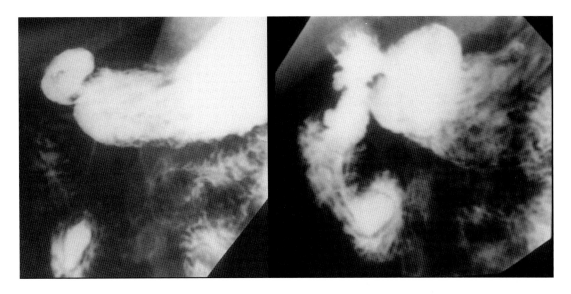

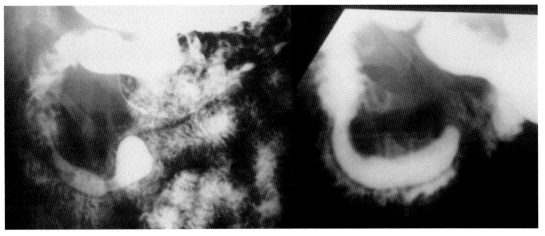

1. What is the correct diagnosis based on all images?

2. What is the origin of a windsock diverticulum and what portion of the duodenum is involved?

3. What are the symptoms of windsock diverticulum and what age do they occur?

4. What is the preferred treatment of windsock diverticulum?

5. What are the complications of windsock diverticulum that can be seen in adults?

Case ranking/difficulty: **Category:** Duodenum

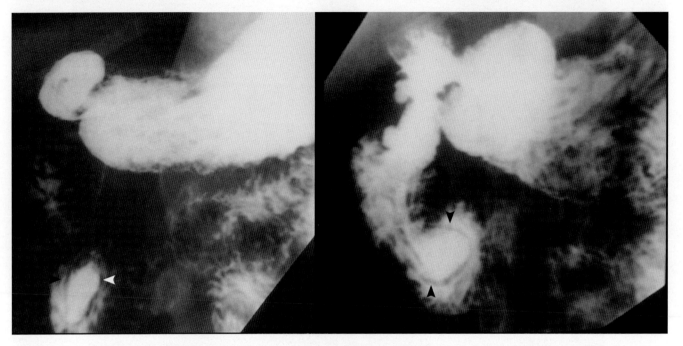

AP spots from an UGI show variable filling and distention of a tubular barium collection starting in the second portion of duodenum extending into the third. Note the halo sign (*arrowheads*).

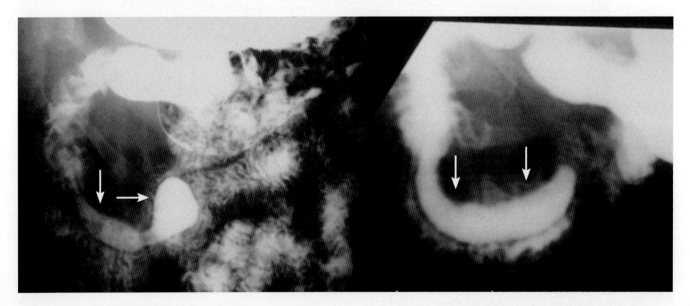

Oblique spots show a tubular barium collection (*arrows*) with distal dilatation that changes size and shape with peristalsis. It begins in the second portion of duodenum and extends into the third.

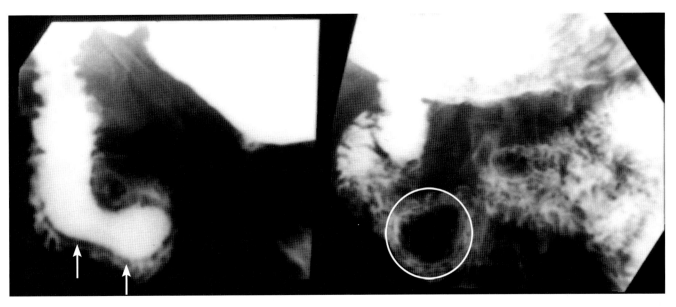

Supine (*left*) and prone (*right*) show the tubular collection of barium (*arrows*) replaced by a circular collection of air (*circle*).

Answers

1. The elliptical intraluminal barium collection that changes size, shape, and position with peristalsis and is surrounded by a halo is pathognomonic of windsock diverticulum.

2. The windsock (intraluminal) diverticulum results from incomplete recanalization of the duodenum during embryological development. The duodenal web is stretched over time by peristalsis, resulting in the development of an intraluminal diverticulum. Most cases originate near the ampulla and lie in an isoperistaltic direction. Rarely, it may arise in the third portion of the duodenum or extend in an antiperistaltic direction.

3. Symptoms of intraluminal duodenal diverticulum are nonspecific: epigastric pain, vomiting, and abdominal fullness. They usually do not appear until 20 to 30 years of age, although they do occur in childhood in 20%.

4. Endoscopic incision is the best treatment and surgery is done if it fails.

5. Complications of intraluminal duodenal diverticulum in adult patients (20%-25%) include duodenal obstruction, peptic ulcer disease, bleeding from ulceration within the diverticulum, and cholangitis or pancreatitis.

Pearl

• Intraluminal duodenal diverticulum is usually diagnosed on upper gastrointestinal series. Its typical appearance is that of a windsock being blown into the duodenum. It originates in the second part of the duodenum and usually extends into the third. It changes size and shape with peristalsis and filling and emptying. It is soft and compressible. The thin radiolucent stripe surrounding the diverticulum has been described as the halo sign. The classic radiographic findings above are pathognomonic. Should the diverticulum be filled with fluid and/or other material and not fill with barium it can be confused with a pedunculated polyp, submucosal tumor, or choledochocele.

Suggested Readings

Clemente G, Sarno G, Giordano M, De Rose AM, Nuzzo G. Intramural duodenal diverticulum mimicking a periampullary neoplasm. *Am J Surg*. October 2008;196(4):e31-e32.

Johnston P, Desser TS, Bastidas JA, Harvin H. MDCT of intraluminal "windsock" duodenal diverticulum with surgical correlation and multiplanar reconstruction. *AJR Am J Roentgenol*. July 2004;183(1):249-250.

Materne R. The duodenal windsock sign. *Radiology*. 2001;218:749-750.

68-year-old diabetic male with right upper quadrant pain and elevated white blood cell count

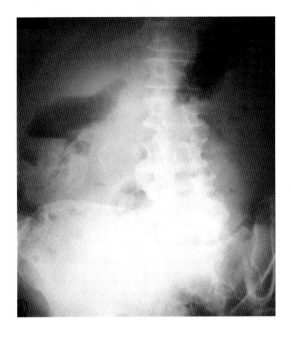
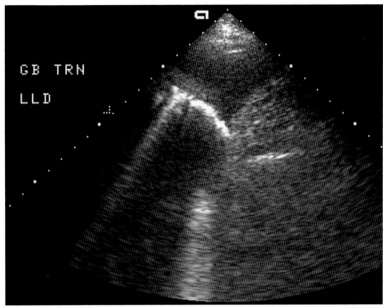

1. What is the most likely diagnosis based on the history and images?

2. Approximately what percentage of patients with emphysematous cholecystitis have diabetes mellitus?

3. Is emphysematous cholecystitis more common in men or women?

4. What entity might be confused with emphysematous cholecystitis on ultrasound examination?

5. Is a nuclear medicine HIDA scan useful in making the diagnosis of emphysematous cholecystitis?

Case ranking/difficulty:

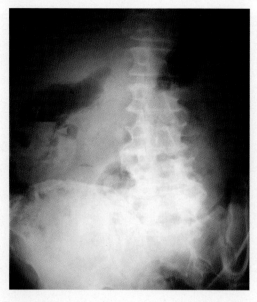

AP upright image of the abdomen shows an air fluid level (*red arrowhead*) within the gallbladder and irregular lucencies within the wall of the gallbladder (*green arrowheads*).

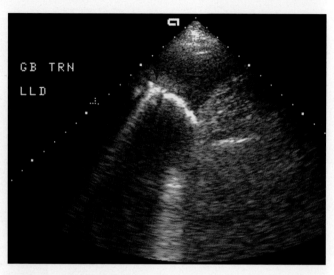

Transverse ultrasound image of the gallbladder shows irregular echogenic line corresponding to the anterior wall of the gallbladder (*red arrowheads*) with dirty shadowing, suggesting that this represents air rather than the calcification within the wall.

Answers

1. The plain radiograph is almost more useful than the ultrasound in this case in that one can see an air fluid level within the gallbladder lumen and a curvilinear collection of air within the gallbladder wall, indicating a diagnosis of emphysematous cholecystitis.

   There are no calcifications within the gallbladder wall to suggest porcelain gallbladder, there are no images of the liver to suggest hepatitis, there are no images of a mass in the gallbladder to suggest gallbladder carcinoma, and the colon is grossly normal, ruling out toxic megacolon.

2. Diabetes mellitus is a significant risk factor for the development of emphysematous cholecystitis. Approximately 40% of patients have underlying diabetes mellitus, which can cause ischemia, small vessel disease, and impaired immunity.

3. Most gallbladder disease is more common in women. Emphysematous cholecystitis is an exception in that it is more common in men, with reported ratios varying but on the order of 7:3. Emphysematous cholecystitis is thought to be related to underlying ischemia as seen in diabetes mellitus and vascular disease.

4. Emphysematous cholecystitis can have hyperechoic foci in the gallbladder wall and sometimes within the gallbladder lumen. In emphysematous cholecystitis the shadowing produced has reverberation artifact ("dirty shadowing"), whereas shadowing in porcelain gallbladder should be cleaner and crisper. In equivocal

cases plain radiography or CT can be used to make the diagnosis, although treatment should not be delayed due to the potential for complications.

5. A HIDA scan is not particularly useful. It may help make the diagnosis of acute cholecystitis, but it is not helpful in making the specific diagnosis of emphysematous cholecystitis. One needs to demonstrate air within the gallbladder wall or gallbladder wall and lumen. Plain film, US, CT, and MRI can make that diagnosis, with CT the most specific and comprehensive, although most patients have an ultrasound examination performed initially.

Pearls

- Insidious onset.
- Association with diabetes mellitus.
- More common in males. Most other gallbladder disease is more common in women.

Suggested Readings

Carrascosa MF, Salcines-Caviedes JR. Emphysematous cholecystitis. *CMAJ.* 2012 Jan;184(1):E81.

Garcia-Sancho Tellez L, Rodriguez-Montes JA, Fernandez de Lis S, Garcia-Sancho Martin L. Acute emphysematous cholecystitis. Report of twenty cases. *Hepatogastroenterology.* 1999;46(28):2144-2148. Epub 1999/10/16.

Grayson DE, Abbott RM, Levy AD, Sherman PM. Emphysematous Infections of the Abdomen and Pelvis: A Pictorial Review. *Radiographics.* 2002;22(3):543-561. doi: doi:10.1148/radiographics.22.3.g02ma06543.

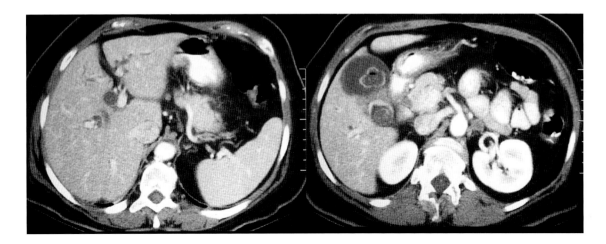

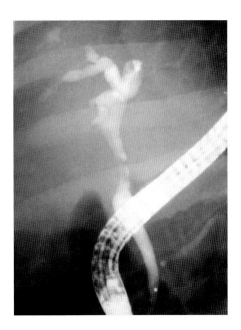

1. What is the most likely diagnosis?

2. What is the approximate M:F ratio for gallbladder carcinoma?

3. At what size should resection of a gallbladder polyp be considered?

4. What is the prognosis for gallbladder carcinoma?

5. Name risk factors for gallbladder carcinoma.

Case ranking/difficulty:

Category: Gallbladder

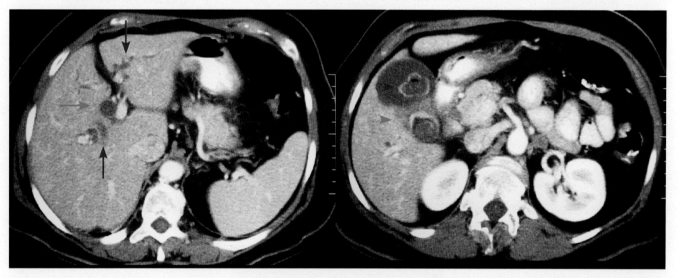

Axial CT (portal venous phase, *left panel*) shows intrahepatic biliary ductal dilatation in the right and left intrahepatic lobe branches (*red arrows*) as well as common hepatic duct dilatation (*green arrow*). The right panel shows a gallstone with air within a fissure (*red arrowhead*) and soft tissue density (*green arrowhead*) corresponding to tumor. There is intrahepatic biliary ductal dilatation.

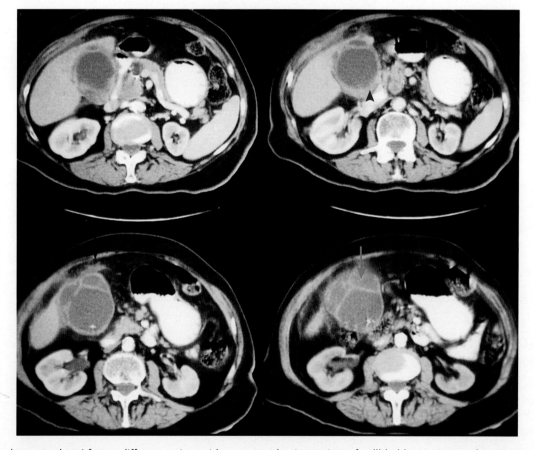

Axial CT (portal venous phase) from a different patient with a neuroendocrine variant of gallbladder carcinoma shows circumferential, somewhat nonuniform, wall thickening (*red arrowheads*), septations versus intramural low density (*green arrow*), soft tissue mass in the perihepatic fat (*blue arrow*), and adenopathy.

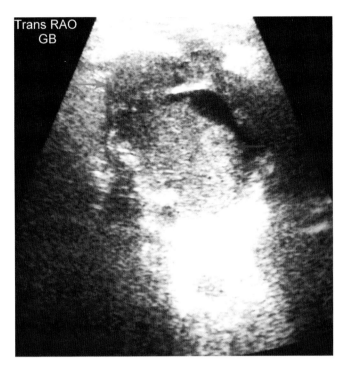

Same patient as above with neuroendocrine variant of GB carcinoma. US shows a homogeneous echogenic mass within the gallbladder (*arrows*) with invasion through the gallbladder wall into the liver (hypoechoic area, top left of image).

Answers

1. Given the stone disease and the focal soft tissue density mass within the gallbladder the most likely diagnosis is gallbladder carcinoma. 65% to 80% of patients with gallbladder carcinoma have gallstones.

   Acute cholecystitis is a thought, but the wall thickening is focal and there is no pericholecystic fluid or Murphy sign.

   Chronic cholecystitis may be present given the stone disease, but it is more often diagnosed by calculating an ejection fraction on nuclear medicine studies.

   Xanthogranulomatous cholecystitis is another consideration. In most such cases, the wall thickening is usually more diffuse, there are hypodense intramural nodules, a continuous mucosal line, luminal surface enhancement and gallstones. Restricted diffusion is more commonly seen in gallbladder carcinoma.

   Hepatitis produces hepatic parenchymal findings and may produce periportal edema, adenopathy in the hepatoduodenal ligament, and gallbladder wall edema, although the gallbladder wall edema/thickening is not focal.

2. The sex ratio varies among populations, but there is a female predilection and reported ratios are in the range of 1:3.

3. In general polypoid lesions greater than 10 mm should strongly be considered for resection, particularly if they are enhancing lesions on CT or MRI or demonstrate vascularity on US examination. These are more likely to represent adenomatous polyps or gallbladder carcinoma. One should also be cognizant that metastatic disease (ie, melanoma) occurs to the gallbladder. Lesions that have the classic appearance of cholesterol polyps are not concerning.

4. Due the advanced stage of disease at the time of diagnosis, the prognosis is generally very poor in that patients often have unresectable disease. Cases found incidentally during imaging or at surgery for benign disease have a better prognosis.

5. Cholelithiasis, female gender, Native American and Chilean Mapuche Indian ancestry, porcelain gallbladder, and a common channel involving the pancreaticobiliary junction are recognized risk factors for gallbladder carcinoma. There are reports that porcelain gallbladder is not as strongly associated as once thought, but there is still an increased risk.

Pearls

- Strong association with cholelithiasis (>65%).
- Typically diagnosed incidentally, on pathologic specimens resected for benign disease, or at a late stage of the disease (most common).
- Prognosis is generally poor secondary to late stage of disease at diagnosis.

Suggested Readings

Duffy A, Capanu M, Abou-Alfa GK, Huitzil D, Jarnagin W, Fong Y, et al. Gallbladder cancer (GBC): 10-year experience at Memorial Sloan-Kettering Cancer Centre (MSKCC). *J Surg Oncol.* 2008;98(7):485-489. Epub 2008/09/20. doi: 10.1002/jso.21141.

Furlan A, Ferris JV, Hosseinzadeh K, Borhani AA. Gallbladder carcinoma update: multimodality imaging evaluation, staging, and treatment options. *AJR Am J Roentgenol.* 2008;191(5):1440-14447. Epub 2008/10/23. doi: 10.2214/ajr.07.3599.

Kang TW, Kim SH, Park HJ, Lim S, Jang KM, Choi D, et al. Differentiating xanthogranulomatous cholecystitis from wall-thickening type of gallbladder cancer: added value of diffusion-weighted MRI. *Clin Radiol.* 2013;68(10):992-1001. Epub 2013/04/30. doi: 10.1016/j.crad.2013.03.022.

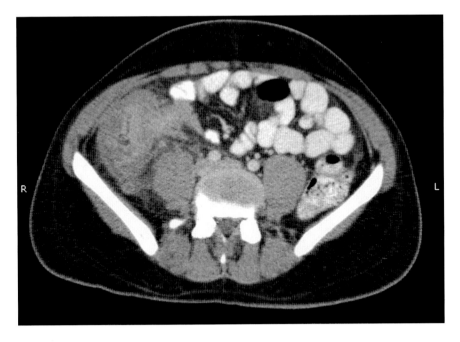 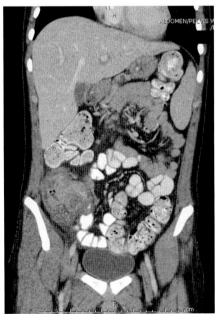

1. What is the most likely diagnosis?

2. What comprises conservative therapy for neutropenic colitis?

3. Into what demographic does the plurality of patients with neutropenic colitis fall?

4. What are the best modalities for evaluation of neutropenic colitis?

5. What entities can be included in the differential diagnosis?

Case ranking/difficulty:

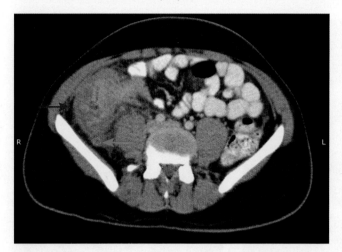

Axial contrast-enhanced CT (portal venous phase) of the abdomen at the level of the cecum shows marked thickening of the cecal wall (*red arrow*) with loss of normal stratification and some edema within the surrounding pericecal fat. What appears to be the appendix also appears to be involved (*green arrow*).

Answers

1. Location, along with the clinical history, is the key to making the diagnosis of neutropenic colitis. The history of neutropenia along with involvement of the cecum, sometimes with right colon or terminal ileal involvement, strongly suggests the diagnosis.

   Cecal diverticulitis is a thought, but one should be able to identify a diverticulum and it is usually more focal. A diagnosis of appendicitis requires identification of an abnormal appendix in the right clinical setting. Pseudomembranous colitis usually occurs in individuals who have been receiving antibiotics, and there is usually circumferential involvement of the bowel over a fairly long segment. *Yersinia* involves the terminal ileum along with mesenteric adenitis.

2. Bowel rest, total parenteral nutrition, and broad-spectrum antibiotics are part of conservative therapy. Granulocyte colony-stimulating factor (G-CSF) is not routinely used but can be part of the regimen in selected cases.

   Right hemicolectomy is used for more severe cases or in cases of frank perforation.

3. Although patients with HIV, organ transplant recipients, patients with solid organ malignancy on chemotherapy, and patients with immunodeficiency disorders may all be at risk for neutropenic colitis, pediatric oncology patients with leukemia still constitute the plurality of cases. There has been a recent increase in cases seen in patients with solid organ malignancy receiving chemotherapy.

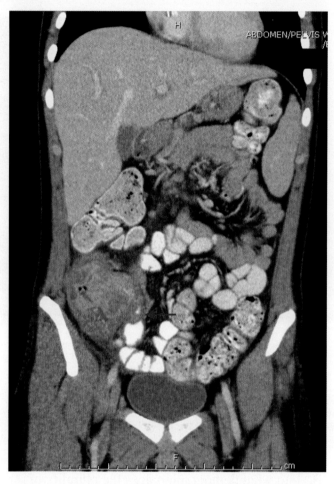

Coronal contrast-enhanced CT (portal venous phase) shows similar findings with marked thickening of the cecal wall, pericecal edema, and some involvement of the terminal ileum (*red arrow*).

4. Multidetector CT (MDCT) and ultrasound are most useful for evaluation. MDCT provides better detail of the bowel, and ultrasound is useful in experienced hands and may be used to follow clinical evolution during treatment without additional radiation exposure. MRI may be useful in selected cases (ie, pregnancy), although there is less experience with MRI and the bowel detail is usually not as crisp with MRI without adequate preparation.

   Colonoscopy and barium may not be diagnostic and carry the risk of bowel perforation.

5. Given an appropriate clinical history and typical radiographic findings one should arrive at the proper diagnosis. In atypical cases one may consider appendicitis, other infectious colitides, ischemic colitis, or Crohn disease. It would be unusual for ulcerative colitis to present with findings isolated to the right colon.

Pearls

- Occurs in profoundly neutropenic patients from multiple etiologies, although the leukemia patient receiving chemotherapy is the most common history. AIDS, organ transplant, and immunodeficiency are other underlying disorders.
- Predilection for the cecum although the terminal ileum, appendix, and more distal large bowel can be involved.

Suggested Readings

Alexander JE, Williamson SL, Seibert JJ, Golladay ES, Jimenez JF. The ultrasonographic diagnosis of typhlitis (neutropenic colitis). *Pediatr Radiol.* 1988 ;18(3):200-204.

Machado NO. Neutropenic enterocolitis: A continuing medical and surgical challenge. *N Am J Med Sci.* 2010 Jul;2(7):293-300.

Thoeni RF, Cello JP. CT imaging of colitis. *Radiology.* 2006 Sep;240(3):623-638.

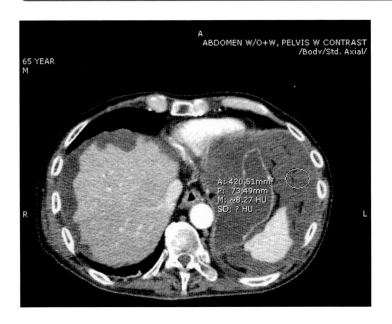
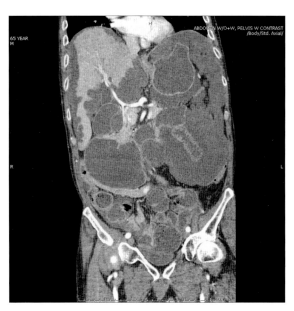

1. What is the most likely diagnosis?

2. Most cases of pseudomyxoma peritonei are thought to arise from neoplasm originating in which organ?

3. What signs are helpful in differentiating pseudomyxoma peritonei from simple ascites?

4. What findings suggest a high-grade tumor?

5. Which are the recommended imaging modalities for evaluation?

Case ranking/difficulty:

Category: Peritoneum

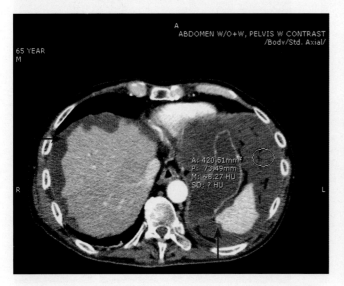

Contrast-enhanced CT (portal venous phase) shows low-density material within the peritoneal cavity insinuating itself around abdominal organs, with scalloping of the borders of the liver and spleen (*red arrows*).

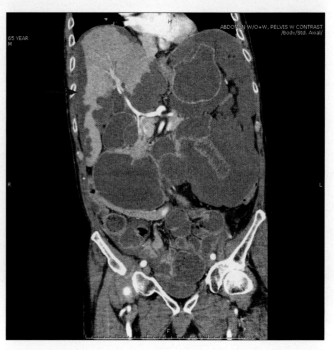

Contrast-enhanced CT (portal venous phase) shows low-density material within the peritoneal cavity insinuating around abdominal organs. Scalloping of the margin of the liver is again seen, and there is mass effect and displacement of bowel (*red arrow*).

Answers

1. Given the scalloping of the margins of the liver and the spleen and the extensive infiltrative low-density material within the peritoneum, the most likely diagnosis is pseudomyxoma peritonei.

2. Most cases of pseudomyxoma peritonei, particularly the lower-grade tumors, are thought to arise from the appendix.

   Some higher-grade cases of pseudomyxoma arise from mucinous adenocarcinomas of other viscera/organs, including the colon, gallbladder, urachal remnant and ovaries.

3. Scalloping of the margins of the liver and spleen is perhaps the most useful sign in differentiating simple ascites from pseudomyxoma peritonei on cross-sectional imaging.

   The density of CT is not always helpful as the mucinous ascites may vary and be near that of simple ascites.

   High signal on MRI DWI has shown to be a useful sign, and a well-performed MRI is a useful modality.

   In experienced hands US is a useful modality and the signs mentioned can be seen with pseudomyxoma peritonei.

4. With low-grade tumors the only sign seen may be mucinous ascites with scalloping of the margins of the peritoneal organs and mass effect.

Lymphadenopathy, distant metastases, frank organ invasion, and omental caking suggest a high-grade neoplasm.

5. Multidetector CT and MRI are the recommended modalities for evaluation. These are more accepted by surgeons as well.

   Ultrasound is still a useful modality in experienced hands, but it is not as useful for surgical planning.

   PET/CT does not provide much incremental value over CT alone, particularly in low-grade tumors.

Pearls

- Scalloped margins of liver and spleen.
- Low-grade and high-grade forms with significantly different prognosis.
- Treated with surgical cytoreduction and intraperitoneal hyperthermic chemotherapy (IPHC).

Suggested Readings

Bevan KE, Mohamed F, Moran BJ. Pseudomyxoma peritonei. *World J Gastrointest Oncol*. 2010 Jan;2(1):44-50.

Carr NJ, Finch J, Ilesley IC, Chandrakumaran K, Mohamed F, Mirnezami A, et al. Pathology and prognosis in pseudomyxoma peritonei: a review of 274 cases. *J Clin Pathol*. 2012;65(10):919-923. Epub 2012/06/22. doi: 10.1136/jclinpath-2012-200843.

Levy AD, Shaw JC, Sobin LH. Secondary tumors and tumorlike lesions of the peritoneal cavity: imaging features with pathologic correlation. *Radiographics*. 2009;29(2):347-373. Epub 2009/03/28. doi: 10.1148/rg.292085189.

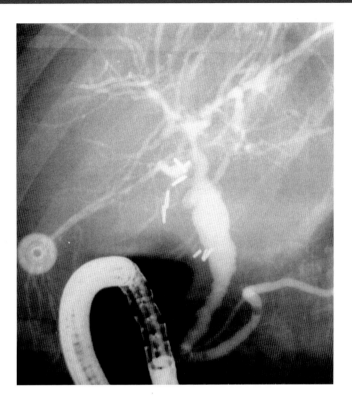

1. What is the best diagnosis based on the history and images?

2. What therapies are there for primary sclerosing cholangitis?

3. Patients with primary sclerosing cholangitis are at risk for the development of what neoplastic diseases?

4. What is a variant of primary sclerosing cholangitis (PSC) which has no imaging correlate called?

5. How does the sex predilection for primary sclerosing cholangitis vary with age?

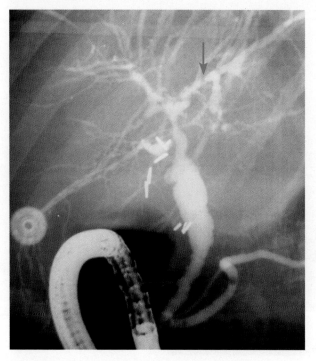

ERCP cholangiogram shows opacification of the biliary ducts and pancreatic ducts. There is marked irregularity with pseudodiverticula (*red arrow*) involving the common bile duct, and there are intrahepatic duct stenoses (*green arrow*), irregularity, and beading.

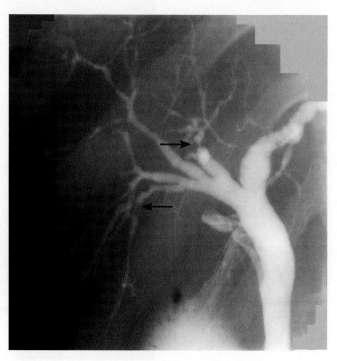

Percutaneous transhepatic cholangiography from a patient with primary sclerosing cholangitis and Crohn disease showing multiple intrahepatic stenoses (*red arrows*).

Answers

1. The best diagnosis given the provided history of concurrent inflammatory bowel disease is primary sclerosing cholangitis (PSC).

   AIDS cholangiopathy can be near indistinguishable from PSC, but checking the HIV status and CD4 counts can help in making the correct diagnosis.

   Cholangiocarcinoma usually has a more focal involvement when compared to PSC.

   Ischemic or infectious cholangitis will have a contributory history that can aid with the diagnosis.

2. Cholangioplasty or stenting, immunosuppressive therapy in selected cases, liver transplant, and antibiotics for cholangitis are all possible therapies for primary sclerosing cholangitis. Strictures and stenoses can be treated via interventional endoscopic retrograde cholangiopancreatography. Immunosuppressive therapy is effective in selected cases, particularly in overlap syndromes and in the pediatric population. Liver transplantation is an option for end-stage disease. Antibiotics are used to treat the complication of cholangitis.

3. Patients with primary sclerosing cholangitis have an 8% to 30% chance of developing cholangiocarcinoma.

   PSC has a strong association with inflammatory bowel disease, which includes both ulcerative colitis and Crohn disease. Approximately 65% to 90% of patients with PSC also have inflammatory bowel disease. The converse association is not as strong. Approximately 5.5% of patients with substantial colitis will develop PSC.

   Consequently, they are also at increased risk of developing colorectal cancer, and by virtue of the development of end-stage liver disease they are at increased risk of developing hepatocellular carcinoma.

   There is no known association with lung cancer or with desmoid tumors.

4. There is a variant of PSC which presents with a cholestatic picture but in which there are no imaging findings on cholangiography. This is called a "small duct" variant. In such cases there are often suggestive pathologic findings with liver biopsy, and clinical and pathologic criteria need to be used to make the diagnosis.

5. The incidence is slightly higher in males in the adult population. Conversely, the incidence is slightly higher in females in the pediatric population.

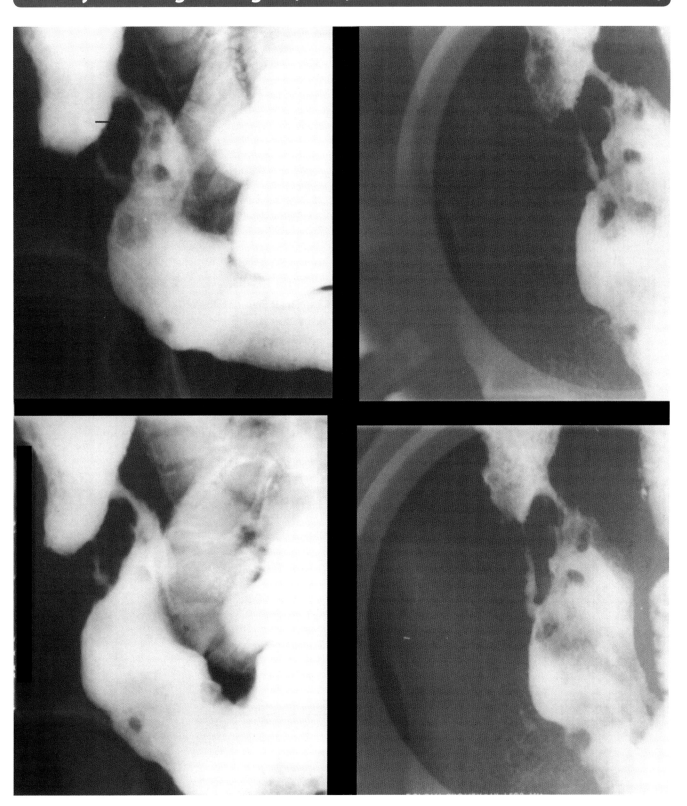

Small bowel follow-through from the same patient whose PTC is shown on previous page top right with Crohn disease showing the diseased terminal ileum with stricturing and pseudopolyps (*red arrow*).

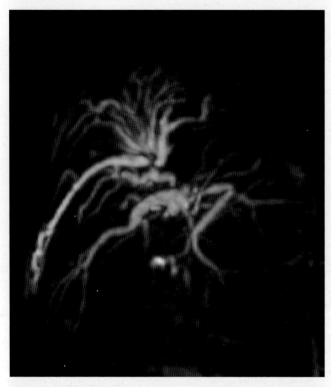

MRCP of a 70-year-old female with primary sclerosing cholangitis shows dilatation of the intrahepatic biliary tree with areas of stenosis and beading.

Pearls

- Strong association with inflammatory bowel disease (65%-90%) of patients develop inflammatory bowel disease.
- At risk for the development of cholangiocarcinoma, colorectal cancer (IBD), and hepatocellular carcinoma (HCC).
- May occur in the pediatric population.
- Some, but minority, may respond to immunosuppressive therapy. Association with other autoimmune disorders.

Suggested Readings

Chapman R, Fevery J, Kalloo A, Nagorney DM, Boberg KM, Shneider B, et al. Diagnosis and management of primary sclerosing cholangitis. *Hepatology*. 2010 Feb;51(2):660-678.

O'Connor OJ, O'Neill S, Maher MM. Imaging of biliary tract disease. *AJR Am J Roentgenol*. 2011;197(4):W551-8. Epub 2011/09/24. doi: 10.2214/ajr.10.4341.

Vitellas KM, Keogan MT, Freed KS, Enns RA, Spritzer CE, Baillie JM, et al. Radiologic manifestations of sclerosing cholangitis with emphasis on MR cholangiopancreatography. *Radiographics*. 2000;20(4): 959-975; quiz 1108-1109, 12. Epub 2000/07/21. doi: 10.1148/radiographics.20.4.g00jl04959.

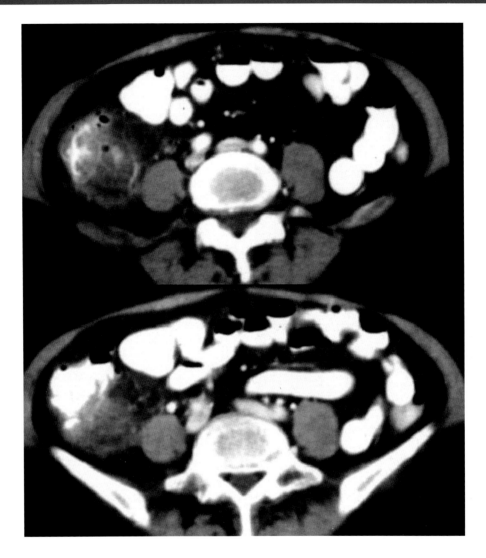

1. What is the most likely diagnosis?

2. What is the most common preoperative diagnosis for patients with cecal diverticulitis?

3. What two findings are useful in distinguishing cecal diverticulitis from cecal adenocarcinoma?

4. What should one exclude when cecal diverticulitis is suspected?

5. Approximately what percentage of diverticular disease is right sided in European and American series?

Case ranking/difficulty:

Category: Colorectum

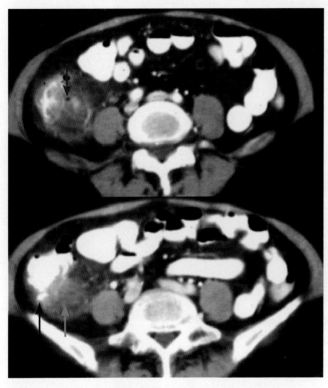

Two contrast-enhanced CT images show what appears to be extraluminal air (*red arrow*), thickening of the cecal wall, phlegmon and inflammatory change in the pericecal fat (*green arrow*), and a collection of contrast which may represent a diverticulum (*blue arrow*).

Answers

1. Typhlitis occurs in patients who are neutropenic and there is usually more circumferential involvement and longer segment involvement of the cecum.

   Pseudomembranous colitis usually occurs in patients who have been receiving antibiotics and longer segments of the bowel are usually involved. There may be an "accordion sign," although this is not specific.

   Appendicitis involves the appendix with an increased diameter, mucosal enhancement, edema in the surrounding fat, and possible complications.

   Cecal diverticulitis is similar to diverticulitis elsewhere in the bowel, with one or more diverticula, wall thickening, edema in the surrounding fat, and possible perforation. In the cecum, one should be cognizant of the possibility of underlying tumor.

Mucocele of the appendix has a distended appendix filled with mucinous material and possible associated tumors.

The findings in this case best fit cecal diverticulitis.

2. The majority (70%) of patients with cecal diverticulitis has a preoperative diagnosis of acute appendicitis.

   In the study cited, of the 15 cases with pathologic confirmation, 8 cases were related to single cecal diverticulum, with or without associated angiodysplasia, and 7 cases were related to multiple diverticulum associated with villous adenomas or adenocarcinomas.

   The single diverticulae tended to occur in a younger population.

3. Inflamed diverticula and a preserved enhancement pattern of the cecal wall are the two statistically significant findings which are helpful in distinguishing a benign cecal diverticulitis from diverticula associated with an underlying malignancy.

4. As already mentioned, cecal diverticulitis is predominantly related to two separate entities. True diverticula and diverticula associated with underlying malignancy or tumor. Both the radiologist and the surgeon should be aware that an underlying malignancy could be present.

   There may be a genetic predisposition in the Asian population for true diverticula.

5. In the paper cited, the percentage is 1% to 2%. This would be expected to be higher in an Asian population.

Pearls

- Cecal diverticulitis appears to be related to two different entities. Development of true diverticula with a higher incidence in the Asian population and diverticula often associated with a tumor, usually villous adenoma or adenocarcinoma of the colon.
- It may be difficult to make the correct diagnosis preoperatively with the preoperative diagnosis usually being acute appendicitis.
- True diverticula tend to be present in a younger population whereas cecal diverticulitis presenting in the older population often have an associated tumor.

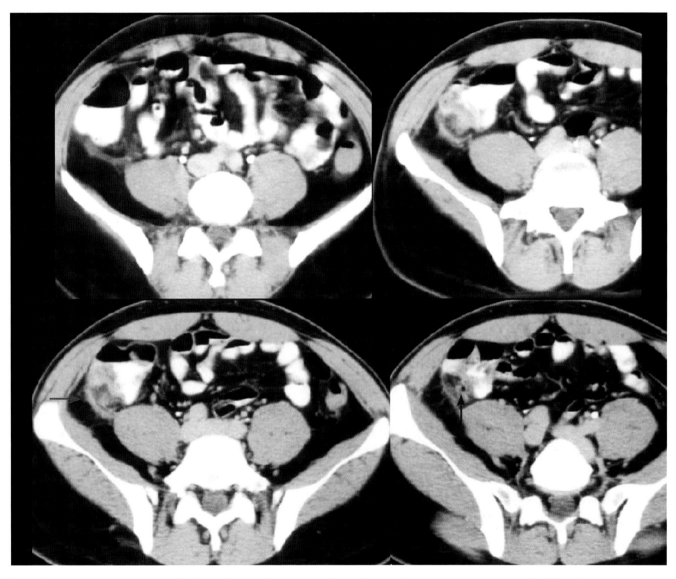

Second case: contrast-enhanced CT collage shows soft tissue density in the lateral portion of the cecum, wall thickening, and soft tissue density and thickening of the lateroconal fascia (*red arrow*). There also appears to be a small pocket of extraluminal air (*blue arrow*).

Suggested Readings

Jang HJ, Lim HK, Lee SJ, Lee WJ, Kim EY, Kim SH. Acute diverticulitis of the cecum and ascending colon: the value of thin-section helical CT findings in excluding colonic carcinoma. *AJR Am J Roentgenol*. 2000 May;174(5):1397-1402.

Karatepe O, Gulcicek OB, Adas G, Battal M, Ozdenkaya Y, Kurtulus I, et al. Cecal diverticulitis mimicking acute Appendicitis: a report of 4 cases. *World J Emerg Surg*. 2008:3(3):16.

Puylaert JB. Ultrasound of colon diverticulitis. *Dig Dis*. 2012;30(1):56-59. Epub 2012/05/11. doi: 10.1159/000336620.

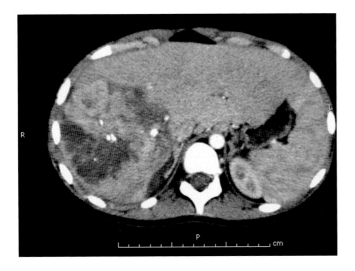 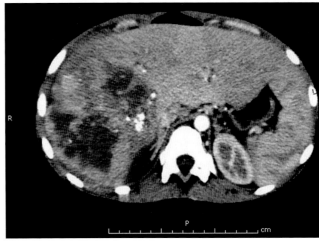

1. What is the most likely diagnosis?

2. What is the best treatment option for
   fibrolamellar carcinoma?

3. What are risk factors for fibrolamellar
   carcinoma?

4. What immunohistochemical stains are positive
   in fibrolamellar carcinoma?

5. How is MR imaging of the liver with a
   hepatobiliary agent such as gadoxetic acid
   (Eovist) helpful when differentiating focal
   nodular hyperplasia from fibrolamellar
   carcinoma?

Case ranking/difficulty:

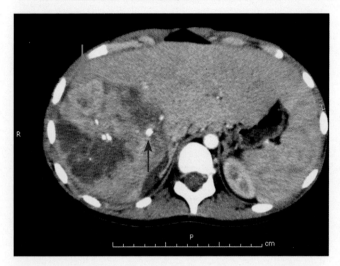

Axial CT (arterial phase) demonstrates a large, approximately 11 cm mass within the right hepatic lobe. Portions of the mass are higher density than normal liver (*green arrow*), and there are portions of the mass that are low density with scattered foci that are very high density (*red arrow*), near that of bone. The margins of the mass are fairly well defined, although a discrete capsule is not seen by CT. The margin is mildly lobulated.

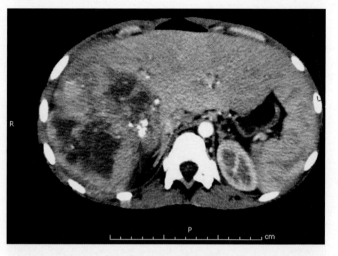

Axial CT (arterial phase) demonstrates findings similar to that noted in image to the left, but shows several other high-density foci with density near that of bone (*red arrow*).

Answers

1. Fibrolamellar hepatocellular carcinoma is the most likely diagnosis, based on the patient's age, otherwise normal liver, heterogeneous appearance of the tumor, and multiple calcifications, some central. A central scar, when present, is usually low signal on T1- and T2-weighted sequence.

   Focal nodular hyperplasia is frequently relatively inconspicuous, except on the arterial phase after the administration of intravenous contrast. A central scar, when present, is most often hypointense on MRI on T1W sequences and variably hyperintense on T2W sequences.

   Hemangiomas tend to follow the density of the abdominal aorta and have enhancement characteristics that are suggestive of the diagnosis.

   Hepatocellular carcinoma tends to occur in patients with underlying cirrhosis. Calcification is rare, and they exhibit arterial phase enhancement with variable washout in delayed phases.

2. Surgical resection in the treatment of choice in resectable tumors, with a 5-year survival of 76%.

   Without resection, the tumor is fatal.

3. Besides a slightly higher incidence in males and the bimodal age distribution, there are no known risk factors for fibrolamellar carcinoma.

4. Cytokeratin 8, cystokeratin 18, chromogranins, and several collagens are positive in fibrolamellar carcinoma. On the other hand alpha-fetoprotein is typically not positive in fibrolamellar carcinoma, with rare positive cases.

5. On MRI images with an agent such as Eovist, the most useful feature in differentiating focal nodular hyperplasia from fibrolamellar carcinoma is delayed enhancement (20-40 minutes) of the tumor in focal nodular hyperplasia. This is related to the presence of functioning hepatocytes in focal nodular hyperplasia.

   Both tumors demonstrate arterial phase enhancement, although it is more heterogeneous and variable in fibrolamellar hepatocellular carcinoma.

   Both tumors may have a central scar.

Pearls

- Malignant hepatic tumor that typically occurs in younger individuals without underlying liver disease, although it can occur in the older population.
- Very often has a central scar, calcifications, and area of necrosis. The central scar on MRI has low signal intensity on T1W and T2W sequences, helping distinguish the tumor from focal nodular hyperplasia in which the scar has high signal on T2W.

Suggested Readings

Eggert T, McGlynn KA, Duffy A, Manns MP, Greten TF, Altekruse SF. Epidemiology of fibrolamellar hepatocellular carcinoma in the USA, 2000–10. *Gut*. 2013. doi:10.136/gutjnl-2013-305164.

El-Serag HB, Davila JA. Is fibrolamellar carcinoma different from hepatocellular carcinoma? A US population-based study. *Hepatology*. 2004 Mar;39(3):798-803.

Smith MT, Blatt ER, Jedlicka P, Strain JD, Fenton LZ. Best cases from the AFIP: fibrolamellar hepatocellular carcinoma. *Radiographics*. 2008;28(2):609-613.

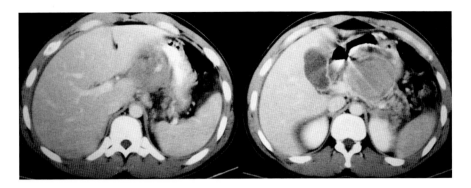

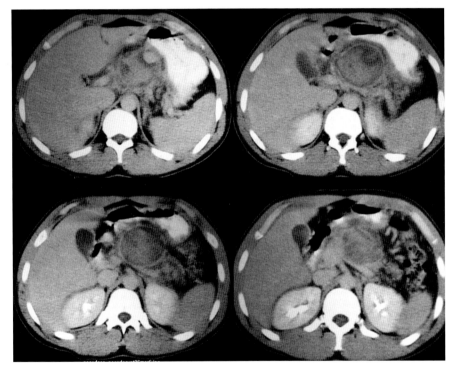

1. The top two images were obtained 2 weeks prior to the bottom 4 images. What are two likely diagnoses?

2. What diagnosis is proven by the sonogram?

3. Where do pseudoaneurysms due to pancreatitis typically rupture?

4. What are the arteries usually affected by pseudoaneurysms due to pancreatitis?

5. What are the CT characteristics of pseudoaneurysms due to pancreatitis?

Case ranking/difficulty:

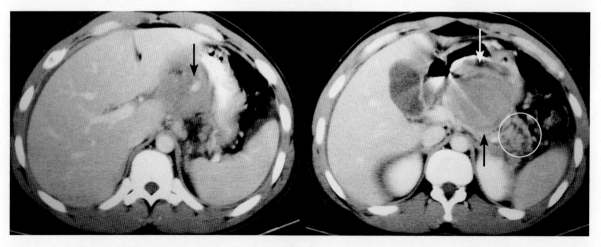

Right: Large round well-circumscribed lesser sac mass (*arrows*) isodense to spleen displacing stomach. Beaded dilated duct in tail of pancreas consistent with pancreatitis (*circle*). Left: Small area of intense enhancement (= to aorta) (*arrow*) at cephalad edge of the mass.

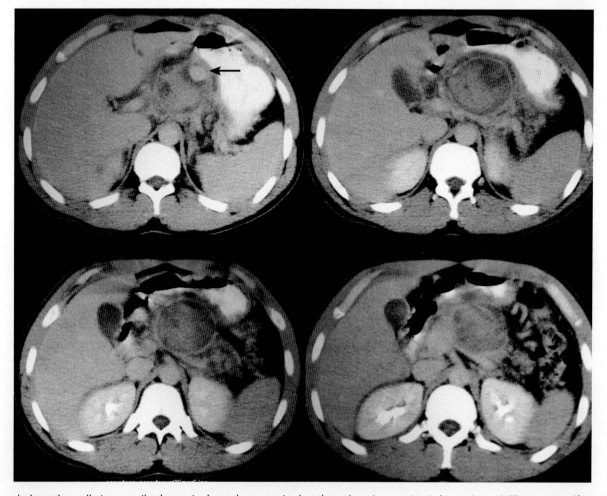

Two weeks later the well-circumscribed mass is about the same size but the enhancing portion is larger (*arrow*). The mass itself now is partially dense and partially hypodense consistent with evolving clot.

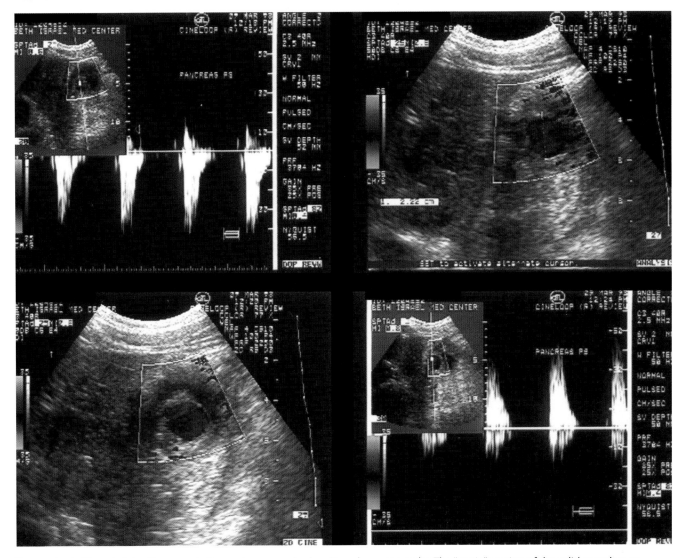

Two-and-a-half weeks later the correct diagnosis was reached on Doppler sonography. The "cystic" portion of the solid mass has an arterial waveform (*top left, bottom right*) and yin-yang color flow (*top right, bottom left*).

Answers

1. Splenic artery pseudoaneurysm due to pancreatitis and active bleeding into a pseudocyst are possible. Even if the latter is correct, pseudoaneurysm must be suspected. Small neuroendocrine tumors and renal cell carcinoma metastases can enhance this intensely but would not have the additional surrounding less enhancing mass. Carcinoma of the pancreas should not have intense arterial enhancement.

2. The yin-yang sign on the color flow images proves the diagnosis of pseudoaneurysm.

3. Pseudoaneurysm rupture can be into the gut (resulting in either upper or lower GI bleeding), can be retroperitoneal or intraperitoneal, or can be into the pancreatic duct eventually making its way into the duodenum.

4. Involved arteries in descending order of frequency include splenic, pancreaticoduodenal, gastric, and hepatic arteries. Any artery in direct contact with pancreatic enzymes can be involved.

5. On noncontrast CT a pseudoaneurysm may be a nonspecific soft tissue mass. Sometimes increased density consistent with blood is seen and then differential is hemorrhagic pancreatitis or bleeding into a pseudocyst. The presence of a homogeneous area of enhancement within a mass contiguous with an artery on portal phase CT should suggest pseudoaneurysm in the appropriate setting. CTA will be diagnostic showing enhancement of the pseudoaneurysm lumen equal to arterial enhancement and display any surrounding thrombus.

Pearls

- Pseudoaneurysm complicating pancreatitis can rupture, leading to exsanguination.
- Self-limited episodes of herald bleeding may precede exsanguination.
- High index of suspicion should be maintained when reviewing imaging examinations of patients with pancreatitis.
- Patients may be asymptomatic as to their pseudoaneurysm or have bleeding (acute or chronic), abdominal pain, or both.
- Imaging findings in addition to the underlying pancreatitis are:
  - Doppler US: Blood flows into the pseudoaneurysm in systole and out of it during diastole.
  - Gray scale US: If the pseudoaneurysm is predominantly filled with clot the aneurysm must then be recognized on gray scale. Old clot is echogenic and fresh clot is sonolucent. Any patent lumen is sonolucent mimicking cyst.
  - CT/MR: On noncontrast CT a pseudoaneurysm may be a nonspecific soft tissue mass. Sometimes increased density consistent with blood is seen.
- On unenhanced MR pseudoaneurysms are small nonspecific T1 hypointense T2 hyperintense structures.
- The presence of a homogeneous area of enhancement within a mass contiguous with an artery on portal phase CT or MR suggests pseudoaneurysm in a pancreatitis patient.
- CTA/MRA is diagnostic, showing enhancement of the pseudoaneurysm lumen equal to arterial enhancement.

Suggested Readings

Ikeda O, Kume S, Torigoe Y, et al. Hemorrhage into pancreatic pseudocyst. *Abdom Imaging*. July 2007; 32(3):370-373.

Smith RE, Fontanez-Garcia D, Plavsic BM. Gastrointestinal case of the day. Pseudoaneurysm of the left gastric artery as a complication of acute pancreatitis. *Radiographics*. June 1999;19(5):1390-1392.

Trout AT, Elsayes KM, Ellis JH, Francis IR. Imaging of acute pancreatitis: prognostic value of computed tomographic findings. *J Comput Assist Tomogr*. July 2010;34(4):485-495.

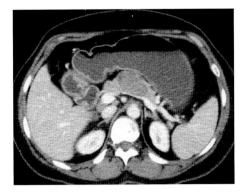
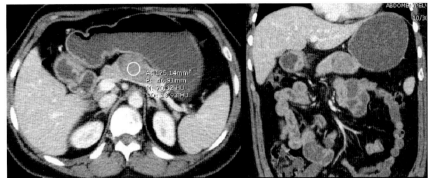

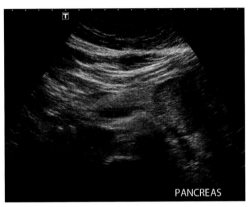
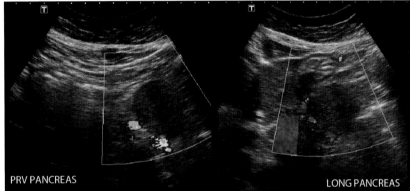

1. What is your differential diagnosis for the mass measuring 70 HU shown on CT and sonography?

2. What is the most likely diagnosis for the mass shown on CT and sonography?

3. What are the characteristics of small solid pseudopapillary tumors?

4. What are the sonographic features of small solid pseudopapillary tumors?

5. What are the CT and MR characteristics of solid pseudopapillary tumors?

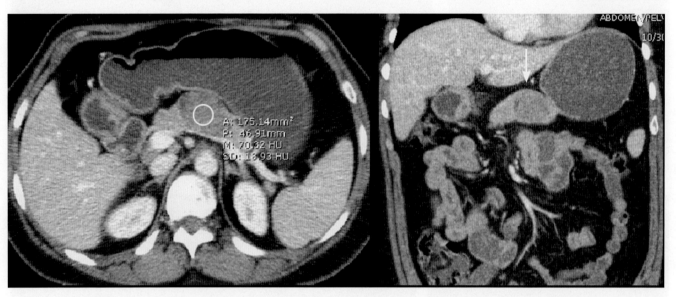

Mass measures 70 HU. Coronal shows a well-circumscribed mass (*arrow*) hypodense to the enhanced pancreatic parenchyma.

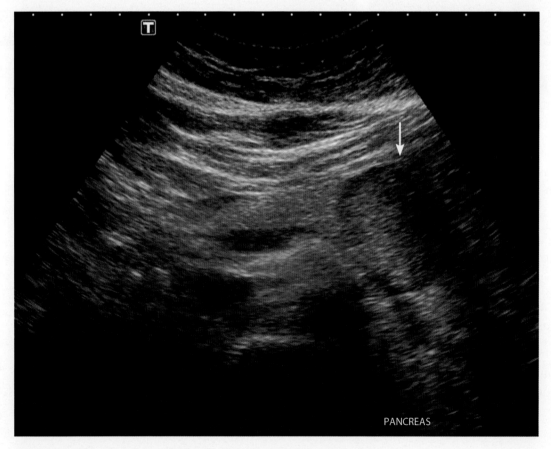

Transverse sonogram shows a solid nearly isoechoic pancreatic mass (*arrow*).

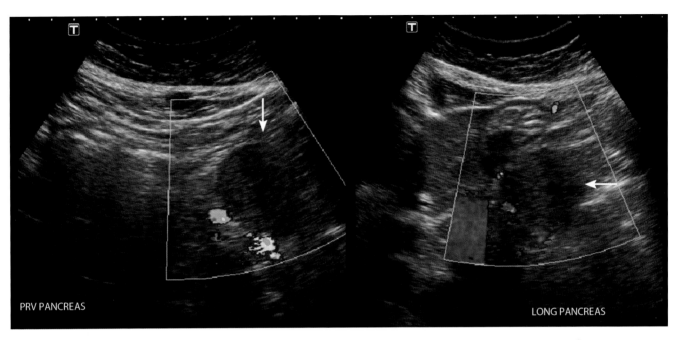

Transverse (*left*) and sagittal (*right*) color images show a slightly hypoechoic solid mass (*arrows*) with no internal color flow.

Answers

1. Adenocarcinoma of the pancreas, islet cell tumor, SPT, metastasis to the pancreas, and acinar cell carcinoma of the pancreas are all possible.

2. Most adenocarcinomas this close to the splenic vein would encase or occlude it. Nonfunctional islet cell tumors often enhance more than what is seen. Most patients with metastasis to the pancreas either have a known primary or their primary is visible on the CT. Acinar cell carcinomas are usually in older men and usually centrally necrotic. Most SPTs are large with hemorrhage, necrosis, or cystic degeneration and in adolescent girls or young women. However, a subset of SPT in asymptomatic middle-aged women consists of small masses without hemorrhage, necrosis, or cystic degeneration. This is the most likely diagnosis.

3. Small solid pseudopapillary tumors are usually asymptomatic and often are incidental findings in middle-aged women. Hemorrhage and necrosis are not common. Although malignant, metastases are uncommon and prognosis after complete resection is good.

4. Small SPTs are solid well-circumscribed hypoechoic masses on US with absent or minimal Doppler flow.

5. On CT and MRI SPTs are well circumscribed and homogeneous. Features on MRI that may be significantly different from islet cell tumor and adenocarcinoma and diagnostic are low SI on T1WI and very high SI on T2WI and early heterogeneous contrast enhancement that slowly, progressively increases over time. This enhancement pattern has been shown on CT as well.

Pearls

- Small pseudopapillary tumors (SPTs) of the pancreas are well-circumscribed solid pancreatic masses usually seen in middle-aged women.
- Both a capsule and intratumoral hemorrhage are classically important in the dx of large SPT in adolescent girls and young women.
- Most small SPTs have neither capsule nor intratumoral hemorrhage.
- Small SPTs are solid well-circumscribed hypoechoic masses on US with absent or minimal Doppler flow.
- They are solid masses hypodense to the enhanced pancreas on CT.
- Features on MRI that may be significantly different from islet cell tumor and adenocarcinoma and diagnostic are:
  - Low SI on T1WI and very high SI on T2WI
  - Early heterogeneous contrast enhancement that slowly, progressively increases over time. This enhancement pattern has been shown on CT as well.

Suggested Readings

Baek JH, Lee JM, Kim SH et al. Small (<or=3 cm) solid pseudopapillary tumors of the pancreas at multiphasic multidetector CT. *Radiology*. 2010 Oct;257(1):97-106.

Coleman KM, Doherty MC, Bigler SA. Solid-pseudopapillary tumor of the pancreas. Radiographics. August 2006;23(6):1644-1648.

Yu MH, Lee JY, Kim MA, et al. MR imaging features of small solid pseudopapillary tumors: retrospective differentiation from other small solid pancreatic tumors. *AJR Am J Roentgenol*. December 2010;195(6):1324-1332.

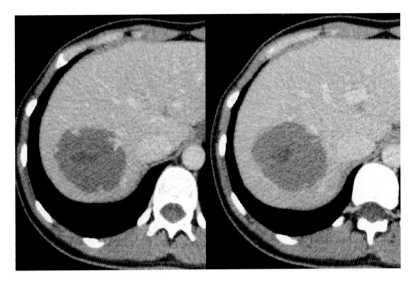

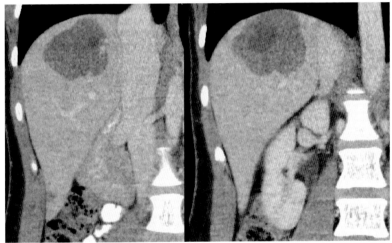

1. Based on the CT scan, what are reasonable choices in a differential diagnosis?

2. What is the proper diagnosis taking the labeled red cell scintigram (next page) into account?

3. Hemangiomas larger than what measurement are considered giant hemangiomas?

4. What are some unusual signs and symptoms of hemangiomas?

5. What are the characteristics of giant hemangiomas on ultrasound?

Case ranking/difficulty:

Category: Liver

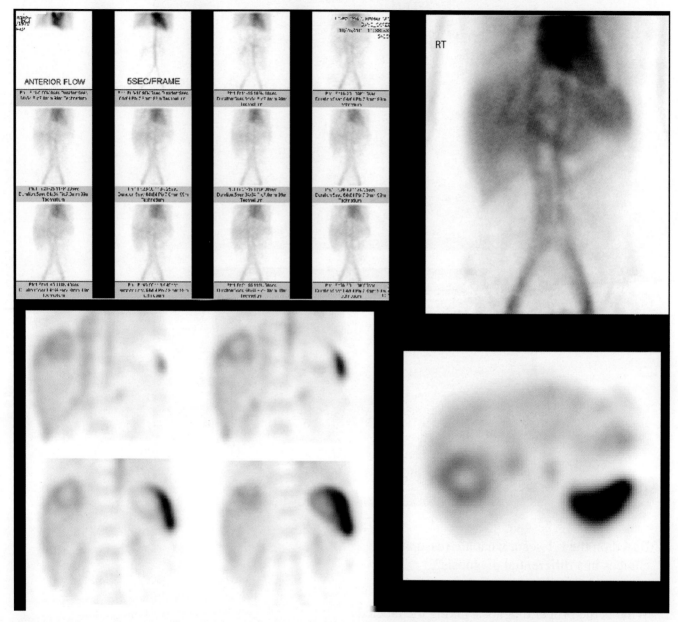

Technetium-99m labeled red cell scintigraphy. Top left: Dynamic flow showing no hypervascular mass. Top right: Early static scan showing no hypervascular mass. Bottom left: 1-hour coronal SPECT (*anterior to posterior, top left to bottom right*) showing a liver mass with peripheral activity and central inactivity. Bottom right: 1-hour axial SPECT showing a doughnut mass in the right liver.

Answers

1. Giant hemangioma, fibrolamellar HCC, and focal nodular hyperplasia all can have central scars and should be considered. Hepatic adenoma is a reasonable suspect in a 31-year-old woman. Angiosarcoma is quite unlikely absent a history of hemochromatosis or exposure to vinyl chloride, radium, Thorotrast, or arsenicals. The discontinuous peripheral enhancement should favor hemangioma.

2. The increased activity on the 1-hour delayed images combined with no increased flow is diagnostic of hemangioma. The ring pattern is seen in giant hemangiomas.

3. Hemangiomas larger than 5 cm are called giant hemangiomas.

4. Most patients with giant hemangiomas are asymptomatic. Right upper quadrant pain or fullness

or symptoms due to mass effect or sudden, severe pain from thrombosis may occur. Thrombocytopenia and hypofibrinogenemia are rare complications. Significant hemorrhage is rare even in large hemangiomas, but does occur. Malignant degeneration does not happen.

5. Smaller hemangiomas are classically homogeneous well-circumscribed echogenic masses. Mixed patterns with hyperechoic and large hypoechoic or anechoic regions and central scars are common in giant hemangiomas due to fibrosis, thrombosis, hemorrhage, or necrosis. Hemangiomas usually do not have flow on Doppler interrogation. When observed over time slow increases or decreases in size may be seen in hemangiomas. Although suggestive of hemangioma when seen behind an otherwise solid mass, posterior acoustic enhancement is uncommon even in small hemangiomas and quite rare in giant ones.

Pearls

- Calcification is unusual in giant hemangiomas; it is usually one or more radiating trabeculae or spicules in the fibrous stroma.
- US: Mixed patterns with hyperechoic and large hypoechoic or anechoic regions and central scars are common in giant hemangiomas that have undergone fibrosis, thrombosis, hemorrhage, or necrosis.
- CT: Early on postcontrast scans of giant hemangiomas there is peripheral, discontinuous enhancement that rarely fills in completely; central cleft-like regions of cystic degeneration or liquefaction or scarring remain hypodense.

- MRI: Giant hemangiomas larger than 3 cm will commonly show heterogeneous low signal areas (both T1 and T2WI) corresponding to thrombosis or fibrosis. They are otherwise hypointense on T1WI and very hyperintense on T2WI. Enhancement pattern same as CT.
- Nuclear medicine: Giant hemangiomas with thrombosis and fibrosis may have atypical scintigraphic findings. Early dynamic images may show hyperperfusion; delayed images may show a ring pattern of increased peripheral activity and decreased central activity.

Suggested Readings

Jhaveri KS, Vlachou PA, Guindi M, Fischer S, Khalili K, Cleary SP, Ayyappan AP. Association of hepatic hemangiomatosis with giant cavernous hemangioma in the adult population: prevalence, imaging appearance, and relevance. *AJR Am J Roentgenol*. April 2011;196(4):809-815.

Prasanna PM, Fredericks SE, Winn SS, Christman RA. Best cases from the AFIP: giant cavernous hemangioma. *Radiographics*. April 2011;30(4):1139-1144.

Shimoji K, Shiraishi R, Kuwatsuru A, Maehara T, Matsumoto T, Kurosaki Y. Spontaneous subacute intratumoral hemorrhage of hepatic cavernous hemangioma. *Abdom Imaging*. April 2011;29(4):443-445.

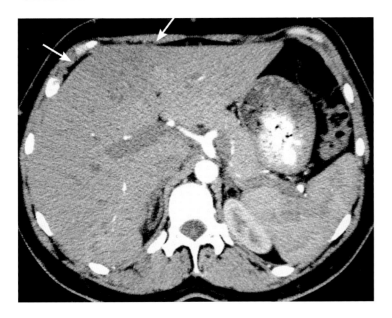
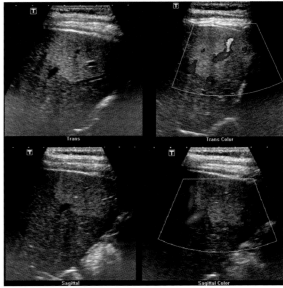
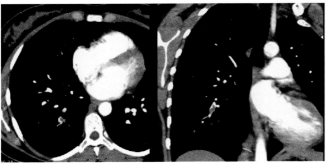
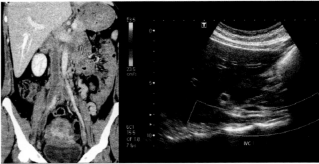

1. Looking at all the images, what is the best diagnosis?

2. What is the best test to clinch the correct diagnosis?

3. What are the causes of fatty liver?

4. What are the characteristics of fatty liver on sonography?

5. What are unusual causes and appearances of multifocal or geographic heterogeneous fatty liver?

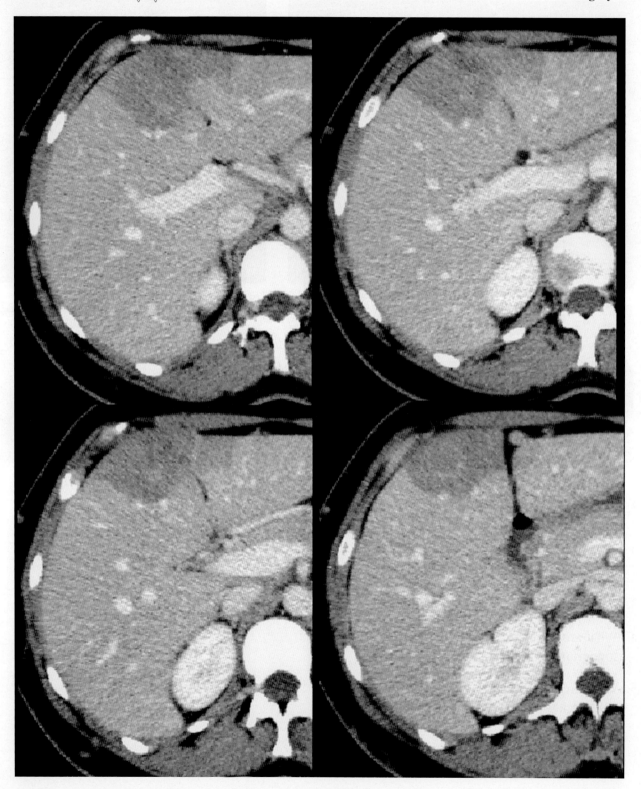

Repeat CT the next day, this time in the portal venous phase, shows a geographic hypodense area adjacent to the falciform ligament. Normal vessels traverse the hypodense area (*best seen lower right*).

Answers

1. The geographic shape, the location adjacent to the falciform ligament, lack of any mass effect, and the normal vessels coursing through the "mass" favor the diagnosis of focal fatty liver. Lymphoma is infiltrative but would not be echogenic. Note the right lower lobe pulmonary emboli and the IVC occlusion.

2. Chemical shift gradient echo MRI will clinch the diagnosis of focal fatty liver by showing isointensity on in-phase images within the focal fatty area and signal drop on out-of-phase images. Spectroscopy would work but is unnecessarily complex. Liver mass biopsy would work but is unnecessarily invasive. Contrast-enhanced MRI with either renally excreted or hepatobiliary excreted gadolinium would add little to chemical shift non contrast MR.

3. Alcoholism, insulin resistance, obesity, hyperlipidemia, viral hepatitis, steroids, drugs (chemotherapy, amiodarone, valproic acid), total parenteral nutrition, rapid weight loss, starvation, jejunoileal bypass, radiation therapy, metabolic and storage disorders, and cystic fibrosis are causes of fatty liver.

4. Fatty liver can be diagnosed if the liver echogenicity is greater than that of renal cortex and spleen and there is poor penetration of the liver and invisibility of the normally echogenic intrahepatic vascular walls.

5. Insulinoma metastases and intrahepatic islet cell transplants are unusual causes of multifocal fat deposition (due to local insulin effects on hepatocyte triglyceride metabolism and storage). Local increased insulin concentration also causes subcapsular fatty liver that appears as multiple discrete fat nodules or a peripheral region of fat in patients with renal failure and insulin-dependent diabetes who may have insulin added to their peritoneal dialysate. Perivascular fat deposition is an unusual pattern of unknown etiology consisting of fat surrounding hepatic and/or portal veins.

Pearls

- Diffuse Fatty Liver
  - US: Liver echogenicity >renal cortex and spleen, poor penetration of the liver, loss of echogenicity of intrahepatic vascular walls.
- Noncontrast CT: Density of the liver is at least 10 HU <spleen or if the liver is <40 HU.
- Contrast-enhanced CT: The liver is subjectively too hypodense to the spleen in a portal predominate image.
- MRI: Signal drop on chemical shift opposed-phase images.
- Focal Fatty Liver
  - Focal fatty liver and focal sparing: Focal fat deposition typically adjacent to the falciform ligament or ligamentum venosum. Focal sparing typically in the porta hepatis or the gallbladder fossa. Focal fat deposition adjacent to insulinoma metastases or intrahepatic islet cell transplants is due to local insulin effects on hepatocyte triglyceride metabolism and storage.
- The lack of mass effect on traversing vessels, geographic configuration, and contrast enhancement similar to or less than normal liver suggest the correct diagnosis on US and CT. Chemical shift MR is more straightforward.

Suggested Readings

Borra RJH, Salo S, Dean K, et al. Nonalcoholic fatty liver disease: rapid evaluation of liver fat content with in-phase and out-of-phase MR imaging. *Radiology*. January 2009;250(1):130-136. Published online November 18, 2008, doi:10.148/radiol.501071934.

Hamer OW, Aguiree DA, Casola G, et al. Fatty liver: imaging patterns and pitfalls. *Radiographics*. 2006;26:1637-1653.

Tang A, Tan J, Sun M, et al. Nonalcoholic fatty liver disease: MR imaging of liver proton density fat fraction to assess hepatic steatosis. *Radiology*. May 2013;267(2):422-431. Published online February 4, 2013, doi:10.148/radiol.2120896.

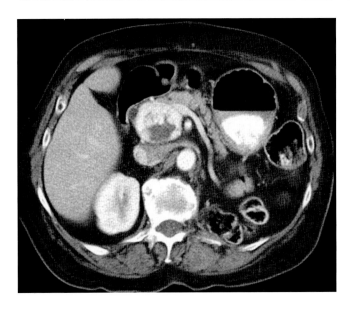 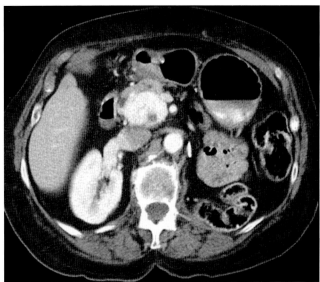

1. What is the most likely diagnosis?

2. In radiology series, what are the two most common sources of pancreatic metastasis?

3. Compared to pancreatic duct cell adenocarcinoma, what is the survival of patients with renal cell carcinoma metastatic to the pancreas?

4. What are imaging features of renal cell carcinoma metastatic to the pancreas?

5. What is in the differential diagnosis of hypervascular pancreatic mass?

Case ranking/difficulty:

Answers

1. The common adenocarcinoma of the pancreas would not enhance in this fashion. Solid pseudopapillary tumor, neuroendocrine tumor, and giant cell carcinoma are all plausible diagnoses with this degree of enhancement and central necrosis, but the absence of the left kidney is strong evidence for s/p resection of renal cell carcinoma and metastatic RCC to the pancreas.

2. In radiologic series, renal cell carcinoma and bronchogenic carcinoma are the two most common primaries to metastasize to the pancreas. In autopsy series breast carcinoma, bronchogenic carcinoma, and melanoma are the most common sources.

3. Although the prognosis of patients with metastatic renal cell carcinoma is poor, cases of isolated pancreatic renal cell carcinoma metastasis treated surgically have 5-year survival rates of up to 75%. No significant differences in survival were observed among patients with single or multiple pancreatic metastases.

4. Renal cell carcinoma metastatic to the pancreas is usually hypervascular and best detected in the arterial phase.

   Masses larger than 1.5 cm may exhibit hypodense central areas of necrosis. Other features are calcifications, pancreatic ductal and biliary obstruction, vascular extension, and cystic degeneration.

5. The differential diagnosis of hypervascular pancreatic mass includes neuroendocrine tumor, metastasis to the pancreas, solid pseudopapillary tumor, intrapancreatic accessory spleen, and vascular lesions, such as arteriovenous fistula or aneurysm of the splenic artery, as well as unusual sarcomatoid pancreatic neoplasms.

Pearls

- Prognosis of renal cell carcinoma metastatic to the pancreas is better than adenocarcinoma of the pancreas.
- Management of isolated renal cell carcinoma metastasis to the pancreas consists of aggressive treatment with complete resection whenever possible.
- Renal cell carcinoma metastatic to the pancreas is usually hypervascular and best detected in the arterial phase.
- Masses larger than 1.5 cm may exhibit hypodense central areas of necrosis. Other features are calcifications, ductal and biliary obstruction, vascular extension, and cystic degeneration.
- Differential diagnosis of hypervascular pancreatic mass includes neuroendocrine tumors, breast or melanoma metastasis, intrapancreatic accessory spleen, and vascular lesions, such as arteriovenous fistula or aneurysm of the splenic artery, as well as unusual sarcomatoid pancreatic neoplasms.

Suggested Readings

Coakley FV, Hanley-Knutson K, Mongan J, Barajas R, Bucknor M, Qayyum A. Pancreatic imaging mimics: part 1, imaging mimics of pancreatic adenocarcinoma. *AJR Am J Roentgenol.* August 2012;199(2):301-308.

Mechó S, Quiroga S, Cuéllar H, Sebastià C. Pancreatic metastasis of renal cell carcinoma: multidetector CT findings. *Abdom Imaging.* June 2009;34(3):385-359.

Shah S, Mortele KJ. Uncommon solid pancreatic neoplasms: ultrasound, computed tomography, and magnetic resonance imaging features. *Semin Ultrasound CT MR.* October 2007;28(5):357-370.

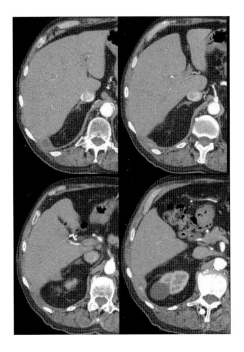 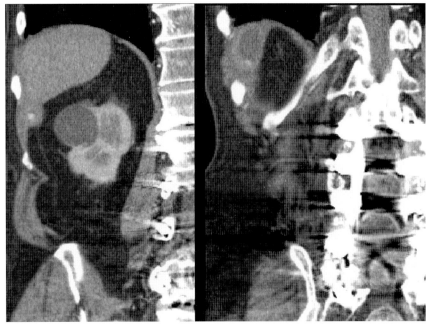

1. What is the most likely diagnosis?

2. How does laparoscopic cholecystectomy
   compare to traditional open cholecystectomy?

3. What are some locations of dropped
   gallstones?

4. What is the most common type of dropped
   gallstone to cause infection?

5. What is the best imaging modality for dropped
   gallstone associated abscess?

Case ranking/difficulty:

Category: Peritoneum

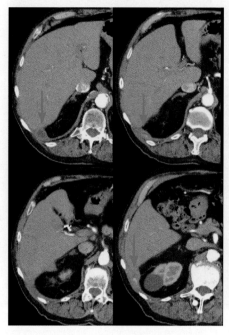

In the hepatorenal fossa there are small slightly enhancing low-density masses (*arrows*) with central hyperdensities and thickening of tissue planes. The patient is s/p cholecystectomy (*laparoscopic*).

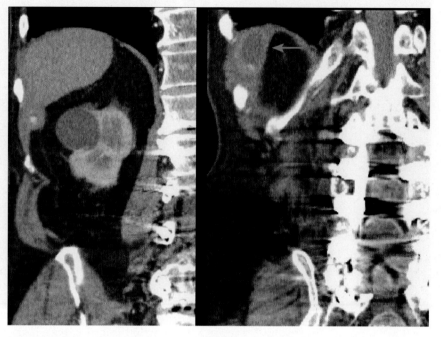

The low-density masses with central calcifications (*arrows*) are demonstrated on the coronal images.

Answers

1. Peritoneal carcinomatosis, pseudomyxoma peritonei, actinomycosis, and mesothelioma are tenable diagnoses, but the calcifications within the small masses and the clips in the gallbladder fossa merit a diagnosis of dropped gallstones.

2. Laparoscopic cholecystectomy is generally associated with fewer complications than traditional open technique.

   There are at least two operative complications that occur with increased frequency with the laparoscopic technique. One is an increased incidence of bile duct injury or leakage, and the other is late (months to years) infection caused by dropped gallstones.

3. Subsequent abscesses or inflammatory masses containing gallstones or stone fragments are generally confined to the subhepatic space or the retroperitoneum below the subhepatic space. Unusual locations include the right thorax, the subphrenic space, the abdominal wall at trocar sites, the sites of incisional hernias, and the pelvic intraperitoneal space.

4. Infectious complications are more likely to occur with spilled bilirubinate stones because these stones often

contain viable bacteria. Most bilirubinate stones have increased CT density.

5. CT gives a nonoperator-dependent overall view of anatomy and will detect most dropped stones within abscesses since most have increased CT attenuation. US may not depict dropped stones due to their unusual locations. MRI will show dropped stones as signal voids but may not show them well due to small size. PET cannot depict dropped stones but the abscesses will have increased SUV and may be mistaken for neoplasms. Hepatobiliary scintigraphy can delineate bile leaks but not dropped stones.

Pearls

- Although the diagnosis of an abscess associated with dropped opaque (on CT) gallstones can easily be made, the abscess can be misdiagnosed as a simple abscess or a neoplasm when the gallstones are nonopaque, leading to inadequate or delayed treatment. Dropped stones with associated abscess formation can be mistaken for simple abscess, actinomycosis, soft tissue sarcoma, or peritoneal neoplastic implants. Often patients with dropped stones and abscess formation can be afebrile and have a normal WBC, and the unusual sites of abscess formation coupled with the lack of awareness of a previous laparoscopic cholecystectomy can lead to an inaccurate or delayed diagnosis.

- The stone fragments are usually diagnosable on CT due to their radiopacity, but are occasionally demonstrated by virtue of fat content or even gas content. Sonography will show shadowing echogenic foci. MR will depict low signal fragments on all sequences, but since the fragments are often quite small MR may be the least effective of the three cross-sectional modalities.

Suggested Readings

Cherif-Idrissi N, El Hajjam M, Acharki M, Chagnon S, Penna C, Lacombe P. [Dropped stone: a case report]. *J Radiol*. June 2010;91(6):717-718.

Karabulut N, Tavasli B, Kiroğlu Y. Intra-abdominal spilled gallstones simulating peritoneal metastasis: CT and MR imaging features (2008: 1b). *Eur Radiol*. April 2008;18(4):851-854.

Singh AK, Levenson RB, Gervais DA, Hahn PF, Kandarpa K, Mueller PR. Dropped gallstones and surgical clips after cholecystectomy: CT assessment. *J Comput Assist Tomogr*. April 2008;31(5):758-762.

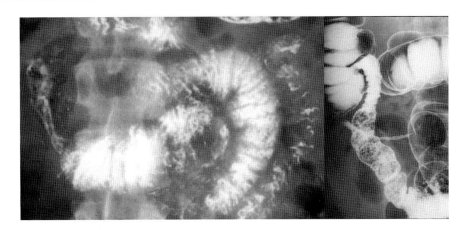

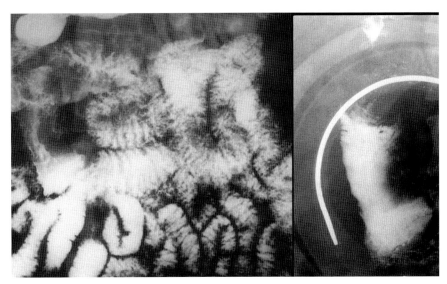

1. What is the most likely explanation for the diffuse small bowel abnormality?

2. What is the most likely explanation for the abnormal descending duodenum?

3. What is nodular lymphoid hyperplasia (NLH) associated with?

4. For what are common variable hypogammaglobulinemia (CVH) patients at risk?

5. What is the treatment of NLH?

Case ranking/difficulty:

Category: Small bowel

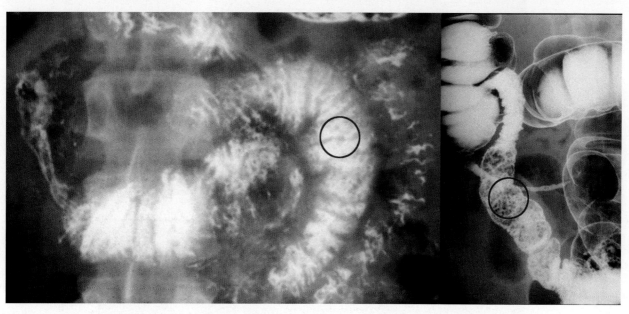

The left film is of the duodenum and proximal jejunum demonstrating multiple tiny jejunal nodules (*circle*) all the same size. The right film is from a double-contrast BE showing even more numerous similar nodules (*circle*) in the distal ileum.

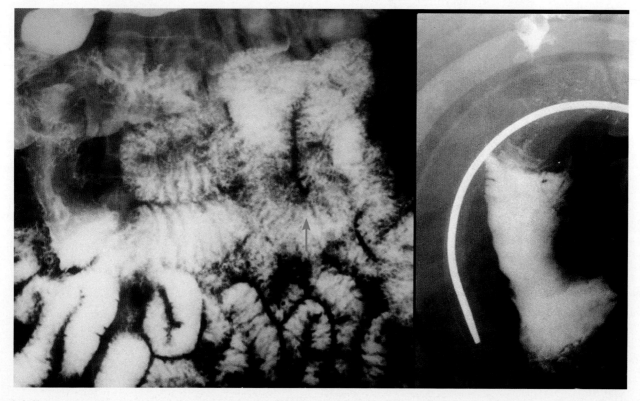

The left film is on overhead showing a formless descending duodenum (*red arrow*) with complete mucosal destruction but no obstruction. The right film is a spot with compression better illustrating the same findings as well as mild dilatation. Careful inspection of the jejunum on the left shows nodules (*green arrow*) but they are less obvious than top-left image.

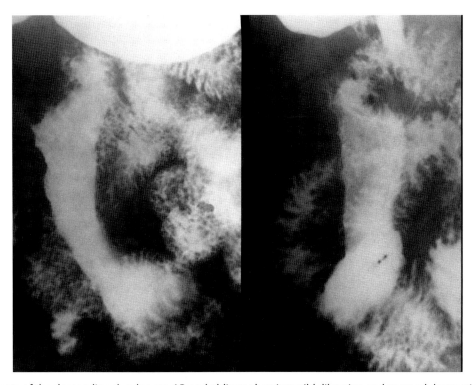

Additional spots of the descending duodenum, AP, and oblique showing mild dilatation and mucosal destruction.

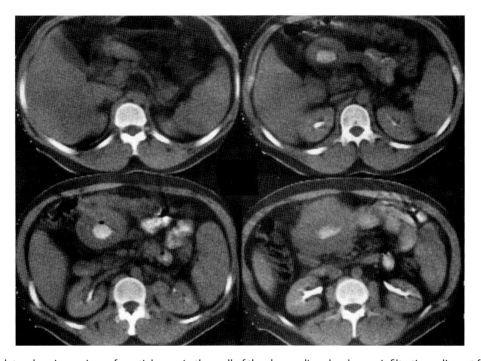

CT scan a few days later showing a circumferential mass in the wall of the descending duodenum infiltrating adjacent fat.

Answers

1. The tiny round polyps throughout the small bowel and most numerous in the distal ileum are characteristic of nodular lymphoid hyperplasia (NLH). Lack of wall thickening, fold thickening, and uniform smooth appearance argue against lymphoma.

2. The complete mucosal destruction and mild dilatation with absence of obstruction is diagnostic of lymphoma. This happened to be a Burkitt lymphoma. There is an increased incidence of small bowel lymphoma in NLH patients.

3. NLH is associated with common variable immune deficiency, selective IgA deficiency, hypogammaglobulinemia, and giardiasis but may be seen with normal immune function. In addition to small bowel lymphoma there is an increased incidence of gastric carcinoma.

4. Common variable hypogammaglobulinemia (CVH) is the usual adult primary immunodeficiency, its main characteristics being impairment to different degrees of immunoglobulin synthesis. Most frequent abnormality is an increased suppressor T-cell activity, which suppresses B-cell maturation and immunoglobulin synthesis. CVH patients are prone to recurrent bacterial infections of respiratory tract—sinusitis, bronchitis, pneumonia. Sixty percent have diarrhea with or without giardiasis or malabsorption. Small bowel histology in CVH has three patterns: diffuse nodular lymphoid hyperplasia (DNLH), hypogammaglobulinemic sprue, or combined.

5. Nodular lymphoid hyperplasia in cases with no complications does not require any special treatment; however, due to the associated increased risk of malignancy the patients should undergo periodic surveillance examinations for small bowel lymphoma and gastric carcinoma.

Pearls

- Nodular lymphoid hyperplasia (NLH) is a rather rare lymphoproliferative disease whose cause still remains unknown.
- NLH usually affects the small intestine; colon and stomach are less commonly involved.
- NLH associated with common variable immune deficiency, selective IgA deficiency, hypogammaglobulinemia, and giardiasis but may be seen with normal immune function.
- NLH requires differentiation from causes of polyps especially malignant lymphoma and familial adenomatous polyposis.
- NLH presents as innumerable round smooth polyps, 1 to 5 mm, usually in the small bowel, especially the terminal ileum.
- NLH in cases with no complications does not require treatment, but periodic surveillance examinations for small bowel lymphoma and gastric carcinoma are recommended.

Suggested Readings

Castellano G, Moreno D, Galvao O, et al. Malignant lymphoma of jejunum with common variable hypogammaglobulinemia and diffuse nodular hyperplasia of the small intestine. A case study and literature review. *J Clin Gastroenterol*. September 1992;15(2):128-135.

Chiaramonte C, Glick SN. Nodular lymphoid hyperplasia of the small bowel complicated by jejunal lymphoma in a patient with common variable immune deficiency syndrome. *AJR Am J Roentgenol*. November 1994;163(5):1118-1119.

Mansueto P, Iacono G, Seidita A et al. Review article: intestinal lymphoid nodular hyperplasia in children—the relationship to food hypersensitivity. *Aliment Pharmacol Ther*. 2012 May;35(9):1000-1009.

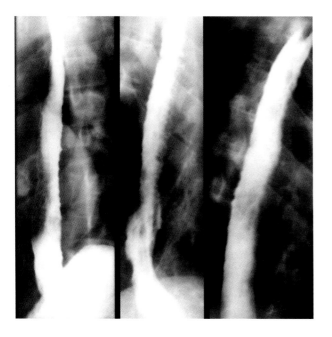 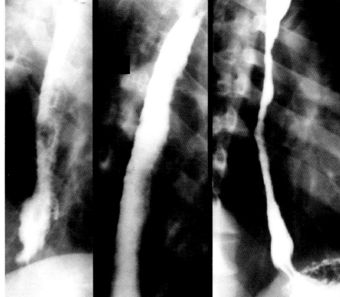

1. What are the diagnostic possibilities on the esophagram (the image on the right is a follow-up exam 1 month later)?

2. What is the best diagnosis?

3. What parts of the GI tract are the most severely injured after alkaline caustic ingestion?

4. What are the mechanisms of alkaline injury?

5. What are some complications of alkaline caustic ingestion?

Case ranking/difficulty:

Category: Esophagus

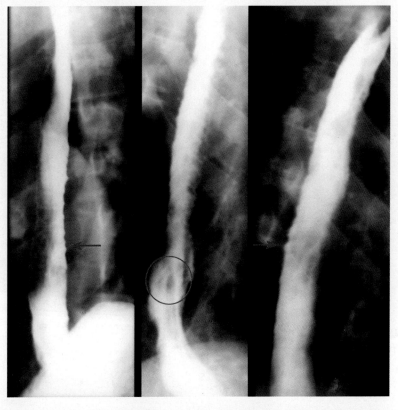

Three films from an esophagram in a male patient presenting to the ER with acute odynophagia. The esophageal contour is shaggy (*arrows*). There is en face evidence of mucosal edema/swelling (*circle*).

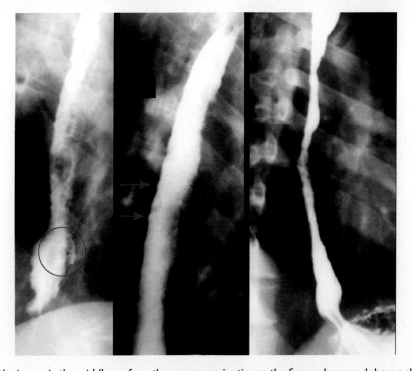

The image on the left and the image in the middle are from the same examination as the figure above and show a shaggy esophagus (*arrows*) and en face mucosal edema (*circle*). The image on the right is from a follow-up examination 1 month later and shows a long stricture.

Answers

1. This esophagram is similar in appearance to the "ringed esophagus" seen in eosinophilic esophagitis. Severe reflux esophagitis can manifest as widespread superficial ulceration. The en face mucosal lucencies could be due to *Candida*, but presence of ulceration and absence of plaques is against it. Both alkali and acid caustic ingestions can cause acute esophagitis as we see here.

2. The acute esophagitis followed by stricture in 1 month is typical of alkaline caustic ingestion. The patient was given a Drano-containing cocktail by his girlfriend. His offense is left to your imagination.

3. The most severely injured tissues are those that first contact the alkali, which are the oropharynx, hypopharynx, and esophagus. The esophagus is the most commonly involved organ with the stomach much less frequently involved. In part, this may be due to neutralization by stomach acid. The immediate effect of the alkali on the encountered tissue proximal to the stomach may be so severe that the liquid does not make it into the stomach.

4. Severe injury occurs rapidly after alkaline ingestion, within minutes of contact. It is characterized by liquefactive necrosis, saponification of fat, and solubilization of protein.

5. Airway obstruction may occur in the first 48 hours due to severe tissue edema. Full-thickness burns may result in esophageal perforation. Given sufficient injury granulation tissue replaces necrotic burned tissue. During the 2 to 4 weeks after injury, scar tissue remodels and may thicken and contract enough to form strictures. Gastric bullae have been reported with alkaline injury to the stomach. There is an increased incidence of carcinoma for 10 to 25 years after esophageal injury and stricture.

Pearls

- If performed acutely the esophagram will show diffuse ulceration and possibly spasm. Endoscopy is now usually performed acutely. Esophagrams are more likely to be performed 2 to 4 weeks after the acute event because of stricture formation. The extensive circumferential narrowing will be more severe than the run of the mill reflux stricture.
- Injury and stricture formation predispose to esophageal carcinoma, with an estimated increase in risk by a factor of 1000, which continues for 10 to 25 years after injury and requires careful follow-up. Routine screening, however, is not currently recommended.

Suggested Readings

Levitt R, Stanley RJ, Wise L. Gastric bullae. An early roentgen finding in corrosive gastritis following alkali ingestion. *Radiology*. June 1975;115(3):597-598.

Song HY, Han YM, Kim HN, Kim CS, Choi KC. Corrosive esophageal stricture: safety and effectiveness of balloon dilation. *Radiology*. August 1992;184(2):373-378.

Temiz A, Oguzkurt P, Ezer SS, Ince E, Hicsonmez A. Predictability of outcome of caustic ingestion by esophagogastroduodenoscopy in children. *World J Gastroenterol*. March 2012;18(10):1098-1103.

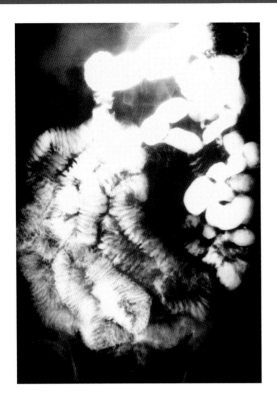 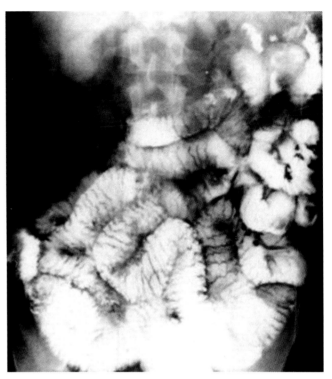

1. What are the findings? Two different patients, same diagnosis.

2. What would you consider in the differential diagnosis?

3. What is the best diagnosis?

4. What are the complications of long-standing, poorly controlled celiac disease?

5. What does the small bowel malabsorption pattern include?

Case ranking/difficulty:

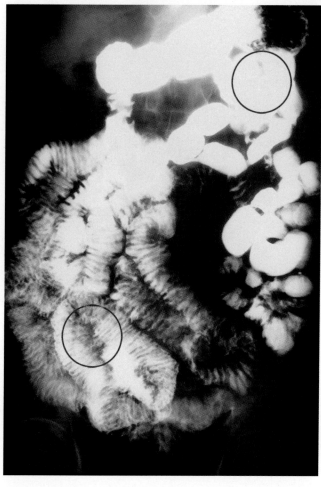

Two-hour film from a small bowel follow through (*circles*).

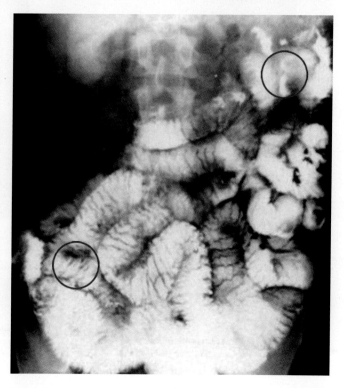

Different patient, same diagnosis (*circles*).

Answers

1. Jejunal folds are absent (moulage sign). There is jejunization of the ileum with too many folds per inch. The small bowel is mildly dilated and the barium is mildly diluted especially in case one on the left. The folds are not nodular.

2. The findings are most compatible with celiac disease CD. Scleroderma is a possibility with dilatation and increased ileal folds per square inch. Whipple disease is a cause of malabsorption pattern and merits consideration. There are no findings to suggest small bowel lymphoma. ZE syndrome is a cause of malabsorption pattern in which there may be dilution of barium due to hypersecretion so it deserves consideration.

3. The findings are almost pathognomonic for celiac disease. Scleroderma should not cause jejunal fold atrophy. Whipple disease causes fold thickening. Small bowel lymphoma should cause fold nodularity, nodules, or masses. ZE should not cause jejunal fold atrophy and may cause visible ulcers in unusual locations.

4. Lymphoma of the small bowel is more frequent in CD patients than adenocarcinoma, but both may occur. CD is a risk factor for the development of squamous cell carcinoma of the pharynx or esophagus. Cavitary lymph node syndrome is a serious but rare complication of CD. Hyposplenism can occur in conjunction with cavitary lymph node syndrome or by itself. Ulcerative jejunoileitis is a serious complication difficult to differentiate from lymphoma by imaging.

5. Delayed transit is part of the malabsorption pattern, not rapid transit. Flocculation, dilated loops, dilution of barium and intussusception are all features of the malaborption pattern.

Pearls

- Duodenojejunal biopsy study showing subtotal villous atrophy with appropriate histologic evidence of mucosal injury and a favorable clinical and morphologic response to a gluten-free diet will establish the diagnosis of CD.

- The mucosa in CD is abnormal from the duodenal bulb for a variable distance into the jejunum. The intensity of the change need not be uniform, and areas of flat mucosa may alternate with patches of only partial villous atrophy. Single suction biopsies may, therefore, produce atypical mucosa and are subject to sampling error.
- Villous atrophy has a DDx particularly in patients with atypical clinical presentations: Whipple disease, Z-E syndrome, eosinophilic gastroenteritis, lymphoma, and parasitic diseases. Radiologic study may be helpful.
- Treatment failure: Imaging indicated to exclude intestinal ulceration and lymphoma.
- Possibly indicated: Surveillance by imaging for lymphoma and other malignancy.

Suggested Readings

Bova JG, Friedman AC, Weser E, Hopens TA, Wytock DH. Adaptation of the ileum in nontropical sprue: reversal of the jejunoileal fold pattern. *AJR Am J Roentgenol.* February 1985;144(2):299-302.

Herlinger H, Maglinte DD. Jejunal fold separation in adult celiac disease: relevance of enteroclysis. *Radiology.* March 1986;158(3):605-611.

Rubesin SE, Herlinger H, Saul SH, Grumbach K, Laufer I, Levine MS. Adult celiac disease and its complications. *Radiographics.* November 1989;9(6):1045-1066.

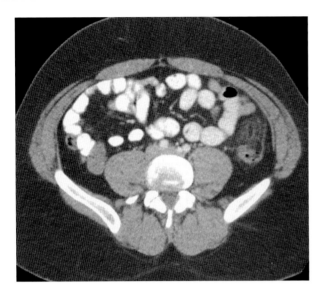
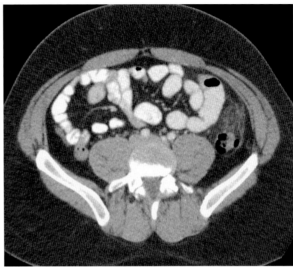
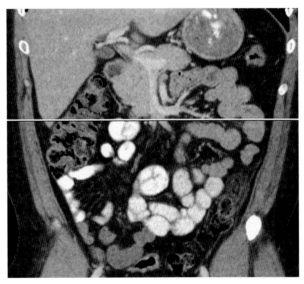

1. What is the most likely diagnosis?

2. What are the characteristics of epiploic appendages and where are they located?

3. What are the characteristics of epiploic appendagitis?

4. What are the possible outcomes of epiploic appendagitis?

5. What are the imaging characteristics of epiploic appendagitis?

Case ranking/difficulty:

Category: Colorectum

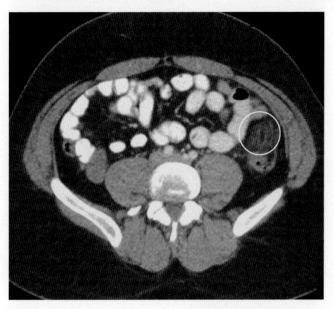

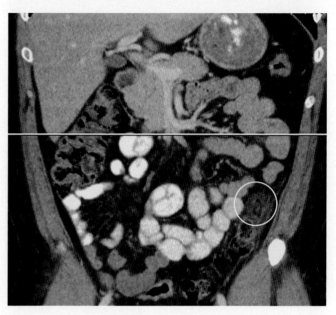

Anterior to the descending colon is a small elliptical mass (*circle*) with fat infiltration. Its center is fat density. It has a hyperattenuating ring around its center. The colon wall is normal.

Coronal image of the mass (*circle*) with central fat density and surrounding infiltration of pericolic fat. Around the central fat is a hyperattenuating ring and within the fat is a linear hyperattenuating focus.

Answers

1. Pericolic mass with central fat and peripheral rim with adjacent fat infiltration and without colonic wall thickening is typical of epiploic appendagitis. Segmental omental infarction is larger and involves omental fat. Diverticulitis, carcinoma, and Crohn disease should thicken the colonic wall.

2. Epiploic appendages are 50 to 100 pedunculated fatty structures extending from the cecum to the rectosigmoid junction covered by the peritoneum. They are most numerous in the cecum and sigmoid colon. They are between 1 and 2 cm thick, 0.5 and 5 cm long, and larger on the left side of the colon than on the right side.

   Supplied by one or two small end arteries and drained by one vein epiploic appendages are prone to torsion and ischemic or hemorrhagic infarction.

3. Primary epiploic appendagitis is caused by torsion or spontaneous thrombosis of the central draining vein, resulting in vascular occlusion and inflammation. It occurs more frequently in the sigmoid colon than in the cecum or ascending colon and is uncommon in the transverse colon.

   It presents as an abrupt onset of focal abdominal pain in the region of the offending appendage with localized tenderness without guarding or rigidity. Low-grade fever is common and the WBC count is usually normal or slightly elevated.

4. Primary epiploic appendagitis usually resolves within 5 to 7 days without treatment. Potential but uncommon complications are adhesions, bowel obstruction, intussusception, intraperitoneal loose bodies, peritonitis, and abscess.

5. US: Incompressible hyperechoic small ovoid mass at site of maximal tenderness. Mass is frequently surrounded by a hypoechoic halo. No Doppler flow.

   CT: Epiploic appendagitis is a 1- to 4-cm ovoid pericolic mass with central fat density surrounded by inflammatory changes and no colonic wall thickening. A 2- to 3-mm hyperdense rim (ring sign) surrounds the ovoid mass. Central, hyperattenuating, ill-defined round (central dot sign), or linear area within mass is common.

   MRI: Epiploic appendagitis is hyperintense on unenhanced T1WI but less intense than normal fat. The thin peripheral rim and the adjacent fat stranding are hypointense on T1WI, hyperintense on T2WI, and enhance on postgadolinium T1W fat sat images.

Pearls

- Epiploic appendagitis occurs more frequently in the sigmoid colon than in the cecum or ascending colon and rarely in transverse colon.
- US: Incompressible hyperechoic small ovoid mass at site of maximal tenderness. Mass is frequently surrounded by a hypoechoic halo.
- CT: Epiploic appendagitis is a 1- to 4-cm ovoid pericolic mass abutting the anterior colonic wall with central fat density surrounded by inflammatory changes. A 2- to 3-mm hyperdense rim (ring sign) surrounds the ovoid mass. Fat stranding is more pronounced than colonic wall thickening. Central, hyperattenuating, ill-defined round (central dot sign) or linear area within mass is common.
- MRI: Epiploic appendagitis is hyperintense on unenhanced T1WI but less intense than normal fat. It will drop in signal on fat suppressed T2WI. The thin peripheral rim and the adjacent fat stranding are hypointense on T1WI, hyperintense on T2WI, and enhance on postgadolinium T1W fat sat images. The central draining vein usually has low signal on both T1WI and T2WI.

Suggested Readings

Almeida AT, Melão L, Viamonte B, Cunha R, Pereira JM. Epiploic appendagitis: an entity frequently unknown to clinicians—diagnostic imaging, pitfalls, and look-alikes. *AJR Am J Roentgenol*. November 2009;193(5):1243-1251.

Singh AK, Gervais DA, Hahn PF, Rhea J, Mueller PR. CT appearance of acute appendagitis. *AJR Am J Roentgenol*. November 2004;183(5):1303-1307.

Singh AK, Gervais DA, Hahn PF, Sagar P, Mueller PR, Novelline RA. Acute epiploic appendagitis and its mimics. *Radiographics*. September 2006;25(6):1521-1534.

Myeloproliferative disease

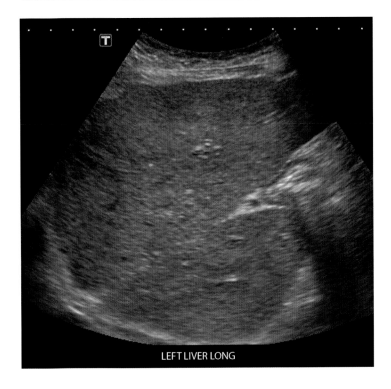

LEFT LIVER LONG

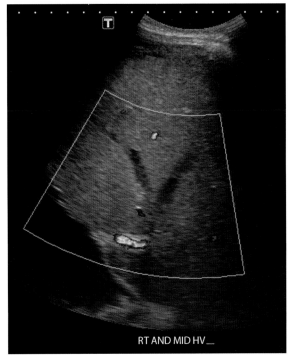

RT AND MID HV

1. Based on the US and the CT next page, what is the most likely diagnosis?

2. What are the causes of primary (intravascular origin) Budd-Chiari?

3. What are the causes of secondary (extravascular origin) Budd-Chiari?

4. What are the sonographic findings in Budd-Chiari syndrome?

5. What are the CT/MRI findings in Budd-Chiari syndrome?

Case ranking/difficulty:

Category: Liver

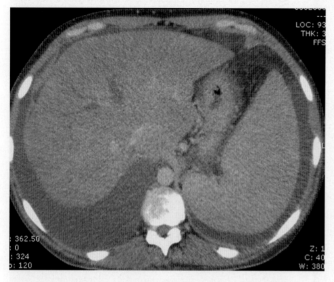

Hepatosplenomegaly, caudate lobe enlargement, ascites, and right pleural effusion seen on CT. Hepatic veins are unenhanced consistent with thrombus.

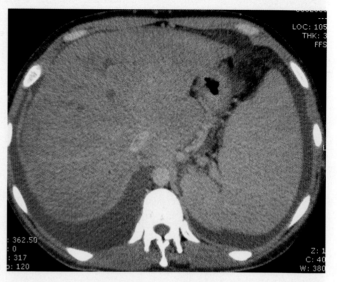

Hepatosplenomegaly, ascites, and right pleural effusion seen on CT. Some hepatic veins are unenhanced consistent with thrombus. Clot (*arrow*) is seen within the IVC. There are varices in the gastrohepatic ligament.

Answers

1. Hepatomegaly with relative caudate lobe enlargement, ascites, and occlusion of hepatic veins with IVC clot are diagnostic of Budd-Chiari syndrome. The right pleural effusion is probably from the ascites.

2. Intravascular thrombosis is the most common mechanism of primary BCS. Almost always a hypercoagulable state exists.

   Acquired: polycythemia vera, essential thrombocythemia, myelofibrosis, paroxysmal nocturnal hemoglobinuria, malignancy, anti-phospholipid antibody syndrome, Behçet disease, pregnancy, and oral contraceptive use

   Inherited: factor V Leiden deficiency, others causing elevations of prothrombin, factors VII and VIII, and homocysteine and deficiencies of antithrombin, protein C, and protein S

   Other causes of primary BCS: neoplasms of the IVC and fibrous webs/membranes of the inferior vena cava, hepatic veins, or both

3. Intravascular spread of hepatocellular carcinoma, renal cell carcinoma, adrenal cortical carcinoma, Wilms tumor, and hepatic angiosarcoma are the common causes of secondary BCS.

   Secondary BCS is sometimes seen when an intrahepatic or juxtahepatic mass compresses venous structures. Examples are hematomas, hepatic abscesses, hydatid cysts, and polycystic liver.

4. Ascites, hepatomegaly, mild splenomegaly, and caudate lobe hypertrophy, and either right atrophy and left hypertrophy or vice versa are common.

   Acute: Abnormalities are seen in at least one of the three major hepatic veins and/or the IVC, stenosis, proximal dilatation, intraluminal echoes, lack of Doppler flow, absent, flattened, or reversed waveforms, abnormal vascular course, or extrahepatic anastomosis.

   Chronic: Collaterals from obstructed segments to the caudate lobe (comma-shaped or curled tubular sonolucencies). Hepatic vein-to-hepatic vein collaterals and portosystemic collaterals. Sometimes the only findings are reduced size or nonvisualization of hepatic veins. Flow in the portal vein may be abnormal.

   Caval: Any responsible mass is usually depicted. Membranous obstruction—narrowed or disappearing IVC at the intrahepatic level or between the liver and right atrium.

5. CT/MR acute: Liver enhances heterogeneously and relative hypoenhancement of the periphery is characteristic. The caudate lobe hyperenhances in the arterial phase. This central hyperdense peripheral hypodense enhancement pattern may reverse on delayed-phase imaging. Occluded veins show lack of intraluminal enhancement.

   Acutely the periphery of the liver has high SI on T2W MRI and low attenuation on noncontrast CT.

CT/MR chronic: Liver fibrosis may be visible as reticular increased signal/low attenuation at unenhanced MR/CT and increase enhancement on delayed images. The liver atrophies, particularly in the periphery. Compensatory hypertrophy of the caudate lobe due to direct venous drainage into the IVC occurs if the IVC is not obstructed.

Regenerating nodules common in chronic BCS.

Pearls

- US: Ascites and hepatomegaly, mild splenomegaly, caudate lobe hypertrophy.
- Acute: Signs of thrombosis in at least one of the three major hepatic veins and/or the IVC.
- Chronic: Hepatic venous collaterals sometimes seen as comma-shaped or curled tubular sonolucencies. Portosystemic collaterals. Sometimes the only findings are reduced size or nonvisualization of hepatic veins. Flow in the portal vein may be abnormal in regions affected by hepatic venous occlusion.
- If BCS is primarily caval, any responsible mass is usually depicted. If membranous obstruction, the IVC seems to narrow or disappear either at the intrahepatic level or between the liver and right atrium. Web itself is rarely seen. Waveforms in the IVC and hepatic veins will be abnormal.
- CT acute: Periphery of enlarged liver is hypodense on unenhanced CT. The liver enhances heterogeneously and relative hypoenhancement of the periphery is characteristic. The caudate lobe (or other areas of the liver with preserved venous drainage) hyperenhances in the arterial phase. This central hyperdense peripheral hypodense enhancement pattern may reverse on delayed-phase imaging. Occluded hepatic veins may be nonvisualized or may show lack of intraluminal enhancement.

- CT chronic: Liver fibrosis may be visible as reticular low attenuation at unenhanced CT. The liver atrophies, particularly in the periphery. Compensatory hypertrophy of the caudate lobe due to direct venous drainage into the IVC occurs if the IVC is not obstructed.
- MRI: Acutely the periphery of the liver has high SI on T2WI. In chronic BCS, atrophic parenchyma may be seen as reticular high signal on T2WI. The enhancement pattern is the same as that of CT.
- Regenerating nodules common in chronic BCS.

Suggested Readings

Diehl K, Sarwani NE, Tulchinsky M. PET/CT in primary hepatic lymphoma with hepatic vein thrombus that extended into the inferior vena cava. *Clin Nucl Med.* February 2013;38(2):153-156.

Ferral H, Behrens G, Lopera J. Budd-Chiari syndrome. *AJR Am J Roentgenol.* October 2012;199(4):737-745.

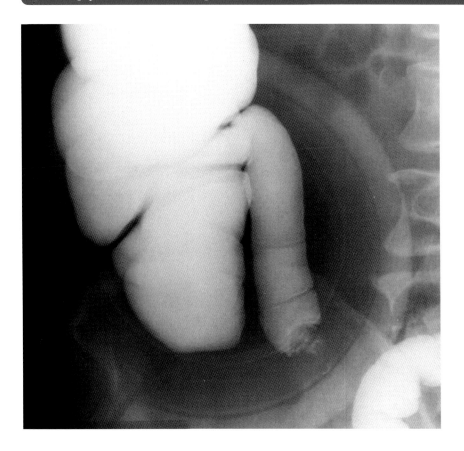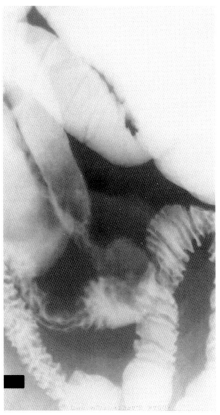

1. What is a reasonable differential diagnosis for the barium enema above and the barium enema on the next page of a different patient with the same diagnosis?

2. Looking at the CT scan on the 2nd following page and knowing it is the same diagnosis as the barium enemas, what is the best diagnosis?

3. What are some complications of ileal carcinoid tumors?

4. What is the appearance of small ileal carcinoids on barium studies?

5. What is the appearance of small ileal carcinoids on CT or MR?

Case ranking/difficulty: **Category:** Small bowel

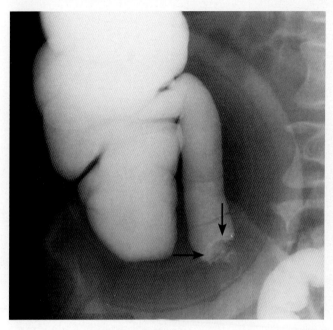

Spot film of a barium enema with reflux into the terminal ileum shows a small mass (*arrows*) with intact folds.

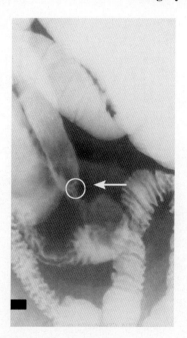

Second spot film shows the same mass (*arrow*) with angles of near 90° with the bowel wall. Note intact mucosal folds (*circle*).

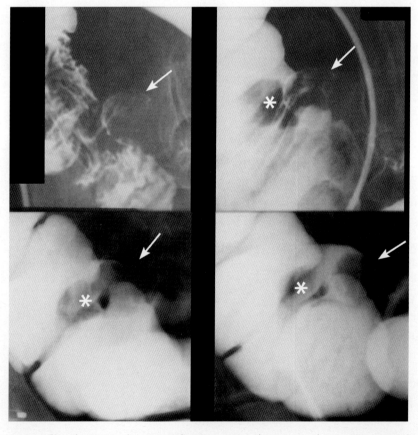

Second case, same diagnosis. Spot films from a single-contrast barium enema show a round, smooth mass in the terminal ileum (*arrows*) medial to the ileocecal valve (*asterisks*).

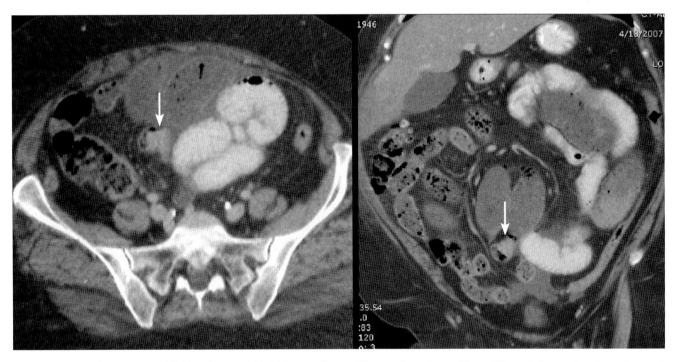

Third case, same diagnosis. Axial (*left*) and coronal (*right*) images from a CT scan of a patient with small bowel obstruction show the small enhancing tumor (*arrows*) that is responsible.

Answers

1. The mass is likely submucosal due to angle of about 90°. Common submucosal ileal masses are carcinoid, lymphoma, or mesenchymal tumor (such as leiomyoma). Sometimes extrinsic masses such as metastasis (intraperitoneal) or endometrioma (in females) look like submucosal masses. Metastases (hematogenous) can be submucosal.

2. Carcinoid is the likeliest small submucosal mass (not lymphoma or leiomyoma) to produce small bowel obstruction. Metastasis can do it but is less common than carcinoid in this location and there is no history of a primary. Even in females this is not a common location for endometrioma (which can produce obstruction even if small).

3. Lymph node, mesenteric and liver metastases may be quite large, overshadowing the small (<3.5 cm) primary. The primary sometimes serves as intussusception lead point. The release of serotonin and other substances causes a desmoplastic reaction in the submucosa extending into the mesentery, causing kinking, retraction, and angulation of bowel. Mesenteric vessels near to and far from the tumor may be thickened and/or accordioned with or without multifocal stenoses/occlusions. Intestinal ischemia may result.

4. Small nodular carcinoids are very difficult to detect with a conventional small bowel series. They are best evaluated with enteroclysis or even barium enema with reflux. When identified, they are characteristically solitary or multifocal, smooth, rounded nodules, or mucosal elevations in the distal ileum. The mucosa overlying the nodule of carcinoid may ulcerate, producing a barium-filled crater on the surface of the lesion.

5. Larger primary masses may be identified on CT by their enhancement. Neutral bowel contrast (as opposed to barium) helps. A small bowel obstruction or intussusception facilitates small primary mass detection on CT. Larger primary masses can be seen on Gd-enhanced T1 fat sat MRI as nodules with moderately intense gadolinium enhancement. The primary tumor may also manifest on CT or MRI as focal, asymmetric, or concentric mural thickening.

Pearls

- Barium studies of carcinoid tumor:
  - Small polypoid carcinoids located in the submucosa can be detected (but it is difficult) by enteroclysis or small bowel series or barium enema with reflux. Characteristically they appear as solitary or multifocal, smooth, rounded nodules in the distal ileum. The mucosa overlying the nodule of carcinoid may ulcerate, producing a barium-filled crater on the surface of the lesion. Obstruction or intussusception facilitates small primary mass detection.
  - Larger small bowel carcinoids may produce a kink or curvature of the intestinal wall called a hairpin turn that is the result of tumor infiltration and fibrosis between two adjacent loops. Fluoroscopic barium evaluation of the small bowel reveals a fixed, rigid, curved segment of small intestine.

Suggested Readings

Kamaoui I, De-Luca V, Ficarelli S, Mennesson N, Lombard-Bohas C, Pilleul F. Value of CT enteroclysis in suspected small-bowel carcinoid tumors. *AJR Am J Roentgenol.* March 2010;194(3):629-633.

Levy AD, Sobin LH. From the archives of the AFIP: gastrointestinal carcinoids: imaging features with clinicopathologic comparison. *Radiographics.* June 2009;27(1):237-257.

Masselli G, Polettini E, Casciani E, Bertini L, Vecchioli A, Gualdi G. Small-bowel neoplasms: prospective evaluation of MR enteroclysis. *Radiology.* June 2009;251(3):743-750.

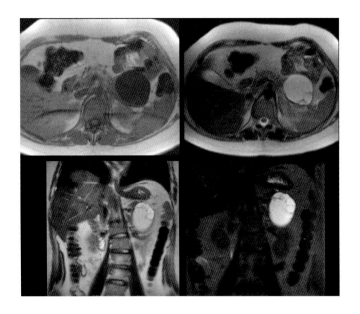 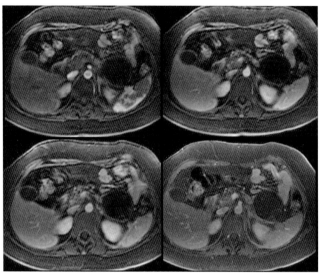

1. What is a reasonable differential diagnosis given the findings on sets of both images?

2. What is the best diagnosis?

3. What is true about the calcifications in cystic pancreatic neoplasms?

4. What are the signal intensity (SI) characteristics of mucinous cystic neoplasms (MCN) on MR?

5. What is the correct treatment of pancreatic mucinous cystic neoplasms (MCN)?

Case ranking/difficulty:

Category: Pancreas

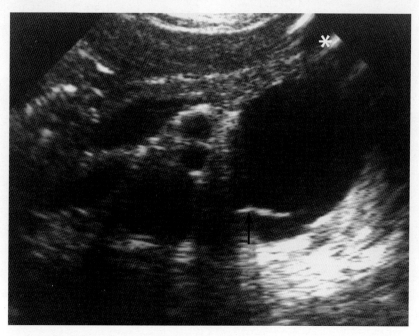

Different case—typical sonogram of mucinous cystic neoplasm—large anechoic (*except for one septum, arrow*) externally smooth mass, increased through transmission. Middle-aged female, tail of pancreas. No malignancy found.

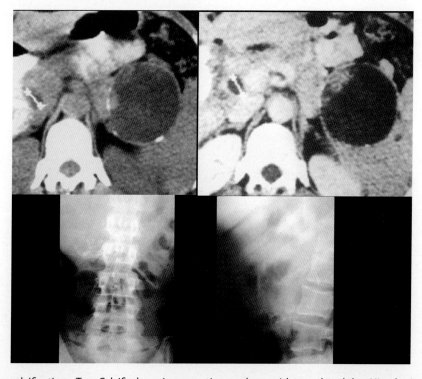

Different cases illustrating calcifications. Top: Calcified mucinous cystic neoplasm with mural nodules. Histologically malignant. Noncontrast CT (*left*) shows a mostly water density mass with a thin wall and arcuate wall calcification and a mural nodule. Nodular excrescences and the wall enhance after contrast (*right*). Bottom: AP and lateral plain films showing wall calcification in a pancreatic head MCN that overlaps the spine. Some of the calcification is arcuate in profile and some of the wall calcification is seen en face.

Answers

1. Pseudocyst of the pancreas, mucinous cyst neoplasm, cystic islet cell tumor, and oligocystic serous cystadenoma comprise a reasonable differential diagnosis. The mass is too large to be an IPMN.

2. The externally smooth cystic intrapancreatic mass with daughter cysts is typical of mucinous cystic neoplasm, which is the correct (and best) diagnosis. Malignancy was not found at pathologic evaluation. Lack of history and intrapancreatic origin are against pseudocyst. Lack of any hormonal activity and presence of daughter cysts are against cystic islet cell tumor. External smoothness and young age is against oligocystic serous cystadenoma. Lymphoepithelial cysts are very rare and usually do not have daughter cysts.

3. Mucinous cystic neoplasms calcify in the wall (periphery) whereas serous cystadenomas calcify in central fibrous tissue. Calcifications obvious on CT are often invisible on MR.

   Wall calcifications in mucinous cystic neoplasms seen en face on plain films were incorrectly described as being central.

   Cystic neoplasm calcification is hard to demonstrate on sonography.

4. SI of MCN cystic compartments can be variable. On T1WI SI can be either less than or greater than that of liver and it varies from much greater to slightly greater than fat on T2WI. Papillary excrescences, old blood, debris, and proteinaceous fluid will cause regions of relatively increased signal on T1WI and decreased signal on T2WI.

5. All MCNs must be treated as at least potentially malignant by local complete excision (unless surgery contraindicated). If MCNs are incompletely resected or treated by cystoenterostomy, recurrence is inevitable even in apparently benign tumors. Malignant behavior may occur as late as 12 years after the initial operation.

Pearls

- 85% tail or body/tail 9:1 F:M, 50% 40-60 years old.
- Uni- or multilocular large cysts with or without smaller cysts, externally smooth, wall calcification, and papillary excrescences may be present, often correlating with frank malignancy.
- Lined by mucin-producing columnar cells, single rows to stratification, and papillary formation to frank adenocarcinoma.
- Benign and malignant epithelium may coexist in the same tumor.
- Malignancy may be small, isolated; all treated as potentially malignant.
- US and CT: Externally smooth, uni- or multiloculated >2 cm cyst(s), solid excrescence(s), near water density, CT enhancement limited to wall, and any septa or excrescences.
- MR: T1WI—hypo- to slightly hyperintense depending on protein. T2WI—hyperintense, any septa or excrescences less intense. Gd enhancement is the same as CT enhancement.
- Liver metastases can be confused with cysts.

Suggested Readings

Hammond NA, Miller FH, Day K, Nikolaidis P. Imaging features of the less common pancreatic masses. *Abdom Imaging*. June 2013;38(3):561-572.

Kucera JN, Kucera S, Perrin SD, Caracciolo JT, Schmulewitz N, Kedar RP. Cystic lesions of the pancreas: radiologic-endosonographic correlation. *Radiographics*. February 2013;32(7):E283-E301.

Sahani DV, Kambadakone A, Macari M, Takahashi N, Chari S, Fernandez-del Castillo C. Diagnosis and management of cystic pancreatic lesions. *AJR Am J Roentgenol*. February 2013;200(2):343-354.

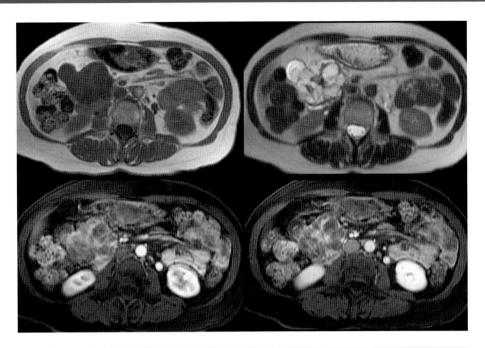

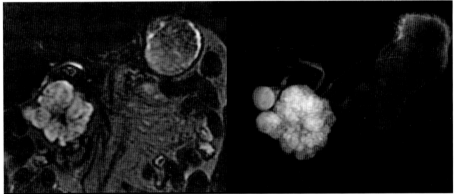

1. Looking at all images what is the most likely diagnosis?

2. What important finding in this entity can be shown by CT but is usually invisible on MRI?

3. What are some clinical characteristics of serous cystadenoma of the pancreas?

4. What are the pathologic features of serous cystadenoma of the pancreas?

5. What are the imaging features of serous cystadenoma of the pancreas?

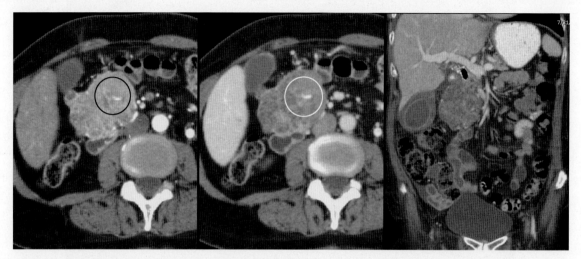

Arterial phase (*left*) and portal phase (*middle*) images from a CT 3 years before the MR, which was unchanged from the prior appendicitis CT. There is some central calcification (*circles*) that was invisible on MR. The mass is coming from the pancreatic head and externally lobulated with a Swiss-cheese enhancement pattern. The coronal portal venous phase image on the right from about the same time as the MR shows the pancreatic origin of the mass a little better.

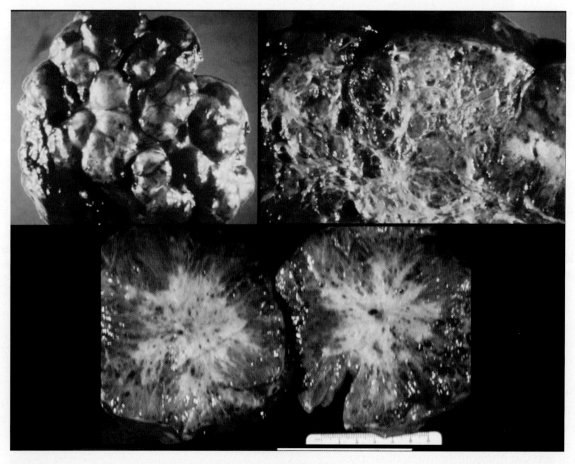

Gross specimen of a serous cystadenoma similar to the clinical case.

Answers

1. The MR features of an externally lobulated mass that is T1 hypointense, T2 bright with a dark stellate central scar that shows delayed enhancement point to a serous cystadenoma of the pancreas.

2. The central calcification shown on CT is characteristic of serous cystadenoma but it cannot be seen on MRI. External lobulation is shown by both modalities, and the delayed enhancement of the central scar was shown better by MRI.

3. Serous cystadenoma may be an incidental finding at imaging, laparotomy, or postmortem. Jaundice is uncommon. Serous cystadenomas occur with increased frequency in patients with von Hippel Lindau disease, but this disease is rarely found in a population of patients with serous cystadenomas. Hemorrhage (from a ruptured vessel within the tumor) from serous cystadenomas has been reported. Serous cystadenomas of the pancreas are virtually always benign but case reports of serous cystadenocarcinoma do exist.

4. Serous cysstadenomas are externally lobulated usually large masses (4-25 cm, mean 13 cm) composed of innumerable small (1 mm-2 cm) cysts. The cysts are filled with proteinaceous fluid which may contain glycogen but not mucin and are lined by cuboidal or flattened epithelium with clear cytoplasm often containing glycogen.

5. The calcification in serous cystadenomas is central. The central scar is dark on T2WI and often has delayed enhancement. The external border is lobulated. Swiss-cheese enhancement is commonly seen on CT.

Pearls

- 82% aged >60 weak female predilection, anywhere in gland, externally lobulated, innumerable small cysts 1 mm to 2 cm, occasionally larger cysts, central fibrotic scar which may calcify.
- Cysts filled with proteinaceous fluid that may contain glycogen, lined by cuboidal or flattened epithelium with clear cytoplasm often with glycogen, thin, nearly acellular connective tissue network, no mucin, nearly always benign.
- US: Solid, mixed hypoechoic/echogenic.
- CT: Hypodense, Swiss-cheese enhancing. Central calcification, central scar, external lobulation, mostly small cysts.
- MR: Low intensity T1WI, occasionally higher intensity if proteinaceous fluid; hyperintense T2WI. Septa/central scar best seen as hypointense areas on T2WI.
- Gd enhancement of connective tissue component and delayed enhancement.
- ERCP/MRCP: if large drape and/or gently narrow pancreatic ducts, obstruction rare, no communication with pancreatic duct.

Suggested Readings

Dewhurst CE, Mortele KJ. Cystic tumors of the pancreas: imaging and management. *Radiol Clin North Am*. May 2012;50(3):467-486.

Sahara S, Kawai N, Sato M, et al. Differentiation of pancreatic serous cystadenoma from endocrine tumor and intraductal papillary mucinous neoplasm based on washout pattern on multiphase CT. *J Comput Assist Tomogr*. April 2013;36(2):231-236.

Zaheer A, Pokharel SS, Wolfgang C, Fishman EK, Horton KM. Incidentally detected cystic lesions of the pancreas on CT: review of literature and management suggestions. *Abdom Imaging*. April 2013;38(2):331-341.

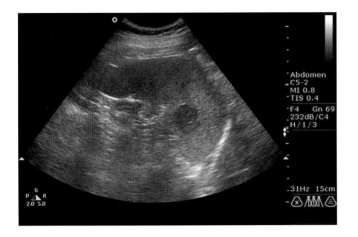 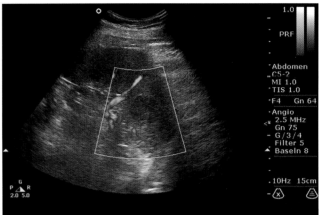

1. What should be in the differential diagnosis?

2. The second case next page is a different patient with the same diagnosis. What is the best diagnosis for both patients?

3. What are clinical features of splenic hamartoma?

4. What are the pathologic features of splenic hamartoma?

5. Which of the following suggest hamartoma in a splenic mass?

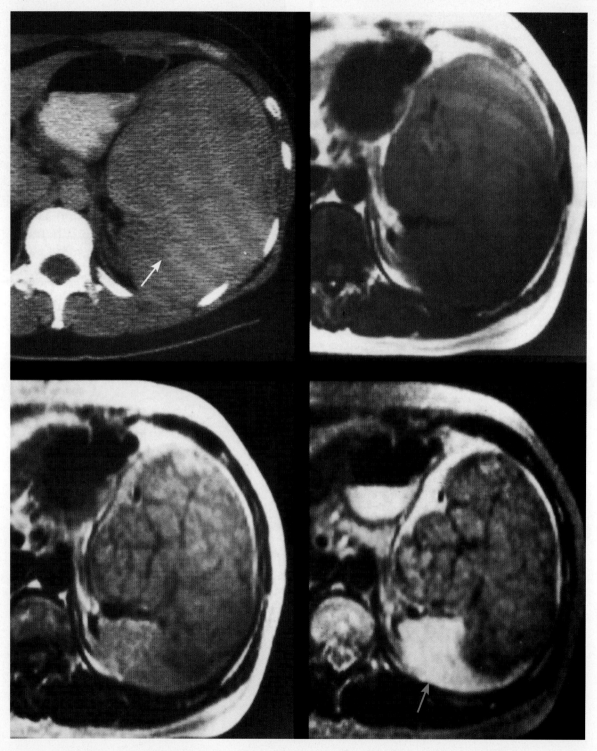

Different case: staging CT for an asymptomatic 39-year-old female for early gastric CA. Contrast-enhanced CT (*top left*) shows marked splenomegaly due to a large mass with slightly increased attenuation. Stippled calcification was seen at a different level (*not shown*). T1WI (*top right*) shows splenomegaly due to an isointense mass. Proton density image (*bottom left*) shows an intermediate signal mass nearly isointense to normal spleen (latter is posteromedial) with dark septa. T2WI (*bottom right*) shows a well-defined lobulated intermediate intensity mass hypointense to the normal posteromedial high SI spleen (*arrow*). Dark septa are redemonstrated.

Answers

1. Lymphoma, metastasis, hemangioma, hamartoma, and angiosarcoma should be considered. Lymphoma is unlikely without adenopathy. Metastasis is unlikely without a known primary. Angiosarcomas are usually larger and more aggressive looking.

2. The T2 dark cords are consistent with fibrous trabeculae and correctly suggest hamartoma. The overall T2 signal is less than the usual hemangioma. Lymphoma is unlikely without adenopathy. Metastasis is unlikely without a known primary. Angiosarcomas are usually without the well-defined borders shown here.

3. Splenic hamartomas are usually asymptomatic incidental findings. Association with tuberous sclerosis or Wiskott-Aldrich syndrome, spontaneous rupture and hypersplenism are all uncommon but possible features.

4. They are usually solitary but may be multiple.

   Most are mixed red and white pulp; some are predominantly one or the other.

   Single layer of endothelial cells lines wide vascular channels filled with lymphoreticular cells. Foci of hemosiderosis, calcification, fibrosis.

   Compresses normal spleen and is sharply demarcated despite lack of true capsule.

   Fibrous trabeculae extending from capsule into the mass may be present.

5. Splenic hamartoma is suggested by:

   a) Increased blood flow on color Doppler images in a homogeneous echogenic mass with well-defined borders.

   b) Attenuation and SI of the mass on unenhanced CT and MR close to normal spleen and diffuse progressive and prolonged enhancement.

Pearls

- Hemangiomas tend to have higher SI on T2WI than hamartomas.
- On arterial phase images, most splenic hemangiomas have nodular peripheral enhancement; hamartomas usually show mild diffuse heterogeneous enhancement.
- Angiosarcomas are heterogeneous masses with irregular, poorly defined contours and have evidence of bleeding. Hamartomas are usually well-defined with smooth borders.
- Splenic lymphoma usually causes multiple splenic masses associated with extrasplenic adenopathy. Primary malignant lymphoma of the spleen without adenopathy is uncommon and often invades adjacent organs.
- Splenic metastases are usually multiple with a known primary.
- Splenic hamartoma is suggested by:
  a) Increased blood flow on color Doppler images in a homogeneous echogenic mass with well-defined borders
  b) Attenuation and SI of the mass on unenhanced CT and MR close to normal spleen and diffuse progressive and prolonged enhancement

Suggested Readings

Elsayes KM, Narra VR, Mukundan G, Lewis JS, Menias CO, Heiken JP. MR imaging of the spleen: spectrum of abnormalities. *Radiographics*. April 2005;25(4):967-982.

Gutzeit A, Stuckmann G, Dommann-Scherrer C. Sclerosing angiomatoid nodular transformation (SANT) of the spleen: sonographic finding. *J Clin Ultrasound*. June 2009;37(5):308-311.

Wang JH, Ma XL, Ren FY, et al. Multi-modality imaging findings of splenic hamartoma: a report of nine cases and review of the literature. *Abdom Imaging*. February 2013;38(1):154-162.

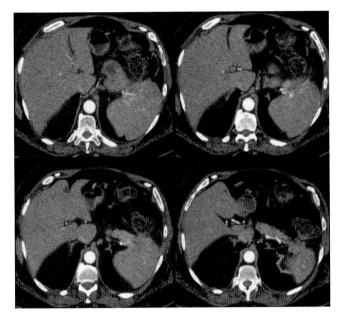
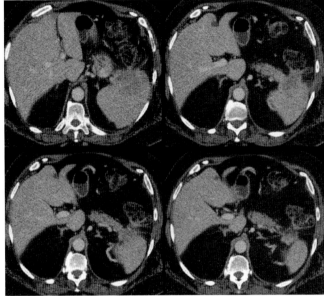

1. Looking at both figures, what should be in your differential diagnosis?

2. What is a reasonable next step to establish a diagnosis?

3. With what signs and symptoms do nonhyperfunctioning pancreatic neuroendocrine tumors present?

4. What hormones do nonhyperfunctioning pancreatic neuroendocrine tumors produce?

5. What are the imaging characteristics of nonhyperfunctioning pancreatic neuroendocrine tumors?

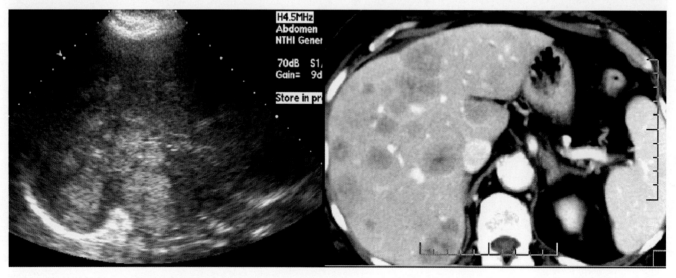

Liver US and portal phase CT in a different patient with metastatic nonhyperfunctioning pancreatic neuroendocrine tumor. Liver mets are echogenic (mitigates against duct cell adenocarcinoma) as does the central necrosis in the larger mets.

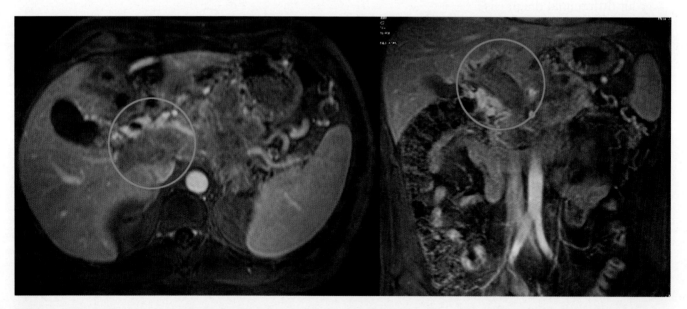

Different patient with malignant nonhyperfunctioning pancreatic neuroendocrine tumor invading the portal vein and occluding the splenic vein. Axial and sagittal MR show expanded portal vein with no intraluminal enhancement and heterogeneous content due to tumor thrombus (*circles*). There is cavernous transformation of the portal vein and gastrosplenic collaterals. Intravenous invasion favors pancreatic neuroendocrine tumor over duct cell adenocarcinoma.

Answers

1. A large mass originating in the tail of the pancreas invading the spleen with nonspecific symptoms is likely to be either a duct cell carcinoma of the pancreas or a nonhyperfunctioning pancreatic neuroendocrine tumor. This mass could be a lymphoma extending from the spleen into the pancreas but it is less likely. The epicenter of the mass is not in the stomach or the colon so gastric and colon carcinomas are not good choices.

2. The mass is near the stomach so EUS-guided biopsy should work. If it does not CT-guided percutaneous biopsy should work. Histologic diagnosis is important since prognosis and treatment are different between pancreatic neuroendorine tumors and duct cell adenocarcinoma.

3. Nonhyperfunctioning pancreatic neuroendorine tumors have a similar presentation to duct cell adenocarcinoma of the pancreas—abdominal pain, jaundice, palpable mass, weight loss, steatorrhea. Size is usually 6 to 20 cm with preference for the tail. Forty percent have liver metastases at presentation and regional lymphadenopathy is common as well.

4. Nonhyperfunctioning pancreatic neuroendorine tumors usually do produce some hormone(s). They are clinically nonfunctioning because they do not produce sufficient hormone, or hormone may be produced but not released, or hormone may be in an inactive form, or the hormone may not produce symptoms even when secreted in large amounts (pancreatic polypeptide).

5. Ultrasound: Larger nonhyperfunctioning pancreatic neuroendorine tumors—complex masses due to hemorrhage and cystic degeneration.

   MRI and CT: Most nonhyperfunctioning pancreatic neuroendorine tumors have higher SI on T2WI than other pancreatic neoplasms and enhance more rapidly and intensely than the normal pancreas on arterial phase imaging. In the portal phase, they may enhance more, the same, or less than the pancreas. They are usually large masses with heterogeneous enhancement. Twenty-five to thirty-three percent central calcification on CT.

   Octreotide scan: Positive in most pancreatic neuroendorine tumors except insulinoma.

   FDG PET: Positive in poorly differentiated nonhyperfunctioning pancreatic neuroendorine tumors, which may be octreotide negative.

Pearls

- Ultrasound: Larger nonhyperfunctioning pancreatic neuroendorine tumors: Complex masses due to hemorrhage and cystic degeneration.
- MRI and CT: Most nonhyperfunctioning pancreatic neuroendorine tumors: Higher SI on T2WI than other pancreatic neoplasms and enhance more rapidly and intensely than the normal pancreas on arterial phase imaging. Nonhyperfunctioning pancreatic neuroendorine tumors are usually large masses and have heterogeneous enhancement. In the portal phase nonhyperfunctioning pancreatic neuroendorine tumors may enhance more, the same, or less than the pancreas.
- Nuclear medicine:
  - Octreotide scan is positive in most pancreatic neuroendocrine tumors but not in insulinoma.
  - FDG PET is positive in poorly differentiated nonhyperfunctioning pancreatic neuroendocrine tumors (which may be octreotide negative).

Suggested Readings

Kim JH, Eun HW, Kim YJ, Han JK, Choi BI. Staging accuracy of MR for pancreatic neuroendocrine tumor and imaging findings according to the tumor grade. *Abdom Imaging.* October 2013;38(5):1106-1114.

Kim KW, Krajewski KM, Nishino M, et al. Update on the management of gastroenteropancreatic neuroendocrine tumors with emphasis on the role of imaging. *AJR Am J Roentgenol.* October 2013;201(4):811-824.

Kim SY, Park SH, Hong N, Kim JH, Hong SM. Primary solid pancreatic tumors: recent imaging findings updates with pathology correlation. *Abdom Imaging.* October 2013;38(5):1091-1105.

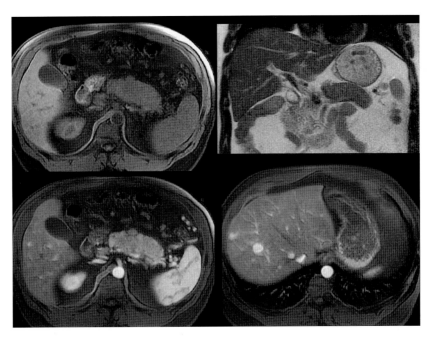

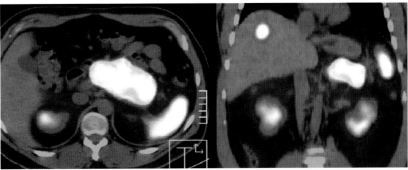

1. Based on MRI on top, what is in your differential diagnosis?

2. Now looking at octreotide scan on the bottom, what is the diagnosis considering the elevated serotonin level?

3. What are the endocrinopathies associated with hyperfunctioning pancreatic neuroendocrine tumors?

4. What are the differences between large and small pancreatic neuroendocrine tumors?

5. What are the differences between pancreatic neuroendocrine tumors and duct cell adenocarcinomas (DCAs)?

443

Case ranking/difficulty:

Category: Pancreas

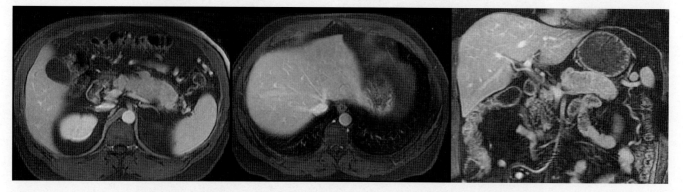

Portal venous phase LAVA postcontrast MRI (*axial, left*) shows mild persistent pancreatic mass enhancement and the gastrosplenic venous collaterals. The liver metastasis (*middle*) is invisible. On a coronal portal venous phase LAVA post-contrast (*right*) there is persistent pancreatic mass enhancement and gastrosplenic collaterals.

Answers

1. This could be a pancreatic neuroendocrine tumor with either a liver metastasis or a flash hemangioma. Pancreatic lymphoma and flash hemangioma are possible, but splenic vein obstruction mitigates against it. Metastatic disease to the pancreas and liver is possible, but pancreatic metastases are usually focal or multifocal. Autoimmune pancreatitis should have some increased T2 signal, but is possible although focal involvement is usually in the head.

2. The octreotide uptake in the pancreas and liver is diagnostic of noninsulinoma pancreatic neuroendocrine tumor with liver metastasis and the elevated serum serotonin level points to carcinoid.

3. Syndromes associated with pancreatic neuroendocrine tumors result from hormone overproduction. Insulinomas, gastrinomas, glucagonomas, somatostatinomas, VIPomas, and ACTH-producing tumors are the most important causes of a clinical syndrome.

4. Small pancreatic neuroendocrine tumors are generally solid and homogeneous; larger pancreatic neuroendocrine tumors are heterogeneous with cystic or necrotic degeneration and sometimes calcification (CT). Malignant tumors tend to be larger than small ones and may show local invasiveness, vascular invasion, liver and/or lymph node metastases. Gastrinomas can be malignant when small.

5. 1) Enhancement: duct cell adenocarcinoma (DCA) is hypovascular; PNET generally has at least some hypervascular component.

   2) Calcification: Rare as hen's teeth in DCA compared to 20% of pancreatic neuroendocrine tumors.

   3) Vascular involvement: DCA encases or obstructs vessels. Pancreatic neuroendocrine tumors extend into vessels, causing tumor thrombus.

   4) Pancreatic duct: DCA commonly causes ductal obstruction. With the exception of carcinoid this finding is uncommon in pancreatic neuroendocrine tumors.

   5) Central necrosis and cystic degeneration: More common in pancreatic neuroendocrine tumors than DCA.

Pearls

- Ultrasound: Larger pancreatic neuroendocrine tumors: complex masses due to hemorrhage and cystic degeneration
- Small pancreatic neuroendocrine tumors: hard to see, round or oval, smoothly marginated hypoechoic solid masses
- MRI and CT: Most pancreatic neuroendocrine tumors: Higher SI on T2WI than other pancreatic neoplasms and enhance more rapidly and intensely than the normal pancreas on arterial phase imaging. Homogeneous enhancement is typical for small <2 cm tumors and larger masses have heterogeneous enhancement. In the portal phase pancreatic neuroendocrine tumors may enhance more, the same, or less than the pancreas.
- Nuclear medicine:
  - Octreotide scan: positive in most pancreatic neuroendocrine tumors but not in insulinoma
  - FDG PET: positive in poorly differentiated pancreatic neuroendocrine tumors (which are usually octreotide negative) and negative in well-differentiated pancreatic neuroendocrine tumors

Suggested Readings

Buetow PC, Miller DL, Parrino TV, Buck JL. Islet cell tumors of the pancreas: clinical, radiologic, and pathologic correlation in diagnosis and localization. *Radiographics.* March-April 1997;17(2):453-472; quiz 472A-472B. Erratum in *Radiographics.* July-August1997;17(4):1010.

Gallotti A, Johnston RP, Bonaffini PA, et al. Incidental neuroendocrine tumors of the pancreas: MDCT findings and features of malignancy. *AJR Am J Roentgenol.* February 2013;200(2):355-362.

Kucera JN, Kucera S, Perrin SD, Caracciolo JT, Schmulewitz N, Kedar RP. Cystic lesions of the pancreas: radiologic-endosonographic correlation. *Radiographics.* January 2013;32(7):E283-E301.

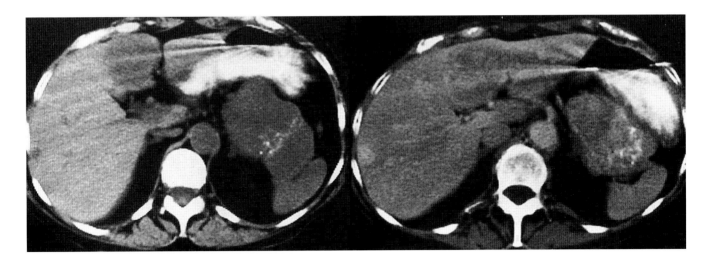

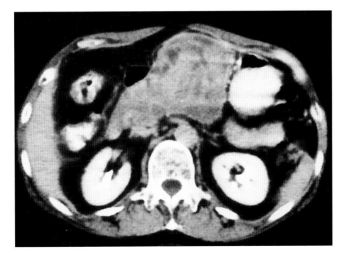

1. What is your differential diagnosis for figure at the top? (left is at presentation, right is 2.5 years later)

2. What is your differential diagnosis for the figure at the bottom?

3. What are the gross characteristics of OGTP (osteoclast-type giant cell tumor of the pancreas)?

4. What are the microscopic characteristics of OGTP?

5. What are the imaging characteristics of OGTP?

Case ranking/difficulty: **Category:** Pancreas

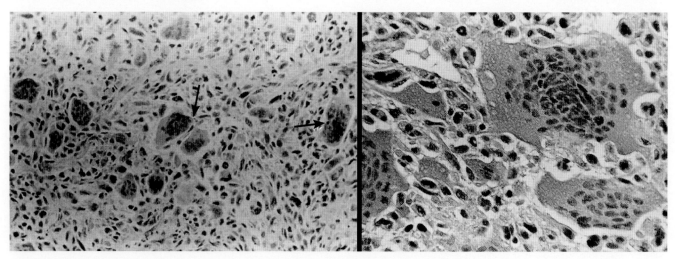

Same patient as top figure previous page. Left-uniform benign-appearing multinucleated giant cells (*arrows*) containing dozens of nuclei and evenly distributed chromatin. Other cells shown are benign-appearing spindle cells. Right-higher power field shows dimorphic population of mononuclear stromal spindle cells and osteoclast-like giant cells, some with >100 nuclei.

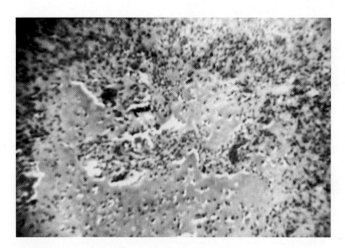

Red/orange material is osteoid in another OGTP.

Answers

1. The powdery osteoid-type calcification and stability of the primary and the liver metastasis with no treatment are consistent with OGTP. Rarely lymphoma calcifies without treatment and lack of progression with no treatment is conceivable although unlikely. Islet cell tumors calcify and one this big is certainly malignant. No growth in 2.5 years with no treatment is conceivable although unlikely. Adenocarcinoma of the pancreas almost never calcifies. Metastasis to the pancreas would not be stable for 2.5 years without treatment.

2. In addition to the correct diagnosis of OGTP, sarcomas, anaplastic carcinoma, pleomorphic giant cell carcinoma, and mucinous adenocarcinoma can be large

partially necrotic aggressive pancreatic malignancies. Neuroendocrine tumors are often large partially necrotic masses but are more indolent.

3. OGTPs are large neoplasms (4-23 cm) with either well-defined or locally invasive margins. On palpation, they are either soft or firm rather than hard, reflecting little desmoplasia. OGTPs are well vascularized by cavernous or sinusoidal blood spaces but some necrosis is common.

4. OGTP has mononuclear stromal spindle cells and osteoclast-like giant cells that resemble benign osteoclasts and may contain up to 100 nuclei but do not exhibit mitotic figures. The presence of zymogen granules within the mononuclear stromal cells suggests an acinar cell origin. It is histologically indistinguishable from giant cell carcinoma of bone.

5. US: large solid component with partially necrotic central areas.

CT: OGTP is heterogeneous with areas of enhancement, cystic necrosis, and sometimes calcification. Some enhancement of solid components may be > normal pancreas in arterial phase.

MRI: solid portion slightly hypointense on T1 and slightly hyperintense on T2 compared to normal pancreas. Necrotic areas are low signal on T1 and hyperintense on T2.

Compared to duct cell adenocarcinomas, liver metastases and extensive local invasion are less likely at presentation.

Pearls

- Osteoclast-type giant cell tumor of the pancreas (OGTP) is characterized by numerous multinucleated osteoclast-like giant cells within a stroma of oval or spindle-shaped mononuclear cells.
- Giant cells may contain up to 100 nuclei but no mitotic figures; they are nonneoplastic.
- Mononuclear cells are neoplastic with mitotic activity.
- Osteoid seen in 20%, can have bone formation, chondroid differentiation.
- Differential diagnosis of benign giant cells in pancreas: granulomatous disease, foreign body reaction, fat necrosis.
- OGTPs may be relatively indolent. They also are:
  - Large (usually 5-8 cm, range 4-23 cm).
  - Soft or firm to palpation rather than hard.
  - Well-circumscribed or locally invasive margins.
  - Hemorrhagic necrosis/cystic degeneration common.
  - Solid portions well vascularized.
- US: large, complex, central necrosis
- CT: large partially or multifocally necrotic masses, some enhancement of solid components which may be greater than pancreas in arterial phase.
- MRI: solid—slightly hypointense T1 and slightly hyperintense T2 compared to normal pancreas. Necrotic areas—low signal T1 and hyperintense T2.

Suggested Readings

Demos TC, Posniak HV, Harmath C, Olson MC, Aranha G. Cystic lesions of the pancreas. *AJR*. December 2002;179(6):1375-1388.

Scott R, Jersky J, Hariparsad G. Case report: malignant giant cell tumour of the pancreas presenting as a large pancreatic cyst. *Br J Radiol*. November 1993;66(791):1055-1057.

Temesgen WM, Wachtel M, Dissanaike S. Osteoclastic giant cell tumor of the pancreas. *Int J Surg Case Rep*. 2014;5(4):175-179.

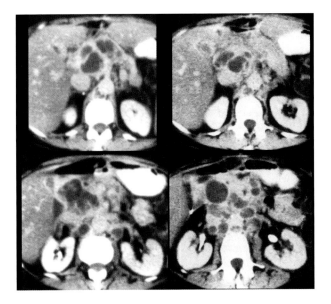 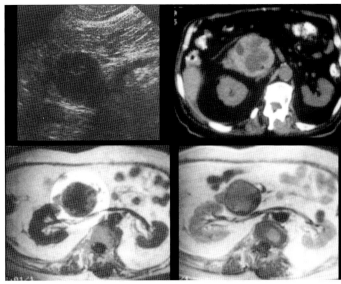

1. What is your differential diagnosis for the left figure?

2. What is your differential diagnosis for the right figure? (Different patient, same diagnosis).

3. What are some clinical and gross pathologic features of pleomorphic giant cell carcinoma of the pancreas?

4. What are the histologic features of pleomorphic giant cell carcinoma?

5. What are the imaging features of pleomorphic giant cell carcinoma?

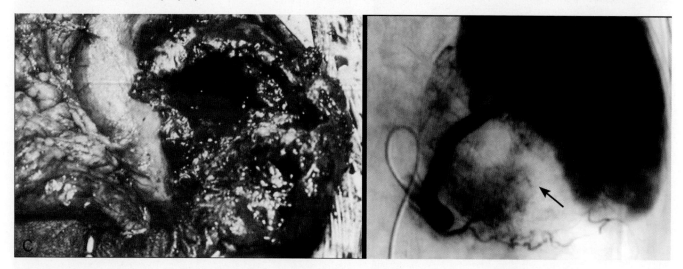

Pleomorphic giant cell carcinoma. Gross specimen (*left*) shows a blood-filled centrally necrotic mass with a thick, nodular wall. Angiography of the same mass shows very good vascularization of the solid portions of the tumor (*arrows*). This is a different patient than previous page.

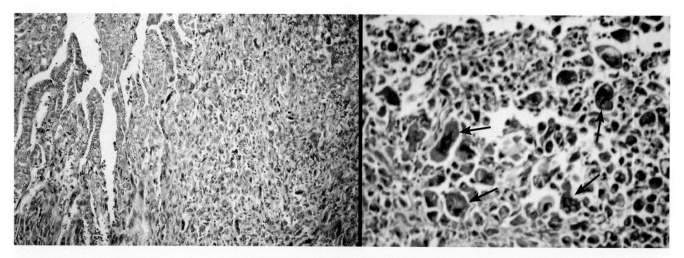

Pleomorphic giant cell carcinoma. Low power field (*left*) shows anaplastic malignant cells on the right and malignant glandular elements on the left. High power of the same neoplasm shows malignant giant cells (*arrows*) with differing but small numbers of nonuniform nuclei. Malignant spindle cells are also present.

Answers

1. Lymphoma, tuberculosis, pleomorphic giant cell carcinoma of the pancreas, neuroendocrine tumor of the pancreas, and malignant IPMN are all reasonable possibilities. I am sure you can come up with a couple more.

2. Neuroendocrine tumor, sarcoma, anaplastic carcinoma, metastasis to pancreas, pleomorphic giant cell carcinoma of the pancreas, mucinous adenocarcinoma, and mucinous cystic neoplasm are all reasonable possibilities. The correct diagnosis for both is pleomorphic giant cell carcinoma. It is suggested in the

left figure previous page by the necrotic adenopathy. Duct cell adenocarcinoma is unlikely for either figure because of the extensive necrosis.

3. Location is evenly distributed between the head, body, and tail. Prognosis is poor with median survival from time of diagnosis of 2 months.

Pleomorphic giant cell carcinomas tend to be large masses (mean 9 cm) of soft consistency often with central hemorrhagic necrosis.

Massive retroperitoneal adenopathy (sometimes necrotic) and hematogenous metastases are common.

4. Large, often bizarre mono- or multinucleated giant cells and obviously malignant spindle cells.

A few osteoclast-like giant cells may be seen, but there is no osteoid.

Small foci of mucin-producing adenocarcinoma can be found with difficulty.

Cytology: Noncohesive mono- and multinucleated pleomorphic malignant giant cells with abundant mitotic figures and only occasional osteoclast-like giant cells.

5. If hemorrhagic necrosis predominates, US, CT, and MR will depict this neoplasm as a large, thick-walled cystic mass with a ragged inner margin.

Otherwise solid or mixed usually well-demarcated masses on US and solid masses sometimes with relatively low-attenuation centers on CT (low T1 signal high T2 signal centers on MR).

Lymphadenopathy (at times centrally necrotic mimicking TB) is often pronounced.

Solid portions enhance more than duct cell adenocarcinoma in arterial and venous phases.

Pearls

- Age and sex distribution same as duct cell adenocarcinoma.
- Median survival 2 months, occasional resectable with long-term survival.
- Epithelial origin.
- Small foci of adenocarcinoma present.
- Retroperitoneal adenopathy, local extension, and liver metastases common at time of diagnosis.
- Large (mean 9 cm). Soft or firm to palpation rather than hard.
- Extensive hemorrhagic necrosis common.
- Nodal metastases may be necrotic.

- Solid portions well vascularized.
- Large, often bizarre, pleomorphic mono or multinucleated giant cells and obviously malignant spindle cells.
- Anaplastic cells and foci of adenocarcinoma usually present, differential diagnosis with anaplastic carcinoma variable.
- US: Can be predominately cystic or complex.
- CT: Often necrotic or central low attenuation with ragged margin.
- MR: Ragged central low T1 high T2 signal.
- On CT and MR solid portions have more arterial and venous phase enhancement than duct cell adenocarcinomas.

Suggested Readings

Moore JC, Bentz JS, Hilden K, Adler DG. Osteoclastic and pleomorphic giant cell tumors of the pancreas: a review of clinical, endoscopic, and pathologic features. *World J Gastrointest Endosc*. January 2010;2(1):15-19.

Scott R, Jersky J, Hariparsad G. Case report: malignant giant cell tumour of the pancreas presenting as a large pancreatic cyst. *Br J Radiol*. November 1993;66(791):1055-1057.

Wolfman NT, Karstaedt N, Kawamoto EH. Pleomorphic carcinoma of the pancreas: computed-tomographic, sonographic, and pathologic findings. *Radiology*. February 1985;154(2):329-332.

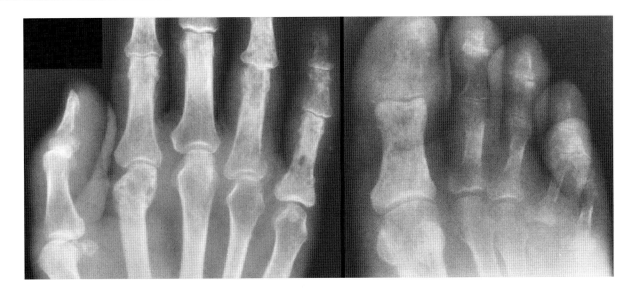

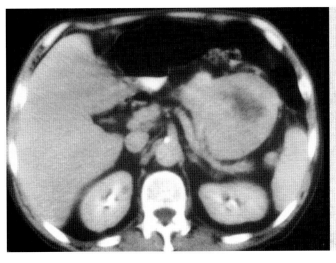

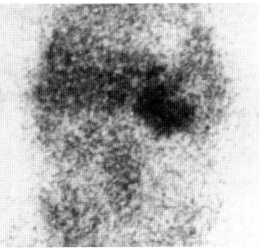

1. What the heck are extremity radiographs doing in a GI book? What is going on with them?

2. What is the best diagnosis for the mass in the bottom 2 images (same patient)?

3. What constellation of clinical findings and lab values comprise metastatic fat necrosis?

4. What is the usual presentation of acinar cell carcinoma (ACC)?

5. What are the imaging findings in ACC?

Case ranking/difficulty:

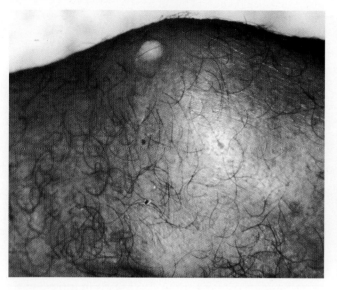

Circumscribed skin nodule in same patient compatible with subcutaneous fat necrosis.

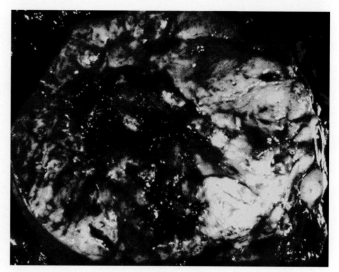

Gross specimen from same patient: large, well-circumscribed yellow mass with central (*bloody*) necrosis.

Answers

1. The permeative osteolysis and multiple lytic lesions combined with the history and physical examination are diagnostic of metastatic fat necrosis also known as lipase hypersecretion syndrome.

2. Just on the images giant cell carcinoma, solid pseudopapillary tumor, neuroendocrine carcinoma, and acinar cell carcinoma are all possible. Duct cell adenocarcinoma is rarely this large, well circumscribed, and this necrotic. Only acinar cell carcinoma (ACC) and solid pseudopapillary tumor are associated with metastatic fat necrosis, but solid pseudopapillary tumor is usually seen in young women and ACC is usually seen in older men so it is the best choice by far. This presentation is unusual for ACC but characteristic.

3. Metastatic fat necrosis is most common in the context of pancreatitis and is caused by systemic release of lipase, hydrolysis of fat in fat cells, and subsequent inflammation. Fat necrosis is manifested by skin lesions (tender erythematous nodules similar to erythema nodosum) and/or lytic bone lesions and/or joint pain, and is frequently accompanied by fever, leukocytosis, and eosinophilia. Elevated serum lipase in the presence of normal serum amylase is characteristic.

4. The usual presentation of ACC is nonspecific with symptoms including abdominal pain, loss of appetite, weight loss, nausea, and vomiting and palpable mass. Jaundice is not common. α-Fetoprotein may be elevated.

5. ACCs are solid when small and centrally necrotic when large.

   Calcifications are seen in a minority on CT and enhancement may be greater or lesser than normal pancreas on the arterial phase but is less on the venous phase when a capsule may be seen. ACC when solid is slightly hypointense on T1WI and hyperintense on T2WI. Larger ones are partially cystic due to necrosis and the central necrotic area has mixed T1 signal intensity and elevated T2W SI. ACCs take up gallium as in this case and 18F-FDG.

Pearls

- Mean age 65, more common in men, seen rarely in children. Nonspecific symptoms usually, bleak prognosis due to high incidence of liver metastases, but may be cured if no liver metastases.
- Large (2-15 cm, mean 11 cm), lobulated, soft, well-demarcated, yellow, frequent necrosis, little desmoplastic response.
- <10% metastatic fat necrosis, identical to that in pancreatitis, due to systemic release of lipase by functioning tumor cells.
- Homogeneous/solid when small (~3.5 cm).
- Cystic/necrotic centers when large (~10 cm).
- Cuboidal or columnar cells in acinar formations and scanty stroma; rare mitotic figures, may have solid pattern with sheets and cords of cells in fibrovascular stroma.

- Positive staining for lipase, trypsin, chymotrypsin, α1-antitrypsin but not amylase.
- PAS+ diastase resistant zymogen granules within cytoplasm (enzyme precursors).
- CT: Enhances < normal pancreas in portal phase.
- May enhance > pancreas in arterial phase.
- Occasional calcification, larger ones have central necrosis.
- MR: Enhances < normal pancreas in portal phase.
- Solid: Slightly hypointense T1 and slightly hyperintense T2 compared to normal pancreas.
- Larger ones have necrotic areas: mixed T1 and hyperintense T2.
- Gallium uptake may occur. PET avid more so than adenocarcinoma.

Suggested Readings

Bhosale P, Balachandran A, Wang H, et al. CT imaging features of acinar cell carcinoma and its hepatic metastases. *Abdom Imaging*. December 2013;38(6):1383-1390.

Bhosale PR, Menias CO, Balachandran A, et al. Vascular pancreatic lesions: spectrum of imaging findings of malignant masses and mimics with pathologic correlation. *Abdom Imaging*. August 2013;38(4):802-817.

Kim HJ, Kim YK, Jang KT, Lim JH. Intraductal growing acinar cell carcinoma of the pancreas. *Abdom Imaging*. October 2013;38(5):1115-1119.

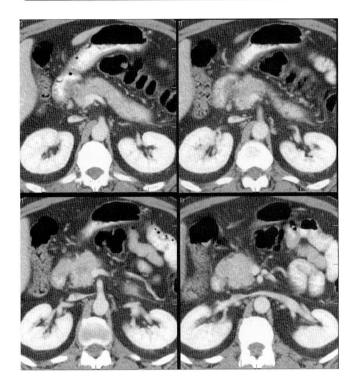 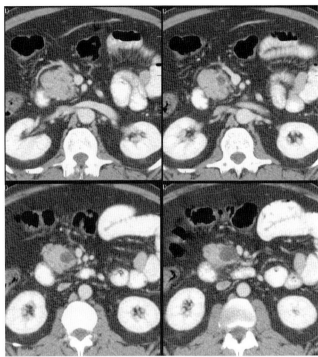

1. What is the best diagnosis on the above figures?

2. What are the types of IPMN?

3. What are the histologic appearances of IPMNs?

4. What imaging features of IPMN increase the likelihood of malignancy?

5. What is the best follow-up study for a side branch type IPMN?

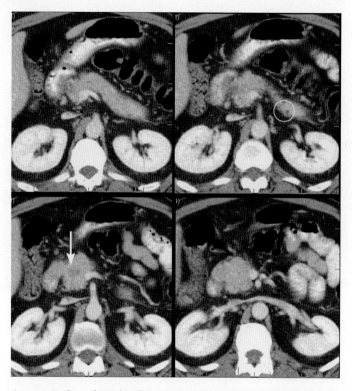

CT through the pancreas shows a tiny cyst in the tail (*circle*). The pancreatic head just above the uncinate process cyst is bulbous and enlarged with subtle central hypodensity (*arrow*).

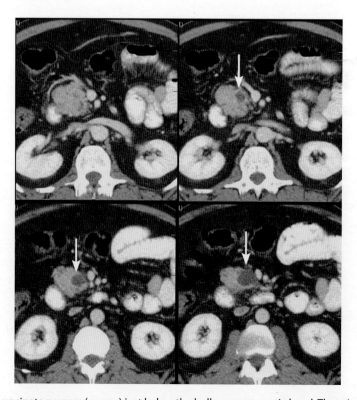

There is large cystic mass in the uncinate process (*arrows*) just below the bulbous pancreatic head. There is bile duct dilatation (*next page*).

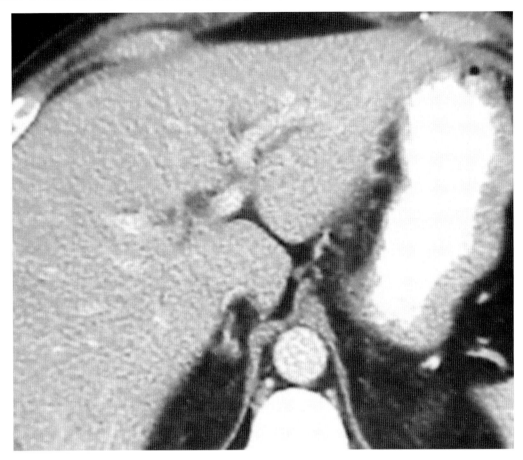

More cephalad CT shows biliary dilatation.

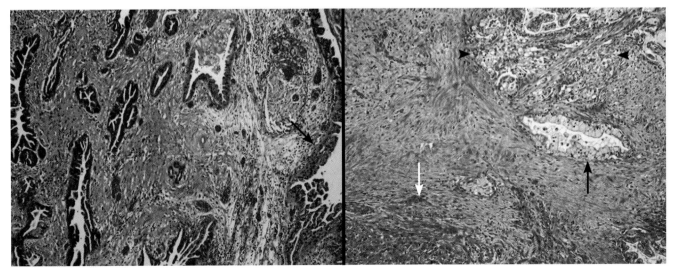

Histopathology in this patient showing both IPMN and frankly invasive adenocarcinoma. Left: Right margin of large cyst-like (*black arrow*) area is lined by borderline featured epithelium. Additional glands are lined by atypical epithelium. Right: Single cell invasion is present (*white arrow*). Gland is lined by mucinous epithelium (*black arrow*). Invasive adenocarcinoma (*between arrowheads*) is infiltrating pancreas.

Answers

1. The bulbous pancreatic head with central hypodensity is diagnostic of adenocarcinoma and the cysts are likely branch duct IPMNs. Both together and in contiguity make the best diagnosis a malignant IPMN or malignant degeneration of IPMN if you prefer.

2. Branch duct type is characterized by cystic or dilated side branches, often in uncinate process but may be anywhere. Main duct type can be segmental or diffuse. When the branch duct type and main duct type occur together it is called the mixed type.

3. The histologic appearances of IPMNs range from adenomas (benign) to adenocarcinomas (malignant), with adenocarcinomas being further subdivided into in situ and invasive lesions.

4. Findings increasing the likelihood of malignancy include solid mass, main pancreatic duct diameter greater than 10 mm, diffuse or multifocal involvement of the main pancreatic duct, presence of calcified intraluminal contents, mural nodules, side branch type IPMN >3 cm.

5. If there is no contraindication MRI with MRCP is best because of reproducibility and lack of ionizing radiation, ability to measure cysts, and lack of need for intravenous contrast. Sonography is an option if the mass is readily visible, but most small branch duct IPMNs are not. Contrast-enhanced CT is a great option if MRI is contraindicated. PET-CT is not useful; the low-dose noncontrast CT will not show the small mass well and increased metabolic activity is a relatively late sign of malignant degeneration of a small branch duct IPMN.

Pearls

- Side branch IPMNs <3 cm are likely benign.
- Main duct IPMNs with >1 cm diameter are likely malignant.
- Mural nodules/thick septa increase likelihood of malignancy.
- When a mass consistent with duct cell carcinoma is seen adjacent to a cystic mass consistent with IPMN the diagnosis of adenocarcinoma coexisting with IPMN can be suggested. This could be the result either of malignant degeneration of IPMN or a manifestation of de novo malignant IPMN.

Suggested Readings

Kang KM, Lee JM, Shin CI, et al. Added value of diffusion-weighted imaging to MR cholangiopancreatography with unenhanced MR imaging for predicting malignancy or invasiveness of intraductal papillary mucinous neoplasm of the pancreas. *J Magn Reson Imaging.* September 2013;38(3):555-563.

Kim JH, Eun HW, Kim KW, et al. Intraductal papillary mucinous neoplasms with associated invasive carcinoma of the pancreas: imaging findings and diagnostic performance of MDCT for prediction of prognostic factors. *AJR Am J Roentgenol.* September 2013;201(3):565-572.

Raman SP, Kawamoto S, Blackford A, et al. Histopathologic findings of multifocal pancreatic intraductal papillary mucinous neoplasms on CT. *AJR Am J Roentgenol.* March 2013;200(3):563-569.

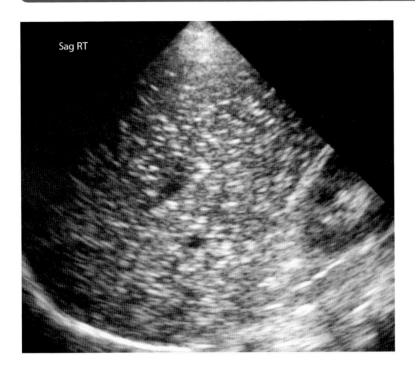
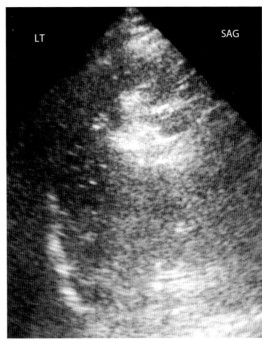

1. What is the name of the organism responsible for the findings in the spleen?

2. In HIV/AIDS, below what CD4 count are patients at increased risk of pulmonary infection by *P carinii*?

3. What pulmonary finding is unusual in pneumocystis pneumonia?

4. How does one make the diagnosis of pneumocystis infection?

5. What findings have been described on US examination of splenic pneumocystosis?

Case ranking/difficulty:

Category: Spleen

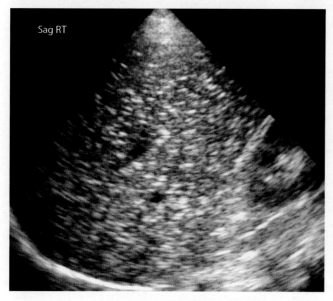

Sagittal ultrasound of the liver shows multiple diffuse, small, echogenic foci within the liver, somewhat randomly distributed (*red arrow*).

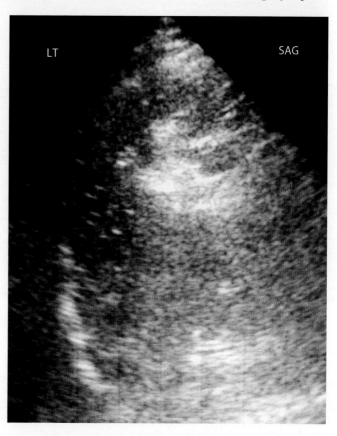

Sagittal ultrasound image of the spleen shows similar small echogenic foci within the spleen (*red arrow*).

Answers

1. Splenic lesions can have a variable appearance, and in general echogenic lesions can be metastases, lymphoma, hemangioma, hematoma or infarct, and inflammatory lesions (eg, granulomas or abscess). One can narrow the differential diagnosis somewhat with so many numerous, small echogenic lesions that do not shadow, suggesting multiple abscesses or foci of infection. Candidiasis is more commonly hypoechoic, and bacterial splenic abscess are also more commonly hypoechoic, sometimes with satellite lesions.

   Pneumocystis jiroveci is somewhat unusual in that it can produce small echogenic lesions on ultrasound, although it can also produce larger hypoechoic abscesses.

   Pneumocystis jiroveci was originally named *P carinii*, and it was also once thought to be a protozoan rather than a fungus. It was later reclassified and renamed based on DNA analysis.

2. A CD4 count less than 200 per microliter is associated with in increased risk of opportunistic infection in HIV/ AIDS.

3. Reticular opacities and ground glass opacities are fairly common findings in pneumocystis pneumonia. Cystic changes and consolidation are a little less common, but might also be seen in patients on pentamidine prophylaxis. Lymphadenopathy can also occur. Pleural effusions are unusual in pneumocystis and might suggest another diagnosis.

4. *Pneumocystis jiroveci* cannot be grown in vitro, so the diagnosis depends upon identification of the organism by histologic stains that make the organism visible, such as a Grocott methenamine-silver stain (GMS), Weigert-Gram, Giemsa, or Wright stains. Some facilities use an immunofluorescence stain. Consequently, infected tissue needs to be obtained to make the diagnosis.

5. Diffuse, small echogenic foci that do not shadow have been described multiple times, although cyst-like lesions, multiple calcified lesions, bull's-eye lesions, and splenomegaly have also been described. In some cases, other organs such as the lymph nodes, liver, and kidneys have also been involved. The appearance of lesions may also change with time, depending on the stage in therapy and the status of the host immune system.

Pearls

- Yeast-like fungus primarily responsible for opportunistic pulmonary infection in immunocompromised patients.
- In HIV/AIDS, CD4+ count less than 200/μL is risk factor.
- Consider diagnosis in the appropriate patient population in diagnostically difficult cases.
- Tissue and histologic analysis required for diagnosis.

Suggested Readings

Anuradha, Sinha A. Extrapulmonary Pneumocystis carinii infection in an AIDS patient: a case report. *Acta Cytol.* 2007;51(4):599-601. Epub 2007/08/28.

Lubat E, Megibow AJ, Balthazar EJ, Goldenberg AS, Birnbaum BA, Bosniak MA. Extrapulmonary Pneumocystis carinii infection in AIDS: CT findings. *Radiology.* 1990;174(1):157-160. Epub 1990/01/01. doi: 10.1148/radiology.174.1.2294543.

Spouge AR, Wilson SR, Gopinath N, Sherman M, Blendis LM. Extrapulmonary Pneumocystis carinii in a patient with AIDS: sonographic findings. *AJR Am J Roentgenol.* 1990;155(1):76-78. Epub 1990/07/01. doi: 10.2214/ajr.155.1.2112868.

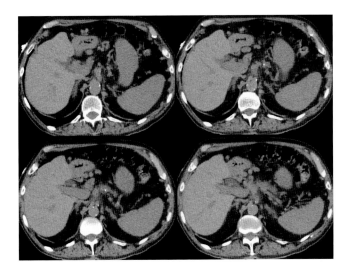
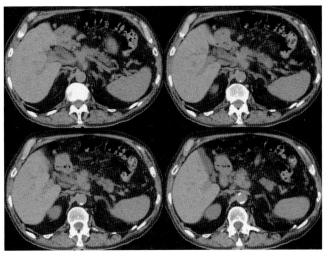

1. After looking at the above CT images what should you do with this patient in the ER?

2. What findings do you see in the contrast-enhanced follow-up CT shown two pages below that are contributory to the correct diagnosis?

3. Why is it important to be able to diagnose carcinoma of the pancreas on noncontrast CT?

4. What are the imaging characteristics of duct cell adenocarcinoma?

5. What should you do if the clinician suspects carcinoma of the pancreas and multiple imaging modalities disagree—some are consistent with carcinoma and some do not show it?

Case ranking/difficulty:

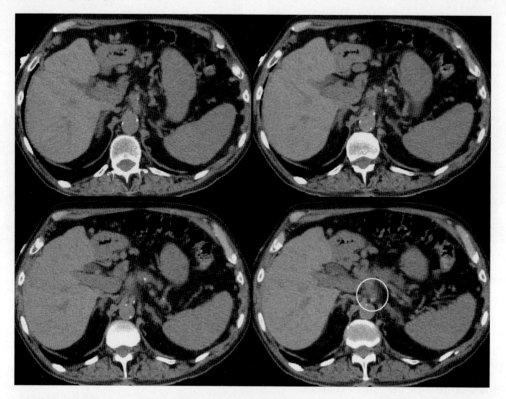

The celiac artery is thickened on all images. There is a little perivascular fat infiltration lower right around the origin of the SMA (*circle*).

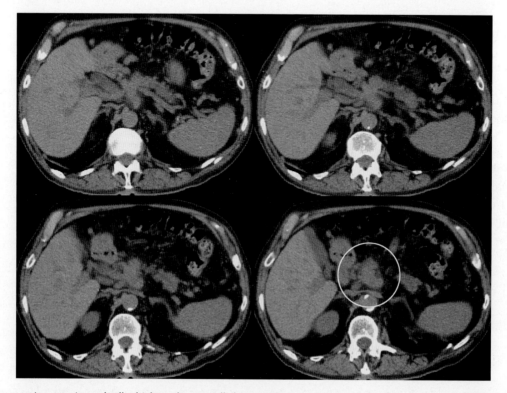

The superior mesenteric artery is markedly thickened, especially lower right (*circle*). There is subtle fat infiltration adjacent to it on all images. No obvious pancreatic mass on either of the above images. Diagnosis of pancreatic carcinoma was not made.

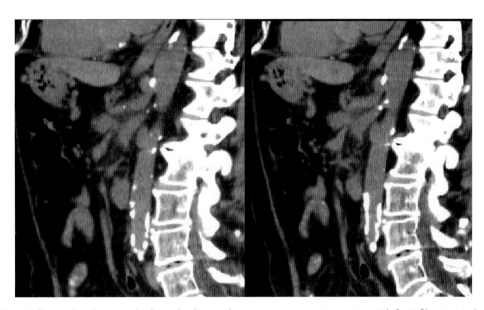

Adjacent sagittal slices, left to right, showing thickened celiac and superior mesenteric arteries with fat infiltration in between them. Diagnosis of pancreatic carcinoma was still not made.

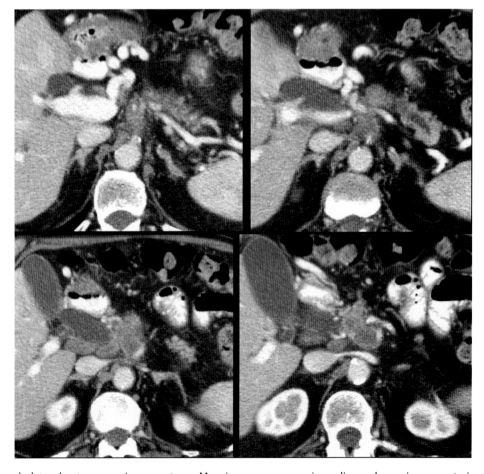

Follow-up scan 6 weeks later due to worsening symptoms. Mass is now seen encasing celiac and superior mesenteric arteries, causing intra- and extrahepatic ductal dilatation. Hypodense mass is seen extending posteromedially from neck of the pancreas with proximal pancreatic ductal dilatation.

Answers

1. The thick vessel sign involving the celiac and superior mesenteric arteries points to the correct diagnosis of carcinoma of the pancreas, which can be confirmed and staged with follow-up postcontrast arterial and venous phase CT.

2. A hypodense mass extending posteriorly from the neck/body of the pancreas encases the celiac and superior mesenteric arteries and causes intra- and extrahepatic biliary ductal dilatation with proximal pancreatic ductal dilatation. Obstruction of the splenic and superior mesenteric veins was seen on other images. Findings are diagnostic of duct cell adenocarcinoma of the pancreas.

3. Patients coming to the ER with back pain may get a stone protocol CT and turn out to have pancreatic cancer.

   Although contrast-induced nephropathy may be a myth and contrast reactions are few and far between some patients with pancreatic carcinoma still get noncontrast CT.

   ER patients with PE protocol CTs may have pancreatic carcinoma either incidentally or their pancreatic carcinoma has caused venous thromboembolism. Because of the bolus timing the pancreas at the bottom of the stack will look like a noncontrast scan of the pancreas.

4. US: usually solid hypoechoic, can be isoechoic

   Noncontrast CT: hypodense or isodense mass, almost never with calcification, little or no necrosis. Abnormal gland contour, loss of marbling and/or loss of lobulation, rounded uncinate process, "normal" head with atrophy body and tail, thick vessel.

   CECT: usually hypoenhancing in arterial and portal venous phases, sometimes isodense (delayed enhancement very helpful in latter case).

   MRI: lack of the normally increased pancreatic gland signal on T1 fat sat. Same postcontrast features as CT.

   Ancillary signs all modalities:

   Dilated biliary and/or pancreatic ducts with abrupt obstruction. Double duct sign (anatomically contiguous stenosis or obstruction of the common bile duct and the pancreatic duct).

   Signs of unresectability such as encased/obstructed vessels, liver metastases usually present.

5. If you suspect pancreatic carcinoma and different imaging examinations yield conflicting results, the examination looking like pancreatic carcinoma is probably correct. Proving it by biopsy or even surgery is reasonable. Follow-up imaging in 6 to 12 months is not reasonable considering the aggressiveness of pancreatic carcinoma. The Tahiti treatment (6 months all expenses paid trip to Tahiti) is really not a bad option—it will save the insurance company money and if the patient does have pancreatic carcinoma at least they will enjoy their last months, but it is facetious.

Pearls

- Thickening of peripancreatic vessels, especially the celiac and superior mesenteric arteries, is a sign suggesting pancreatic carcinoma visible on noncontrast CT. Postcontrast scans of thick vessels show encasement, occlusion, and/or perivascular fat infiltration. Sometimes the pancreatic mass will be invisible or inapparent even when the vessels are thickened. Ability to diagnose pancreatic carcinoma on noncontrast scans is more important in today's era of noncontrast stone protocol CT.
- Other signs of pancreatic carcinoma on noncontrast CT:
  - Focal isodense or slightly hypodense mass, almost never with calcification, little or no necrosis.
  - Abnormal gland contour.
  - Loss of marbling and/or loss of lobulation.
  - Rounded uncinate process.
  - Normal head with atrophy body and tail.

Suggested Readings

Sai M, Mori H, Kiyonaga M, Kosen K, Yamada Y, Matsumoto S. Peripancreatic lymphatic invasion by pancreatic carcinoma: evaluation with multi-detector row CT. *Abdom Imaging*. April 2010;35(2):154-162.

Vikram R, Balachandran A, Bhosale PR, Tamm EP, Marcal LP, Charnsangavej C. Pancreas: peritoneal reflections, ligamentous connections, and pathways of disease spread. *Radiographics*. July 2009;29(2):e34.

Zhang XM, Mitchell DG, Witkiewicz A, Verma S, Bergin D. Extrapancreatic neural plexus invasion by pancreatic carcinoma: characteristics on magnetic resonance imaging. *Abdom Imaging*. April 2010;34(5):634-641.

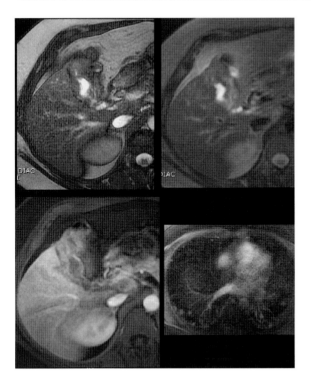

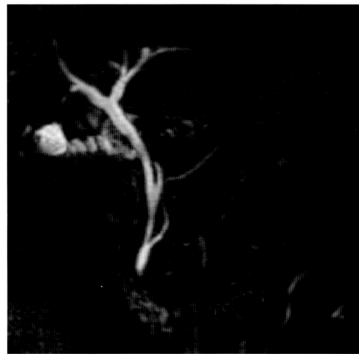

1. Based on the MRI top left, what is the best diagnosis?

2. What is the risk factor for GB carcinoma illustrated in top right MRCP and following CT and ERCP?

3. What are the types of GB carcinoma?

4. What are the three broad clinical scenarios in which GB carcinoma presents?

5. What are the three common imaging manifestations of GB carcinoma?

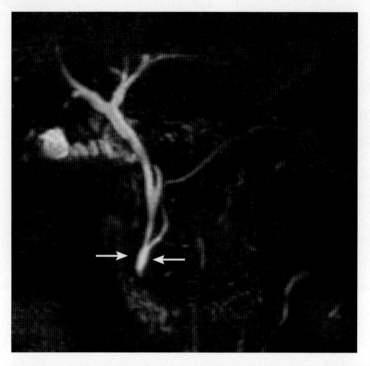

MIP of MRCP 1.4-mm-thick sections shows a long common channel (*arrows*) between the common bile duct and the pancreatic duct (12-17 mm depending on the modality). The cystic duct is seen joining the common hepatic duct cephalad to the junction of the pancreatic duct and the common bile duct.

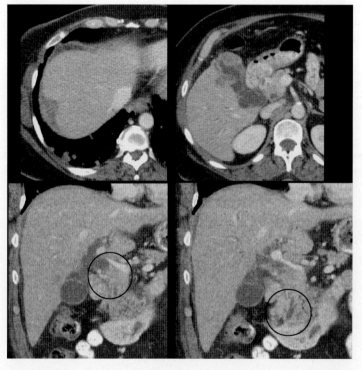

CT scan 6 months later after development of jaundice. Peritoneal implant and lung metastases top left. GB mass invading liver (*top right*). Common duct obstruction due to mass in the hepatoduodenal ligament (*circle*) (*bottom left*) and long common channel between pancreatic duct and common bile duct (*circle*) (*lower right*).

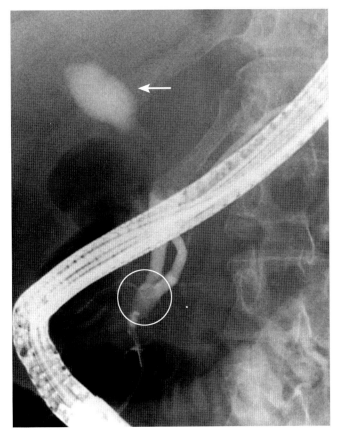

ERCP next day shows very dilated common bile duct (*arrow*) proximal to a long segment high-grade stenosis and a long common channel (*circle*).

Answers

1. The asymmetric irregular GB wall thickening with heterogenous enhancement accompanied by invasion of the liver and lung metastases all point to gallbladder carcinoma.

2. High confluence of the pancreaticobiliary ducts can be defined as a common channel that is 6 mm or greater in length. There is increased risk of GB carcinoma in patients with a common channel which is associated with GB mucosal proliferative changes. Prophylactic cholecystectomy is advised by some.

3. Approximately 80% of GB carcinomas are adenocarcinomas. Subtypes include papillary, nodular, and tubular adenoca.

   Papillary tumors (grow intraluminally) have a better prognosis.

   Less common types of GB carcinomas include squamous cell carcinoma, cystadenocarcinoma, small cell carcinoma, and adenoacanthoma.

4. GB carcinoma is typically detected in one of the following three scenarios:

   1. Incidental finding during or after cholecystectomy for gallstones

   2. Suspected or confirmed neoplasm that appears to be resectable after preoperative evaluation

   3. Advanced, unresectable intra-abdominal malignancy

5. GB carcinoma appears on all imaging techniques as a mass completely occupying or replacing the gallbladder lumen, focal or diffuse asymmetric gallbladder wall thickening, or an intraluminal polypoid mass.

Pearls

- Well known is the increased risk of GB carcinoma due to gallstones and porcelain GB; not so is the increased risk in patients with a common pancreaticobiliary ductal channel.
- GB carcinoma has three imaging presentations:
  - Mass replacing GB (40%-65%): large mass replacing the GB lumen, often with invasion of adjacent liver.
    - US: heterogeneous, predominantly hypoechoic tumor fills much of the GB lumen, echogenic shadowing foci, and wall thickening
    - CT or MRI: intense irregular enhancement at the periphery of large GB carcinomas during the early arterial phase with slow washout
  - Focal or diffuse asymmetric wall thickening (20%-30%):
    - Asymmetric, irregular, or extensive thickening with marked arterial phase enhancement persisting into portal venous phase.
  - Polypoid intraluminal no wall thickening (15%-25%):
    - Malignant GB polyps usually >1 cm; may have thickened implantation base, will enhance with contrast.

Suggested Readings

Furlan A, Ferris JV, Hosseinzadeh K, Borhani AA. Gallbladder carcinoma update: multimodality imaging evaluation, staging, and treatment options. *AJR Am J Roentgenol.* November 2008;191(5):1440-1447.

Hara H, Morita S, Sako S, et al. Relationship between types of common channel and development of biliary tract cancer in pancreaticobiliary maljunction. *Hepatogastroenterology.* March-April 2002;49(44):322-325.

Kamisawa T, Funata N, Hayashi Y, et al. *Gastrointest Endosc.* July 2004;60(1):56-60.

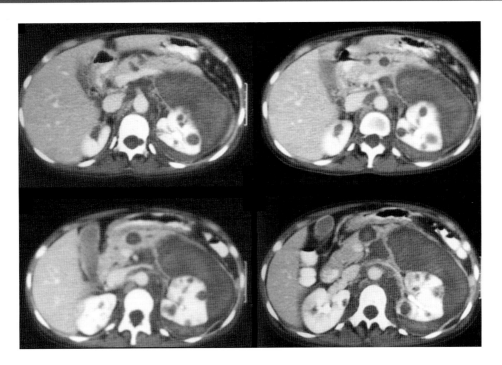

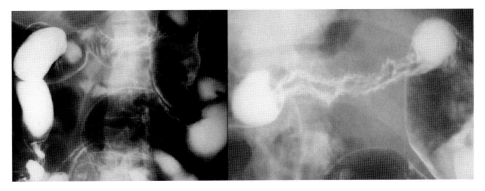

1. What are the some causes of multiple
   pancreatic masses as seen in the CT on top?
   The barium enema is of a different patient with
   the same diagnosis.

2. Combining the perirenal hematoma and the
   findings in the kidneys and pancreas, what is
   the best diagnosis based on the CT scan?

3. What are the gastrointestinal tract
   manifestations of PAN?

4. What are the arteriographic findings in PAN?

5. What are the renal manifestations of PAN?

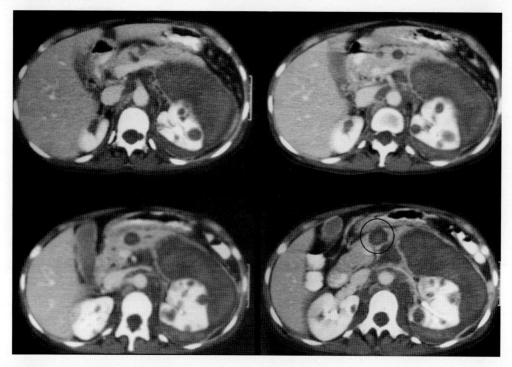

There is a large left perirenal fluid collection with an enhancing rim and higher than water central attenuation due to a large hematoma. Multiple round hypodense masses are present in the kidneys (*left more than right*) and pancreas. In some of the masses central high attenuation is seen (*best in pancreas, circle top right*). These are likely aneurysms with surrounding hematomas. Purely cystic masses could be old hematomas, infarcts, or thrombosed aneurysms.

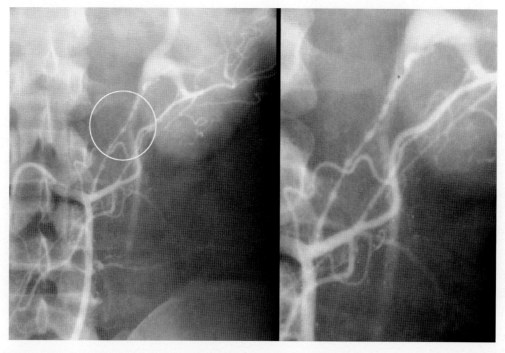

Inferior mesenteric arteriogram on the same patient as Image 2 with colonic disease shows alternating stenosis and ectasia (*circle, left*). Magnification right.

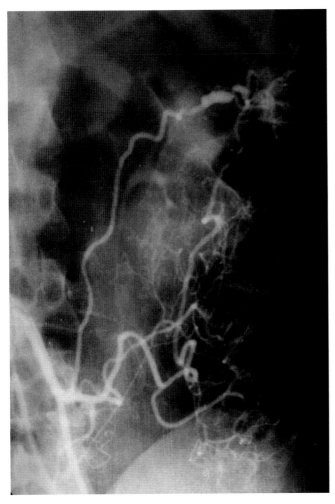

After a course of corticosteroids repeat angiography shows improvement.

Answers

1. Metastases to the pancreas and lymphoma are causes of multiple pancreatic masses. Lung, breast, renal cell, and GI tract carcinomas and melanoma are the common primaries. IPMNs can be multiple. Multiple pancreatic masses are characteristic of Type 1 multiple endocrine neoplasia and von Hippel Lindau syndromes.

2. Absent evidence of renal neoplasm the most common cause of spontaneous perirenal hemorrhage is polyarteritis nodosa (PAN). The low-density masses in the kidneys and pancreas are consistent with aneurysms/pseudoaneurysms/small hematomas due to PAN, which is the best diagnosis.

3. The gastrointestinal tract (50% of patients) may be affected with ulceration, perforation, hemorrhage, or infarction. Imaging findings are small and/or large bowel wall thickening, mesenteric vascular engorgement and haziness, ascites, luminal narrowing with obstruction, or diffuse mucosal fold thickening. The liver, pancreas, or spleen may have infarcts or hematomas.

4. Multiple small aneurysms (2-5 mm commonly at branch points) in the renal and visceral arteries very suggestive of PAN but other vasculitides must be considered.

   Sometimes larger aneurysms are found.

   Ectatic and stenotic arterial segments or occlusions may be seen.

5. Renal manifestations (90% of PAN patients) are acute or chronic renal failure, nephrotic syndrome, proteinuria, hematuria, and perirenal hemorrhage. Renal ischemia and infarcts can occur.

Pearls

- Multiple small aneurysms (2-5 mm commonly at branch points) on abdominal arteriograms are nearly pathognomonic for PAN if it is suspected clinically.
- Renal arteries and visceral arteries can be affected.
- Sometimes larger aneurysms and/or pseudoaneurysms form.
- Ectatic and stenotic arterial segments or occlusions may be seen.
- Differential diagnosis of multiple aneurysms: heroin and methamphetamine abuse, Wegener granulomatosis, systemic lupus erythematosus, diabetes, rheumatoid arthritis, giant cell temporal arteritis, and segmental mediolytic arteriopathy (splenic and hepatic arteries).
- Arterial phase MDCT has been effective in showing some microaneurysms in PAN and is better than MRA due to superior spatial resolution.

Suggested Readings

Baishya RK, Dhawan DR, Sabnis RB, Desai MR. Spontaneous subcapsular renal hematoma: a case report and review of literature. *Urol Ann.* January-April 2011; 3(1):44-46.

Ozaki K, Miyayama S, Ushiogi Y, Matsui O. Renal involvement of polyarteritis nodosa: CT and MR findings. *Abdom Imaging.* November 2011;34(2):265-270.

Rhodes ES, Pekala JS, Gemery JM, Dickey KW. Case 129: polyarteritis nodosa. *Radiology.* January 2008;246(1): 322-326.

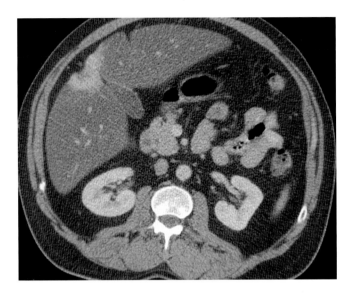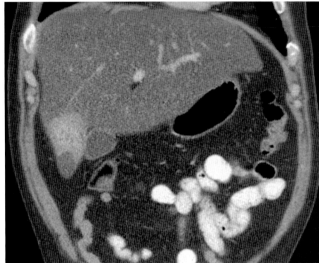

1. What is the differential diagnosis of this finding?

2. What features favor peripheral cholangiocarcinoma rather than hepatocellular carcinoma?

3. What are the causes of delayed persistent enhancement of liver lesions?

4. What is the component of cholangiocarcinoma responsible for central T2 hypointensity on MRI?

5. What are the imaging findings that can differentiate peripheral cholangiocarcinoma from metastasis?

Case ranking/difficulty: **Category:** Biliary tract

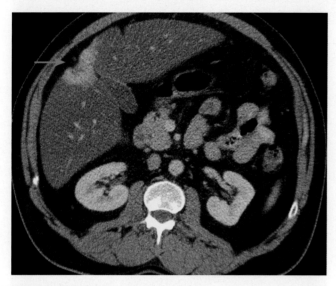

Axial CT in portal venous phase shows peripheral enhancing focal lesion with capsular retraction (*green arrow*).

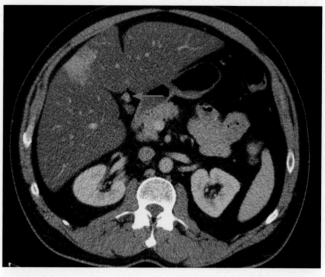

Additional finding is an enhancing lymph node in the porta hepatis (*green arrow*).

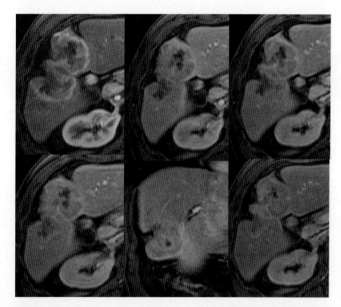

Dynamic contrast-enhanced MR as a follow-up of a CT diagnosis of focal fatty sparing (3 years after the CT) demonstrates peripheral rim enhancement, progressive concentric central filling, and persistent delayed enhancement (fibrous tissue).

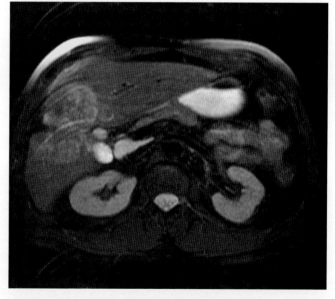

Axial MRI T2W image (3 years after the CT) shows areas of hypo- and hyperintensity (corresponds to the areas of delayed persistent enhancement and non enhancement on DCE study), consistent with fibrosis and necrosis, respectively

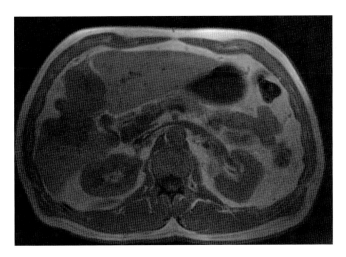

Axial MRI T1 in-phase image (3 years after the CT) shows hypointensity of the lesion.

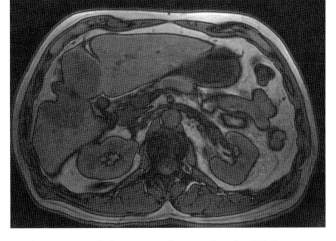

Axial MRI T1 out-of-phase image (3 years after the CT) shows no signal drop in comparison to in-phase image.

Answers

1. Cholangiocarcinoma, focal confluent fibrosis, sclerosing hemangioma, and HCC could be responsible for this liver mass with capsular retraction. Dynamic contrast-enhanced study is necessary for further differentiation between these masses.

2. Central T2 hypodensity, capsular retraction, delayed persistent enhancement, and biliary invasion favor cholangiocarcinoma. T2 hyperintensity, early arterial enhancement with venous washout and delayed capsular enhancement, mass effect, and venous invasion favor HCC.

3. Cholangiocarcinoma, metastasis, and focal confluent fibrosis are all potential causes of delayed persistent enhancement.

4. Fibrosis causes low signal intensity on T2W MR images of cholangiocarcinoma.

5. No imaging finding can differentiate among these two entities. Biliary duct dilatation is helpful for the diagnosis of ICC but it can be seen in metastasis. The central T2 hypointensity is characteristic of cholangiocarcinoma but not diagnostic. It is also common in colorectal metastasis. Rim enhancement and delayed persistent enhancement do not exclude metastasis; indeed the pathologist cannot reliably differentiate ICC from a GI metastasis to the liver.

Pearls

- Salient imaging features are peripheral rim-like enhancement, centripetal filling but not becoming isodense or isointense to vessels (unlike hemangioma), and persistent delayed enhancement.
- Capsular retraction is a classical finding (also seen in sclerosing hemangioma and focal confluent fibrosis).
- Biliary duct dilatation favors the diagnosis of ICC over HCC. Venous invasion favors HCC. ICC presents late, metastasizes early, and has a poor prognosis.

Suggested Readings

Chung YE, Kim MJ, Park YN, et al. Varying appearances of cholangiocarcinoma: radiologic-pathologic correlation. *Radiographics*. 2009 Nov;29(3):683-700.

Maetani Y, Itoh K, Watanabe C, et al. MR imaging of intrahepatic cholangiocarcinoma with pathologic correlation. *AJR Am J Roentgenol*. 2001 Jun;176(6): 1499-1507.

Sainani NI, Catalano OA, Holalkere NS, Zhu AX, Hahn PF, Sahani DV. Cholangiocarcinoma: current and novel imaging techniques. *Radiographics*. 2009 Nov;28(5):1263-1287.

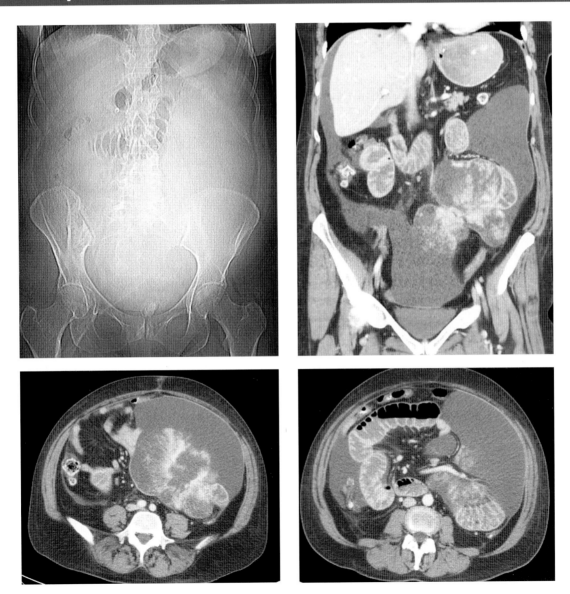

1. What are the imaging findings?

2. What is the differential diagnosis of a mesenteric cyst?

3. What is the most common primary mesenteric neoplasm?

4. What is the most common cause of mesenteric lymphadenopathy?

5. What is the most common primary peritoneal malignant tumor?

Case ranking/difficulty: 🦃🦃🦃

Answers

1. Mesenteric or bowel mass, small bowel obstruction, and ascites are the imaging findings.

2. Lymphangioma, enteric cyst, duplication cyst, and mesothelial cyst are the differential diagnoses of a mesenteric cyst. Lymphangioma is the commonest.

3. Desmoid is the most common primary tumor of small bowel mesentery. Patients with Gardner syndrome are at increased risk of developing a desmoid tumor. It is benign, locally aggressive, and invasive. Postsurgical recurrence is frequent. Metastases are much more common than primary malignant mesenteric tumors. GI and ovarian carcinomas are the most common primaries to metastasize to the omentum and mesentery.

4. Non-Hodgkin lymphoma is the most common cause of mesenteric lymphadenopathy.

5. Mesothelioma. Associated pleural calcifications, thickening, and effusions are common. History of asbestosis exposure may be present. Only minimal ascites are present compared to the bulky soft tissue mass. Treatment is cytoreduction and chemotherapy.

Pearls

- Any solid mesenteric mass, other than reactive lymph node or lymphoma, needs surgical removal.
- Malignant solid tumors are usually located close to the root of mesentery and benign tumors in the periphery of the mesentery.
- Two-thirds of primary mesenteric tumors are mesenchymal in origin (mostly leiomyosarcoma and liposarcoma).
- Mesenchymal origin needs consideration whenever there is no definite bowel origin identified.

Suggested Readings

Eltweri AM, Gravante G, Read-Jones SL, Rai S, Bowrey DJ, Haynes IG. A case of recurrent mesocolon myxoid liposarcoma and review of the literature. *Case Rep Oncol Med.* 2013;2013(2013):692754.

Faria SC, Iyer RB, Rashid A, Ellis L, Whitman GJ. Desmoid tumor of the small bowel and the mesentery. *AJR Am J Roentgenol.* 2004 Jul;183(1):118.

Souza FF, Jagganathan J, Ramayia N, et al. Recurrent malignant peritoneal mesothelioma: radiological manifestations. *Abdom Imaging.* 2010 Jun;35(3):315-321.

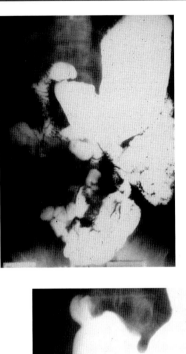
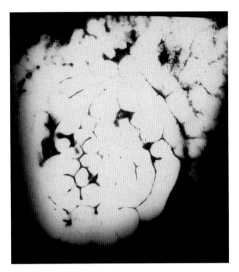
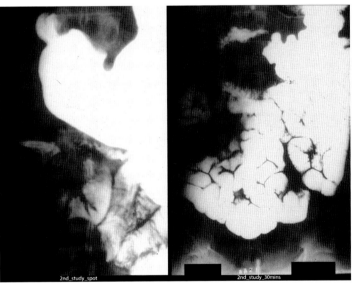

1. What is the most likely diagnosis? The top two images are from the same UGI/SBFT. The bottom two are from a repeat examination for confirmation.

2. What is the location of right paraduodenal hernia?

3. What predisposes to right paraduodenal hernia?

4. What are the small bowel series (SBFT) and CT findings of right paraduodenal hernia (RPDH)?

5. What are the vascular findings of RPDH on CT?

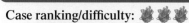
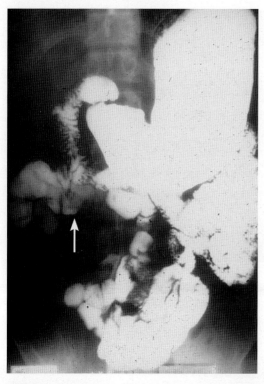

30-minute overhead showing entrance loops (*arrow*) to the right of and inferior to the descending duodenum.

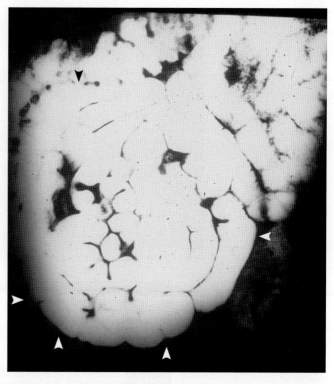

60-minute overhead showing large round encapsulated bowel collection that moved as a unit fluoroscopically (*arrowheads*). It is located just off midline slightly toward the right lower quadrant.

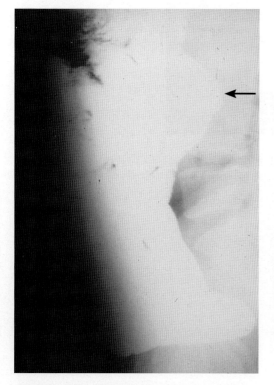

Erect lateral examination showing small bowel overlapping the spine (*arrow*).

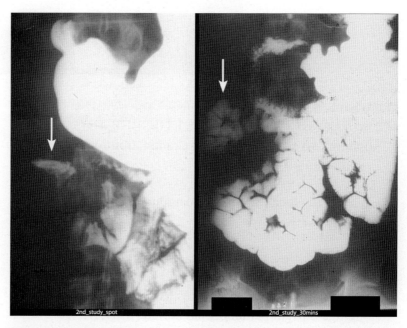

Second (a repeat) study shows the entrance loops again to the right of the descending duodenum (*arrows*). Spot film, left; 30-minute overhead, right.

Answers

1. There is a large round encapsulated bowel collection (located just off midline slightly toward the right lower quadrant) that moved as a unit fluoroscopically. It overlaps the spine on an erect lateral. It has entrance loops to the right of and inferior to the descending duodenum. This was confirmed on a repeat examination. These findings are consistent with right paraduodenal hernia.

2. Right paraduodenal herniated contents are located in the right half of the transverse mesocolon and behind the ascending mesocolon.

3. Waldeyer fossa (representing a defect in the first part of the jejunal mesentery), behind the SMA and inferior to the transverse (third) portion of the duodenum is found in less than 1% of the population and predisposes to right paraduodenal hernia, as does nonrotated small bowel.

4. SBFT: Encapsulated, ovoid collection of bowel loops is noted lateral and inferior to the descending duodenum. Both the afferent and efferent loops of bowel are closely opposed and narrowed. Small bowel overlapping the spine on an erect lateral film is suggestive.

   On CT an encapsulated cluster of small-bowel loops is noted in the right midabdomen, with looping of the small bowel around the SMA and SMV at the root of the small-bowel mesentery being seen occasionally. Small-bowel nonrotation as evidenced by the superior mesenteric vein occupying a more ventral and leftward position and the absence of a normal horizontal duodenum may be present.

5. In RPDH CT may show:

   1. Jejunal branches of the SMA and SMV looping posteriorly and to the right of the parent vessel to supply the herniated loops

   2. Presence of the SMA, ileocolic artery, and right colic vein in the anterior margin of the neck of the hernial sac, sometimes displaced by bowel

   3. Vessel engorgement

Pearls

- Small bowel series: Large ovoid encapsulated collection of bowel loops lateral and inferior to the descending duodenum. Afferent and efferent loops of bowel are closely opposed and narrowed. Small bowel overlapping the spine on an erect lateral film is suggestive.
- CT: An encapsulated cluster of small-bowel loops is noted in the right mid abdomen, with looping of the small bowel around the SMA and SMV at the root of the small-bowel mesentery being seen occasionally. Small bowel nonrotation may be present with cecum in normal position.

Suggested Readings

Abdullah A, Elsamaloty H, Patel Y, Castillo-Sang M. Small bowel obstruction due to a right-sided paraduodenal hernia: a case report. *Abdom Imaging*. October 2010;35(5):571-573.

Liao YH, Lin CH, Lin WC. Right paraduodenal hernia: characteristic MDCT findings. *Abdom Imaging*. April 2011;36(2):130-133.

Takeyama N, Gokan T, Ohgiya Y, et al. CT of internal hernias. *Radiographics*. 2005;5:997-1015. doi: 10.148/rg.54045035.

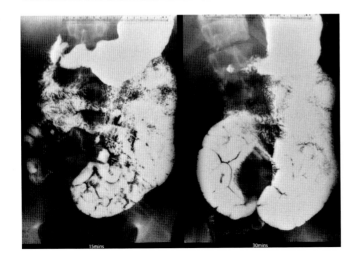 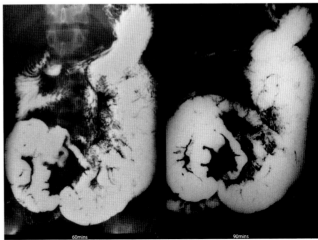

1. What is the best diagnosis based on the four images above as well as the additional images on the next 3 pages?

2. What does a left paraduodenal hernia herniate through?

3. What are the types of congenital internal hernias and their relative frequency?

4. What are the clinical features of left paraduodenal hernia?

5. What vascular changes that can be seen on CT are suggestive of left paraduodenal hernia?

Case ranking/difficulty: **Category:** Small bowel

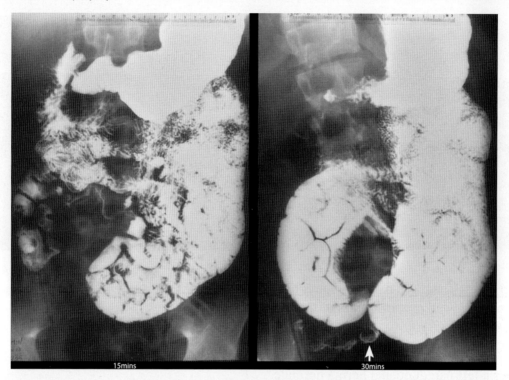

15- and 30-minute overheads show the small bowel loops in one large group with a smooth contour. Fluoroscopically they moved as a unit. The loop leaving the hernia sac is on lower right (*arrow*). Most loops are to the left of the midline.

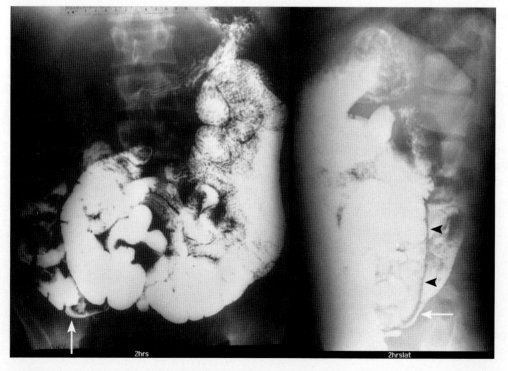

2-hour AP and lateral films show colon and appendix filling (*arrows*). The group of small bowel loops persists. The sac surrounding them is seen as a lucency (*arrowheads*) on the lateral film. Small bowel overlaps the spine on the lateral film, which is abnormal (*erect lateral is better for this sign*).

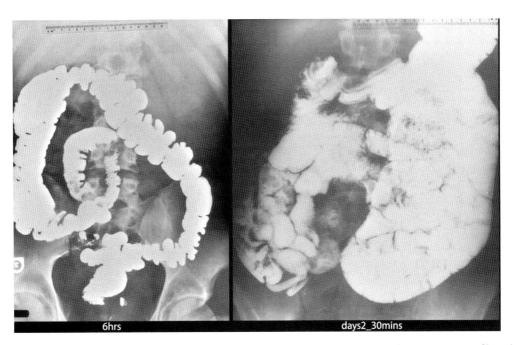

6-hour film (*left*) shows depression of the splenic flexure, a finding seen in this entity. On the right is a 30-minute film taken from a repeat examination the next day recapitulating the group of small bowel loops.

Answers

1. There is a group of loops with smooth border consistent with a sac. A loop exiting the group is seen. The group of loops overlies the lumbar spine (positioned more posterior than normal). Almost entire small bowel is in the hernia. The epicenter is to the left of midline and the splenic flexure is displaced downward. These findings are consistent with left paraduodenal hernia.

2. Left paraduodenal hernias are through Landzert fossa, an aperture seen in about 2% of people. It is located behind the ascending (fourth) part of the duodenum. It is formed by the lifting up of a peritoneal fold by the inferior mesenteric vein and ascending left colic artery as they run along the lateral side of the fossa.

3. Congenital types of internal hernias based on location:
   - Paraduodenal (53%), left 3× as common as right
   - Pericecal (13%),
   - Foramen of Winslow (8%),
   - Transmesenteric and transmesocolic (8%),
   - Intersigmoid (6%),
   - Retroanastomotic (5%)
   - Missing 7% described by Meyers were paravesical hernias, which are no longer considered true internal hernias

4. Left paraduodenal hernia patients often present with chronic postprandial pain. Additional symptoms include nausea, vomiting, and recurrent intestinal obstruction. Severity relates to the duration and reducibility of the hernia and the presence or absence of incarceration and strangulation. Symptoms may be altered or relieved by changes in patient position. Since these hernias often spontaneously reduce, patients are best imaged when they are symptomatic.

5. Mesenteric vessel abnormalities suggesting left paraduodenal hernia (LPDH) are:
   1. Enlargement, stretching, and anterior displacement of the main mesenteric trunks to the left.
   2. Engorged vessels grouped together at the entrance of the hernia sac, with proximal jejunal arteries showing an abrupt change of direction posteriorly behind the IMA.
   3. The IMV and ascending left colic artery lie in the anterior wall of the left paraduodenal hernia above the encapsulated bowel loops.

Pearls

- Since left paraduodenal hernias often spontaneously reduce, patients are best imaged when they are symptomatic.

- Small bowel series:
  - An encapsulated circumscribed group of small bowel loops (usually jejunal) in the LUQ, lateral to the ascending duodenum. May depress the distal transverse colon and/or the duodenojejunal junction inferomedially and/or indent the posterior wall of the stomach.
  - Mild proximal duodenal dilatation and abrupt efferent loop caliber change are additional findings.
  - Fluoroscopically movement of a group of loops as a unit or fixation may be noted. Segmental reversed peristalsis has been seen.
  - On an erect lateral film overlap of the spine by small bowel suggests paraduodenal hernia.
- CT: Similar encapsulated group of small bowel loops seen, either:
  - At the duodenojejunal junction between the stomach and pancreas to the left of the ligament of Treitz
  - Behind the pancreatic tail displacing the inferior mesenteric vein to the left or
  - Between the transverse colon and the left adrenal gland

Suggested Readings

Blachar A, Federle MP, Dodson SF. Internal hernia: clinical and imaging findings in 17 patients with emphasis on CT criteria. *Radiology*. January 2001;218(1):68-74.

Osadchy A, Weisenberg N, Wiener Y, Shapiro-Feinberg M, Zissin R. Small bowel obstruction related to left-side paraduodenal hernia: CT findings. *Abdom Imaging*. 2004;30(1):53-55.

Takeyama N, Gokan T, Ohgiya Y, et al. CT of internal hernias. *Radiographics*. 2005;5:997-1015. doi:10.148/rg.54045035.

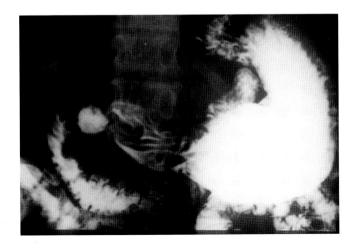 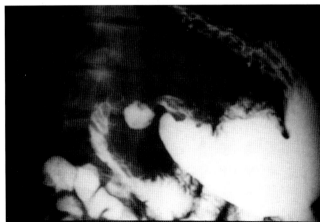

1. Based on the above images, what is your diagnosis?

2. What are the three entities that giant duodenal ulcer is most likely mistaken for?

3. What are some clinical manifestations of giant duodenal ulcer?

4. How does one fluoroscopically differentiate giant duodenal ulcer from a normal or mildly deformed bulb?

5. What is the current treatment for giant duodenal ulcers?

Case ranking/difficulty:

Category: Duodenum

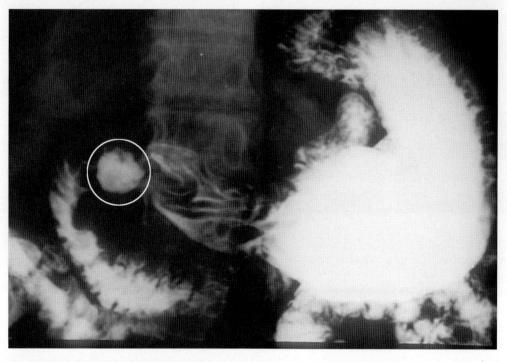

AP: Barium collection (*circle*) with some nodularity but without normal folds in the region of the bulb. Crater is fixed without change over time. Mild mass effect on c-loop. No normal bulb.

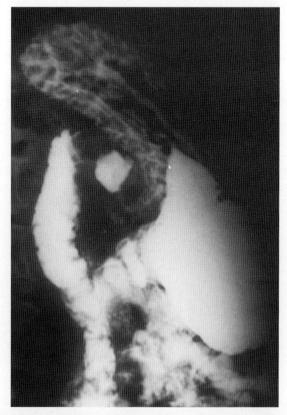

Lateral: persistent large collection of barium. No normal bulb.

Answers

1. The fixed barium collection with no fold pattern and lack of a normal bulb strongly suggest giant ulcer of the duodenum and the history of UGI bleeding and abdominal pain is consistent.

2. Although pancreatic cancer and mesenchymal neoplasm merit some consideration, giant duodenal ulcer (GDU) is most likely to be confused with a normal or deformed bulb or a duodenal diverticulum.

3. Symptoms of GDU are commonly abdominal pain and upper GI bleeding. The latter can be massive. The size of the ulcer and the surrounding inflammatory mass may cause gastric outlet obstruction and weight loss. Perforation and fistula formation may occur.

4. All of the below help differentiate a giant ulcer from a normal bulb:

   1. Consistency in size and shape of crater

   2. Loss of normal mucosal pattern

   3. Constriction of the gastrointestinal tract proximal and distal to the ulcer

   4. Nodularity in the ulcer crater

   5. Prolonged barium retention in the crater

   6. Ulcer within the giant ulcer

   7. Surrounding mass effect

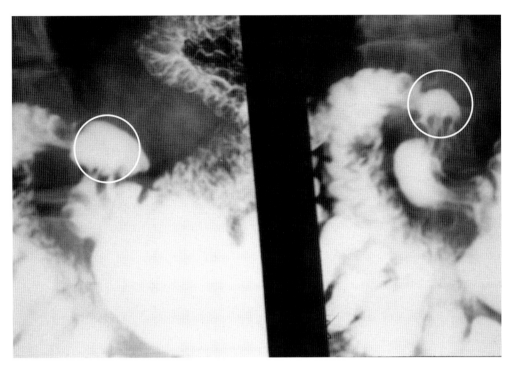

Two months later after maximal medical therapy the ulcer is healed. RAO on the left, AP on the right. Normal bulb seen (*circle*).

The lack of change in shape and size of a GDU is the single feature most useful in distinguishing it from a normal duodenal bulb.

5. GDU was classically treated with surgery and mortality was high. Now aggressive medical therapy with proton pump inhibitors, withdrawal of NSAIDs, and eradication of *H pylori* is usually successful.

Emergent surgery is indicated for uncontrolled hemorrhage or perforation. Elective surgery is indicated for unresolving obstruction, intractable or recurrent bleeding, and fistula formation.

Pearls

- Differentiation of GDU (defined as benign, full-thickness ulcer at least 2 cm in diameter involving a large portion of the duodenal bulb) from a normal bulb:
  - Consistency in size and shape of crater
  - Loss of normal mucosal pattern
  - Constriction of the gastrointestinal tract proximal and distal to the ulcer

- Nodularity in the ulcer crater
- Prolonged barium retention in the crater
- Ulcer within the giant ulcer
- Surrounding mass effect
- The lack of change in shape and size of a GDU is the single feature most useful in distinguishing it from a normal duodenal bulb.

Suggested Readings

Malangoni MA. Commentary: perforated giant duodenal ulcers: what is the best treatment? *Am J Surg*. September 2009;198(3):324.

Newton EB, Versland MR, Sepe TE. Giant duodenal ulcers. *World J Gastroenterol*. 2008; August 28;14(32): 4995-4999. doi:10.748/wjg.4.995.

Thompson WM, Norton G, Kelvin FM et al. Unusual manifestations of peptic ulcer disease. *Radiographics*. 1981;1:1-16.

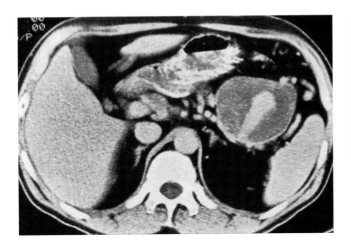 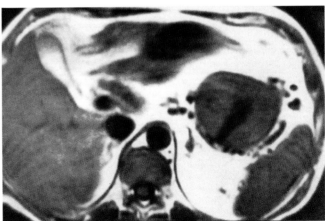

1. On the above images what is your differential diagnosis?

2. Given the history of pancreatitis, what diagnosis is best?

3. What imaging test could confirm the diagnosis of splenic artery pseudoaneurysm?

4. What is the yin-yang sign?

5. What is the preferred treatment of splenic artery pseudoaneurysm?

Case ranking/difficulty: **Category:** Spleen

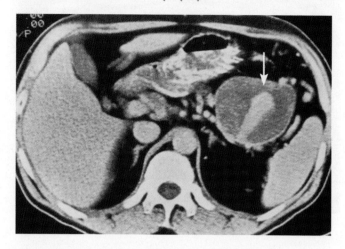

Pseudoaneurysm is seen as a mass in the hilum of the spleen. Most of the mass is low-density thrombus. There is a higher density elliptical enhancing patent central lumen (*arrow*).

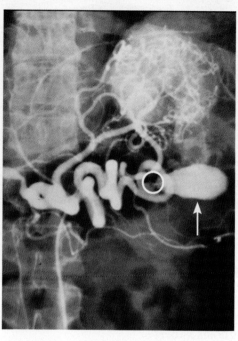

On the celiac arteriogram, the large oval patent lumen (*arrow*) corresponds to the cross-sectional findings. It communicates through a narrow neck (*circle*) with the splenic artery.

Answers

1. Mucinous cystic neoplasm of the pancreas deserves some consideration given this large well-circumscribed mass. The mass is larger than most pseudoaneurysms, but pseudoaneurysm is likely. Islet cell tumors can undergo central necrosis, but the center of this mass seems to be enhancing on CT. Carcinoma of the pancreas this large would not be well circumscribed. Epidermoid cyst in an intrapancreatic spleen is unlikely to be this large.

2. The central enhancement on CT and the corresponding area of signal void on MR consistent with flowing blood point to a splenic artery pseudoaneurysm.

3. Doppler sonography would show the yin-yang sign and confirm the diagnosis. Multiphasic contrast-enhanced CTA or MRA would show arterial enhancement and rapid washout and communication of the patent lumen with the splenic artery diagnostic of pseudoaneurysm. PET-CT would be of no help. Angiography would be diagnostic but should only be needed for therapy.

4. In Chinese philosophy, the concept of yin-yang is used to describe how seemingly opposite or contrary forces are interconnected and interdependent in the natural world and how they give rise to each other as they interrelate to one another. The sign refers to color Doppler when a pseudoaneurysm contains both flow toward the transducer and away from the transducer, giving a picture of half blue and half red.

5. The preferred treatment is intraarterial embolization. Rupture and hemorrhage may be fatal and is to be avoided.

Pearls

- Pseudoaneurysms due to pancreatitis affect the splenic artery most often, followed by the pancreaticoduodenal and gastroduodenal arteries. The left gastric, hepatic, and small intrapancreatic arteries are involved less often.
- Arterial bleeding is a life-threatening complication.
- In patients who have a history of pancreatitis, one should suspect a pseudoaneurysm when transient vascular enhancement is seen in a cystic pancreatic region mass or in the central portion of a solid mass. Smaller pseudoaneurysms are mostly patent and "cystic" whereas large ones can be mostly solid (thrombus) with a small central patent (cystic) portion.
- Therefore on imaging, a pseudoaneurysm can be seen as a completely or partially vascular cystic or solid mass.

Suggested Readings

Ikeda O, Kume S, Torigoe Y, et al. Hemorrhage into pancreatic pseudocyst. *Abdom Imaging*. July 2007;32(3):370-373.

Smith RE, Fontanez-Garcia D, Plavsic BM. Gastrointestinal case of the day. Pseudoaneurysm of the left gastric artery as a complication of acute pancreatitis. *Radiographics*. June 1999;19(5):1390-1392.

Trout AT, Elsayes KM, Ellis JH, Francis IR. Imaging of acute pancreatitis: prognostic value of computed tomographic findings. *J Comput Assist Tomogr*. July 2010;34(4):485-495.

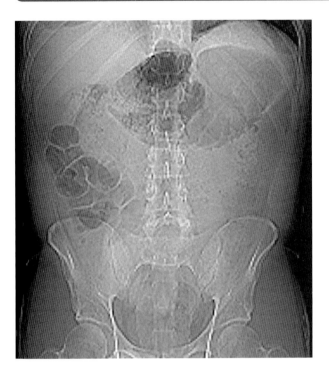

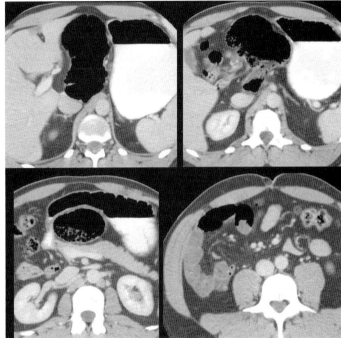

1. What is the most likely diagnosis?

2. What anatomic structures can herniate into the lesser sac via the foramen of Winslow?

3. What are predisposing conditions for foramen of Winslow hernia?

4. What are the imaging findings of foramen of Winslow hernia?

5. What differentiates foramen of Winslow hernia (FofWH) from left paraduodenal hernia (LPDH)?

Case ranking/difficulty:

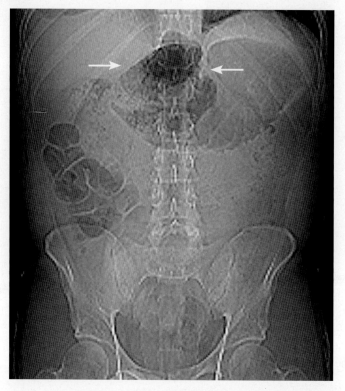

CT scout shows an unusual gas collection (*arrows*) superior to the gastric antrum and medial to the gastric fundus. There is no colon in the right lower quadrant.

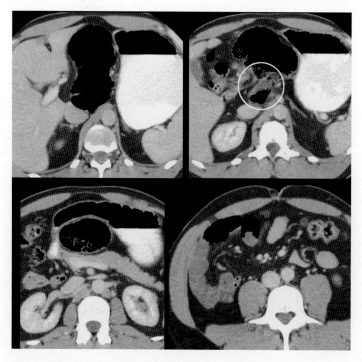

Top left: Colon (*cecum*) in gastrohepatic ligament part of lesser sac. Top right: Colon (*cecum*) and ileum traversing the foramen of Winslow (*circle*) Bottom left: Colon (*cecum*) in lesser sac between stomach and pancreas. Bottom right: There is small bowel but no cecum in the right lower quadrant.

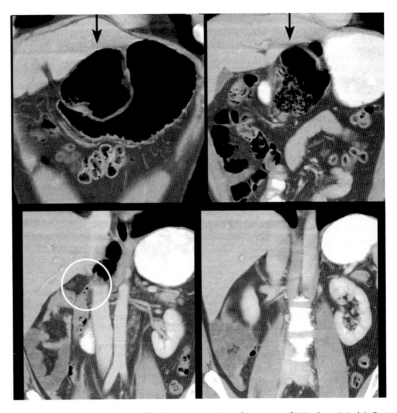

Top left and right: Cecum (*arrows*) in lesser sac. Bottom left: Ileum traversing foramen of Winslow (*circle*). Bottom right: Small bowel in right lower quadrant but no cecum there.

Answers

1. Coupled with a right lower quadrant devoid of cecum, the bowel loop entering the lesser sac via the foramen of Winslow is diagnostic of foramen of Winslow hernia containing cecum.

2. Approximately 2/3 of foramen of Winslow hernias contain small bowel alone. The remainder can additionally or solely contain cecum, ascending colon and/or GB, transverse colon, omentum. The liver cannot herniate into the lesser sac.

3. Predisposing conditions are:
   - Enlarged foramen of Winslow
   - Abnormally long small-bowel mesentery
   - Persistence of the ascending mesocolon allowing marked mobility of bowel
   - Elongated right hepatic lobe (Riedel lobe), which is thought to direct mobile intestinal loops toward the foramen of Winslow

4. Plain film: A circumscribed collection of gas-filled loop(s) in the upper abdomen, medial and posterior to the stomach. When the cecum is herniated a foramen of Winslow hernia can look like a cecal volvulus.

   Barium study: Mass effect with the stomach and the first and second parts of the duodenum shifting anterolaterally.

   CT: Gas-filled loop(s) are located in the lesser sac, posterior to the liver hilum, anterior to the inferior vena cava, and between the stomach and pancreas, with tapering of the herniation through the foramen of Winslow.

5. An encapsulating membrane seen with LPDH not with FofWH. Entry point of LPDH slightly inferior and to the left of the spine, delineated anteriorly by the inferior mesenteric vein and the left colic artery.

   FofWH entry point will be relatively superior and to the right of the spine, delineated by the liver hilum anteriorly.

   Mass effect on the transverse colon and/or prominent, congested blood vessels are more likely with LPDH.

   Small bowel obstruction may be present in either FofWH or LPDH

Pearls

- 2/3 of foramen of Winslow (FofW) hernias contain small bowel alone.
- 1/3 contain cecum, ascending colon and/or GB, transverse colon, omentum.
- Typical patients are middle aged with acute onset of severe, progressive pain, and signs of SBO.
- Plain films: Circumscribed collection of gas-filled loop(s) in the upper abdomen, medial and posterior to the stomach. Small bowel obstruction possible. When the cecum is herniated FofW hernia looks similar to a cecal volvulus.
- Barium studies: Mass effect is likely with the stomach and the first and second parts of the duodenum shifting anterolaterally.
- CT: Gas-filled loop(s) are located in the lesser sac, posterior to the liver, anterior to the inferior vena cava, and between the stomach and pancreas.

Suggested Readings

Azar AR, Abraham C, Coulier B, Broze B. Ileocecal herniation through the foramen of Winslow: MDCT diagnosis. *Abdom Imaging*. October 2010;35(5):574-577.

Izumi J, Hirano H, Kasuya T, et al. Gallbladder hernia into the foramen of Winslow: CT findings. *Abdom Imaging*. November 2009;34(6):734-736.

MacDonald K, Hayward S, Nixon M, Holbrook A. Internal herniation through the foramen of Winslow during pregnancy: MR findings [corrected]. *Abdom Imaging*. June 2011;36(3):318-320.

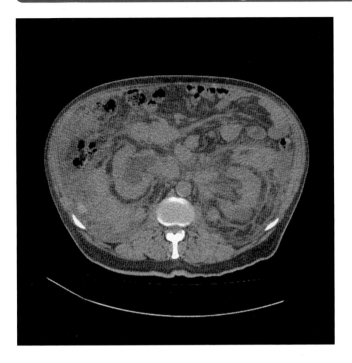 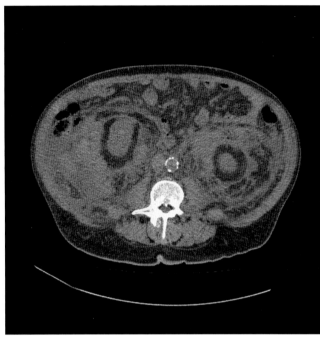

1. What is your differential diagnosis for the abnormalities in the two images above? You may look at the images on the following pages if you want but don't peek at the answer.

2. What is against retroperitoneal fibrosis?

3. What features favor the correct diagnosis of IgG4-related sclerosing disease?

4. What is the treatment of IgG4-related sclerosing disease?

5. What are the imaging manifestations of IgG4-related sclerosing disease?

Case ranking/difficulty:

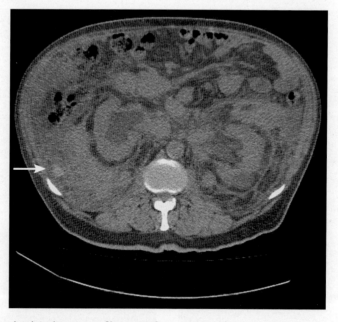

Pararenal masses right >left, bilateral pelvicaliectasis, infiltration of mesentery, pararenal spaces, and paraaortic/paracaval space. Focus of high attenuation (*arrow*) in right pararenal mass.

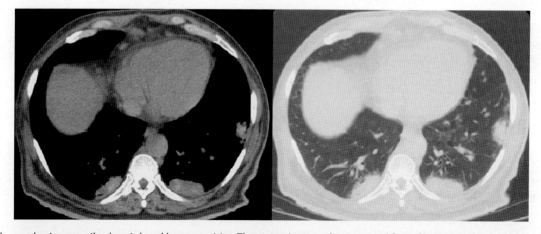

Three slightly poorly circumscribed peripheral lung opacities. The posterior ones have central foci of high attenuation.

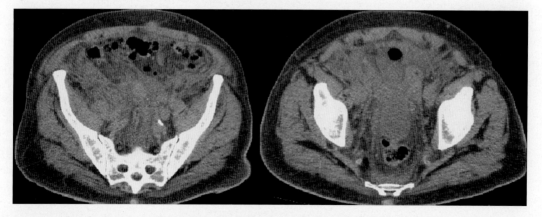

Caudally there is minimal free fluid and extensive infiltration of mesenteric fat and the spaces adjacent to the iliac vessels. There is confluent presacral fat infiltration and mild pararectal fat infiltration.

Answers

1. Lymphoma, carcinomatosis, tuberculosis, retroperitoneal fibrosis, and IgG4-related sclerosing disease comprise a good differential diagnosis.

2. The widespread infiltration of fat in the mesentery and the masses outside the paraaortic/paracaval areas are against retroperitoneal fibrosis.

3. The widespread involvement of both intraperitoneal and retroperitoneal compartments favors IgG4-related sclerosing disease as does the lack of constitutional symptoms such as weight loss and fever. The lung masses would be unusual in lymphoma and tuberculosis and retroperitoneal fibrosis and do not have the typical round and sharply circumscribed appearance of metastases.

4. Corticosteroids are the first-line treatment often producing long-term remission. Relapses can be treated with proteasome inhibitors, immunosuppressive therapy, or anti-CD20 antibodies.

5. Imaging should include whole-body examinations (CT, MRI, PET-CT) to show extent of disease. Anatomic and metabolic imaging are both useful to evaluate response to therapy. In early/active disease marked contrast enhancement and FDG uptake and increased T2 signal are seen. Later fibrosis predominates with little or no enhancement/FDG uptake and decreased T2 signal.

Pearls

- Systemic IgG4-related sclerosing disease is a fibrosclerotic disease with multiorgan involvement difficult to distinguish from other inflammatory diseases and neoplasms.
- Natural history is inflammation morphing into dense fibrosis with deleterious effects on involved sites. Response to steroids in the inflammatory phase is excellent. Risk of eventual malignancy development may be elevated.

- Imaging should include whole-body examinations (CT, MRI, PET-CT) to show extent of disease. Active disease enhances and has high T2 signal and high FDG uptake. Later in the course fibrosis predominates with little or no enhancement/FDG uptake and decreased T2 signal.
- Imaging abnormalities include:
  - Retroperitoneal fibrosis
  - Renal/pararenal nodules and/or infiltration
  - Lymphadenopathy
  - Autoimmune pancreatitis
  - Sclerosing cholangitis
  - Hepatitis
  - Sialadenitis
  - Pulmonary opacities, pleural thickening
  - Paravertebral masses
  - Fibrosing mediastinitis or sclerosing mesenteritis
  - Riedel struma or Hashimoto disease

Suggested Readings

Farsi MM, Sahebari M, Khazaeni K, Rezaieyazdi Z. Immunoglobulin G4-related risease in the head and neck: two case reports and literature review. *Arch Rheumatol.* 2015;30(x):i-v Mar 7, 2015.

Horger M, Lamprecht HG, Bares R, et al. Systemic IgG4-related sclerosing disease: spectrum of imaging findings and differential diagnosis. *AJR Am J Roentgenol.* September 2012;199(3):W276-W282.

Proctor RD, Rofe CJ, Bryant TJ, Hacking CN, Stedman B. Autoimmune pancreatitis: an illustrated guide to diagnosis. *Clin Radiol.* April 2013;68(4):422-432.

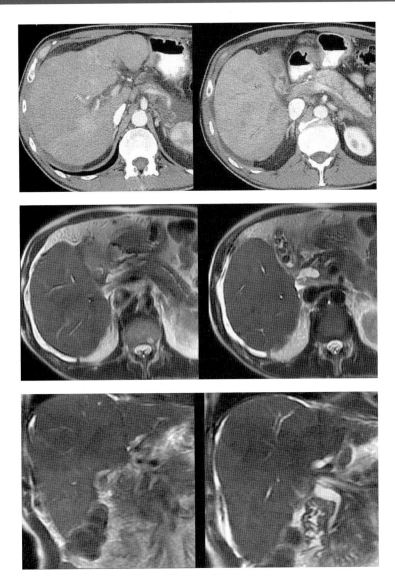

1. Looking at the CT and MRI above, what is in your differential diagnosis?

2. What is the correct diagnosis after the ERCP two pages down?

3. Who was Mirizzi?

4. What comprises Mirizzi syndrome?

5. Why is a correct preoperative diagnosis of Mirizzi syndrome important?

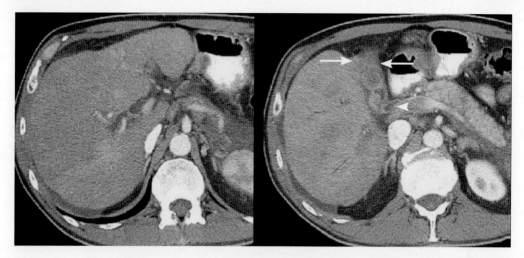

Geographic fatty liver, ascites, chronic hepatocellular disease, pancreatitis, thick-walled gallbladder (*arrows*) with stones and its neck indenting the suprapancreatic duct, ascites, dilated intrahepatic ducts, and dilated common hepatic duct.

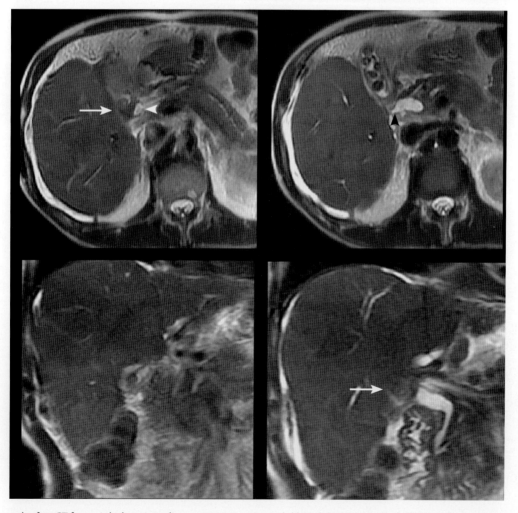

MRCP done 1 month after CT for weight loss, jaundice, nausea, emesis, and dilated ducts (*arrowhead*). Dilated intrahepatic ducts and common hepatic duct. Gallstones with impingement of GB neck on the common hepatic duct (*arrows*).

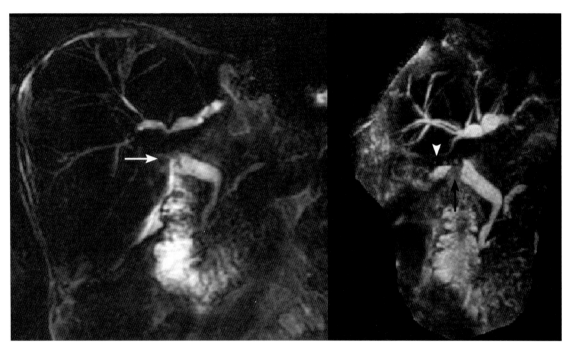

Thick slab (*right*) and 3D MRCP images (*left*) show intrahepatic ductal dilatation and a gap between the porta hepatis and the dilated common duct. There is mass impression on the common duct (*arrows*) and adjacent fluid consistent with bile within an abnormal gallbladder (*arrowhead*) left.

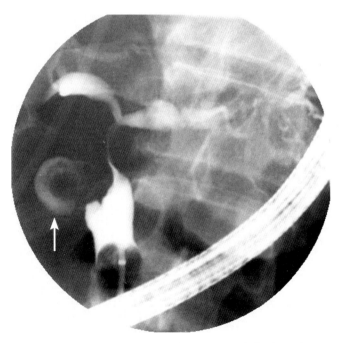

ERCP through a balloon catheter shows a smooth, high-grade stricture of the common hepatic duct extending into the porta hepatis with mass effect on the dilated distal duct (dilated due to prior stone passage?). There is filling of an adjacent abnormal gallbladder (*arrow*) with stones outlined.

Answers

1. Cholangiocarcinoma can produce biliary obstruction and must be considered even without a mass. Gallstones and a thick-walled gallbladder are in the area of the obstruction and Mirizzi syndrome deserves consideration. Periportal metastatic disease is possible. Pancreatic carcinoma is unlikely; the obstruction is remote from the pancreas which is free of apparent mass.

2. The lateral impression on the duct by the gallbladder with stones in its neck and the smooth stricture are consistent with Mirizzi syndrome. It would be very unusual for a gallbladder carcinoma advanced enough to be extending into the porta hepatis not to be associated with a complete cystic duct obstruction.

3. In addition to describing the syndrome named after him, Mirizzi was an Argentine surgeon who developed intraoperative cholangiography in the early 1900s.

4. Mirizzi syndrome is defined as common hepatic duct obstruction caused by a stone impacted in the cystic duct, gallbladder neck, or cystic duct remnant. The obstruction is not merely a result of the mechanical effect of the calculus; the surrounding chronic inflammation is contributory.

5. During retrograde dissection from the fundus to the neck to free the gallbladder, the surgeon usually ligates the first small-caliber, bile-containing duct encountered, which is normally the cystic duct. In Mirizzi syndrome it is the common duct, and ligation of this structure by mistake is a disaster.

An incorrect preoperative diagnosis of carcinoma may be "confirmed" at surgery because the extensive inflammatory adhesions and mass around the gallbladder and hepatoduodenal ligament mimic an unresectable neoplasm. Unidentified fistulas may leak after surgery and an impacted stone may be entirely missed during surgery.

Pearls

- Triad of stone in the gallbladder neck or cystic duct with dilatation of intrahepatic and common hepatic ducts and a normal common bile duct is suggestive of Mirizzi.
- Deviation of the common hepatic duct or tapering at the point of obstruction suggesting an extrinsic impression is supportive of Mirizzi.

- An inflammatory mass can dominate the cross-sectional imaging picture.
- Cholangiography: Smooth, curved segmental stenosis of, or a lateral impression upon, the common hepatic duct in the region of the expected insertion of the cystic duct. Impression upon the medial common duct is less common.
- Offending stone(s) may be outlined at the point of obstruction via either a cholecystobiliary fistula or an incompletely obstructed cystic duct.

Suggested Readings

Menias CO, Surabhi VR, Prasad SR, Wang HL, Narra VR, Chintapalli KN. Mimics of cholangiocarcinoma: spectrum of disease. *Radiographics*. April 2009;28(4):1115-1129.

Turner MA, Fulcher AS. The cystic duct: normal anatomy and disease processes. *Radiographics*. April 2009;21(1): 3-22; questionnaire 288-94.

Yun EJ, Choi CS, Yoon DY, et al. Combination of magnetic resonance cholangiopancreatography and computed tomography for preoperative diagnosis of the Mirizzi syndrome. *J Comput Assist Tomogr*. June 2009;33(4): 636-640.

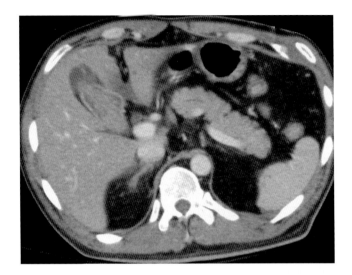
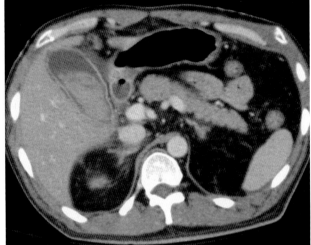
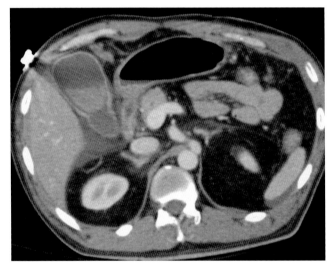

1. Based on the above figures coning in on the gallbladder with no history what is a reasonable differential diagnosis?

2. With the history of trauma and looking at the entire scan what is the best diagnosis?

3. What protects the gallbladder from injury and what predisposes it to injury?

4. What are the sonographic findings of an injured gallbladder?

5. What are the CT findings of an injured gallbladder?

Case ranking/difficulty: 🖤🖤🖤

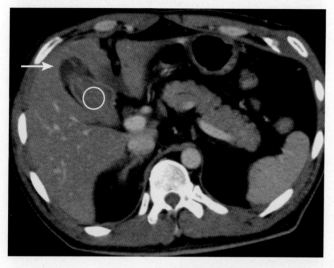

Low-attenuation fluid (*arrow*) displaces the GB away from the liver. High-density material consistent with clot (*circle*) is seen within the GB.

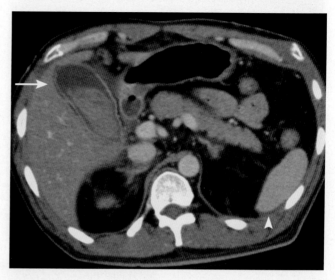

A thin line of fluid (*arrow*) separates the GB from the liver. Medial to the GB is more relatively low attenuating fluid and high-density clot is again depicted in the GB. A small amount of relatively low-density hemoperitoneum (*arrowhead*) is adjacent to the spleen.

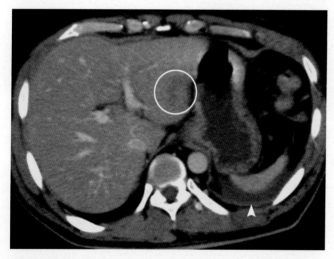

Cephalad to the gallbladder is a low-attenuation left lobe liver contusion (*circle*) and more hemoperitoneum adjacent to the spleen (*arrowhead*).

Answers

1. Looking just at the GB and its immediate surroundings acute cholecystitis, gangrenous cholecystitis, and gallbladder avulsion/injury are a good differential. Carcinoma of the gallbladder is possible but a polypoid carcinoma without wall thickening is unusual. Tumefactive sludge is possible but something else would have to account for the fluid adjacent to the gallbladder.

2. The hemoperitoneum, pericholecystic fluid, liver laceration, and stripping of the gallbladder away from the liver make gallbladder avulsion the best diagnosis.

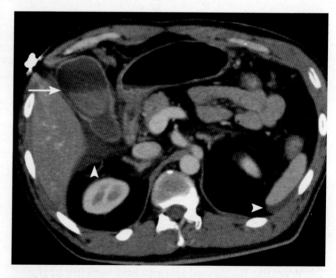

Caudally there is a hematocrit level in the GB (*arrow*) and hemoperitoneum (*arrowheads*) in the hepatorenal space and adjacent to the spleen. There were bilateral small renal lacerations as well (*not shown*).

3. The rib cage and spine shield the GB and the GB is cushioned by the liver and right kidney. Factors that increase the risk of GB injury include a thin-walled normal distended fasting gallbladder, anomalous or abnormal GB position, and alcohol ingestion. The latter elevates biliary pressure and distends the GB by increasing sphincter of Oddi tone.

4. Blood-bile fluid/fluid level in the GB suggests GB injury.

   Focal GB wall thickening, thickening of or fluid in the hepatocholecystic space separating the GB from the liver (pericholecystic fluid), or echogenic nonshadowing clots in the GB suggest GB injury.

   Absence of the GB from the GB fossa without a history of cholecystectomy suggests complete avulsion.

5. Most common but least specific CT finding in GB avulsion is fluid between the GB and the liver.

   More specific CT findings for GB injury include:

   Discontinuous or absent gallbladder wall enhancement (arterial injury)

   Ill-defined contour or focal thickening of the GB wall

   Intraluminal high-attenuation material due to blood

   Active intraluminal arterial extravasation

   Collapse of the gallbladder lumen due to rupture

Pearls

- Types of GB injury are contusion, laceration, avulsion, traumatic cholecystitis, and rupture with bile peritonitis. Avulsion is the second most common type. Ninety percent of GB injuries are associated with other significant injuries such as liver and spleen lacerations.
- US: Blood-bile fluid/fluid level in the GB suggests GB injury. Focal GB wall thickening, thickening of or fluid in the hepatocholecystic space separating the GB from the liver (pericholecystic fluid), or echogenic nonshadowing clots in the GB suggests GB injury. Absence of the GB from the GB fossa without a history of cholecystectomy suggests complete avulsion.

- CT: The most common but least specific finding in gallbladder avulsion is fluid between the gallbladder and the liver. Findings more specific for GB injury include discontinuous or absent gallbladder wall enhancement (arterial injury) ill-defined contour or focal thickening of the GB wall, intraluminal high-attenuation material due to blood, active intraluminal arterial extravasation, and collapse of the gallbladder lumen due to rupture.
- Nuclear medicine: Although rarely used in trauma patients hepatobiliary scintigraphy can show leakage of the agent throughout the peritoneal cavity with or without GB visualization in patients with GB rupture and/or avulsion with tearing of the cystic duct.

Suggested Readings

Chen X, Talner LB, Jurkovich GJ. Gallbladder avulsion due to blunt trauma. *AJR Am J Roentgenol.* October 2001;177(4):822.

Erb RE, Mirvis SE, Shanmuganathan K. Gallbladder injury secondary to blunt trauma: CT findings. *J Comput Assist Tomogr.* October 2001;18(5):778-784.

Gembala RB, Flynn DE, Radecki PD, Friedman AC, Caroline DF. Sonographic diagnosis of traumatic gallbladder avulsion. *J Ultrasound Med.* May 1993;12(5):299-301.

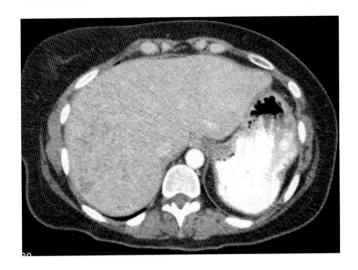 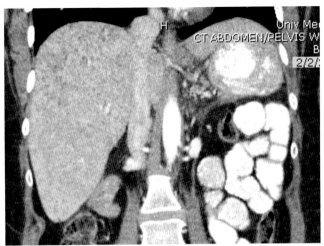

1. Based on the CT scan what would you consider in your differential diagnosis?

2. After examining the sonogram (next page), what is the most likely diagnosis?

3. What does the presence of diffuse multifocal fatty liver after islet cell transplant signify?

4. What is the significance of evolution of diffuse multifocal fatty liver after islet cell transplant into one or two areas of mass-like focal fatty liver?

5. Is diffuse multifocal fatty liver after islet cell transplant normal?

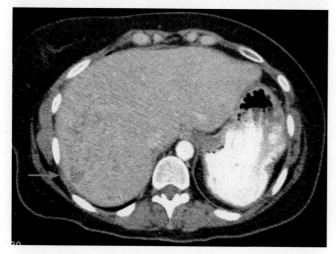

A 51-year-old female 2 months status post islet cell transplant. There are innumerable small patchy hepatic lucencies predominately in the right lobe. The largest lucency (*arrow*) is a known hemangioma. The hemangioma was the only abnormality on preop CT and MR.

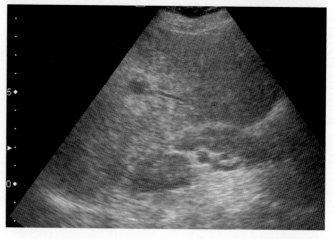

A 51-year-old female 9 months status post islet cell transplant. Ultrasound shows heterogeneous increase echotexture in the upper right lobe.

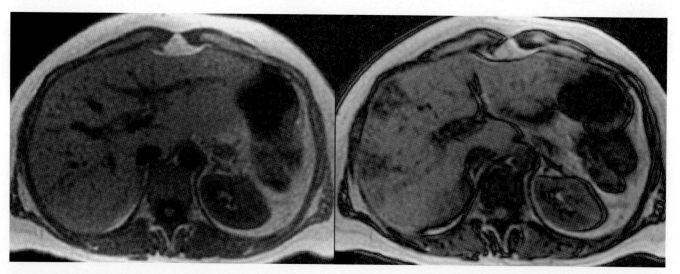

A 51-year-old female 10 months status post islet cell transplant. In (*left*) and out (*right*) of phase gradient echo MR shows two large geographic areas of peripheral right lobe signal drop on out-of-phase image. Development of mass-like focal fatty liver may be a harbinger of graft failure.

Answers

1. The differential diagnosis might include hepatocellular carcinoma (unlikely in the absence of signs of cirrhosis), alveolar echinococcal disease (unlikely absent an exposure history), posttransplant lymphoproliferative disorder (usually larger masses), fungal infection (unlikely without clinical signs of infection), cholangiocarcinoma, diffuse intrahepatic type (unlikely without risk factors), and diffuse multifocal hepatic steatosis following intraportal islet transplantation.

2. Heterogeneous increased echogenicity points toward diffuse multifocal hepatic steatosis following intraportal islet transplantation.

3. Development of diffuse multifocal fatty liver after islet cell transplant requires functioning islet cells.

4. Evolution of the diffuse multifocal pattern toward one or two areas of focal fatty liver on CT, US or MR may be associated with impending graft failure.

5. Although requiring the presence of functioning islet cells diffuse multifocal hepatic steatosis could be an indicator of insulin resistance or graft dysfunction. More studies are needed. It may be a normal finding of a functioning graft.

Pearl

- Imaging:
  - Most common pattern is heterogeneous diffuse increased echogenicity on US and diffuse peripheral predominant multifocal signal drop on GRE T1 out-of-phase images.
  - A fine branching linear, reticular, and beaded pattern of signal loss on opposed-phase imaging has been described.
  - Focal fatty liver on both US and MR may be associated with impending graft failure.
  - Noncontrast CT should show peripheral predominant focal lucencies corresponding to regions of out-of-phase signal drop on MRI. These areas would remain hypodense after contrast.

Suggested Readings

Bhargava R, Senior PA, Ackerman TE, et al. Prevalence of hepatic steatosis after islet transplantation and its relation to graft function. *Diabetes.* 2004;53:1311-1317.

Markman JF, Rosen M, Siegelma ES, et al. Magnetic resonance-defined periportal steatosis following intraportal islet transplantation. A functional footprint of islet graft survival? *Diabetes.* 2003;52:1591-1594.

Venturini M, Angeli E, Maffi P, et al. Liver focal fatty changes at ultrasound after islet transplantation: an early sign of altered graft function? *Diabet Med.* August 2010;27(8):960-964.

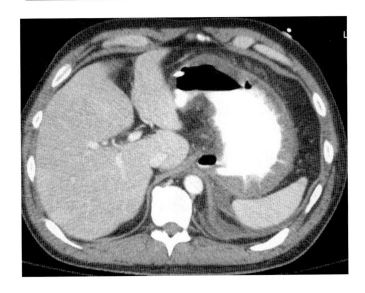 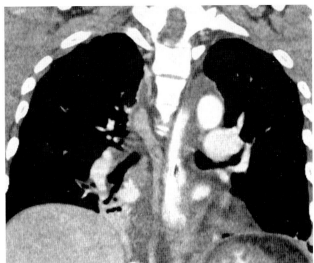

1. What is the most likely diagnosis? You may peek at the images on the next two pages but do not look at the diagnosis.

2. What are the complications of acid caustic ingestion?

3. What is the most common portion of the GI tract injured in acid ingestion and the portion most adversely affected?

4. When does gastric perforation after acid ingestion occur?

5. When does gastric outlet obstruction develop after acid ingestion?

Case ranking/difficulty: **Category:** Stomach

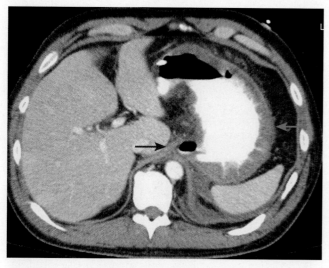

The gastric wall is diffusely thickened (*green arrow*). There is a sealed perforation or ulcer medially near the GE junction (*red arrow*).

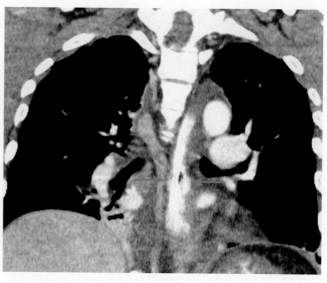

The esophagus (*arrows*) is shaggy.

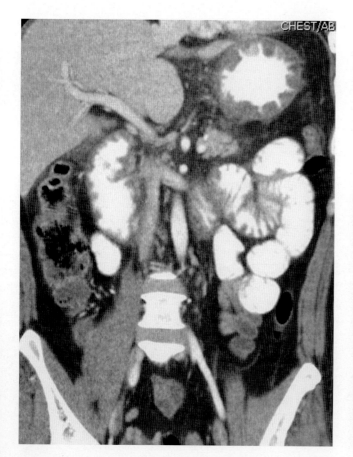

The stomach and descending duodenum are thick walled with thickened folds.

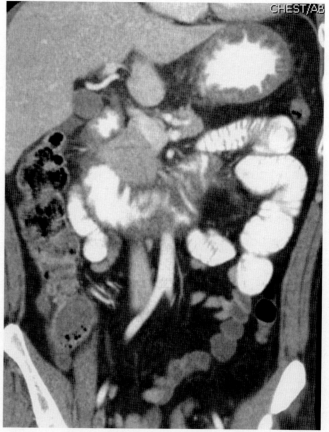

The stomach and duodenum up to the ligament of Treitz are thick walled with thickened folds.

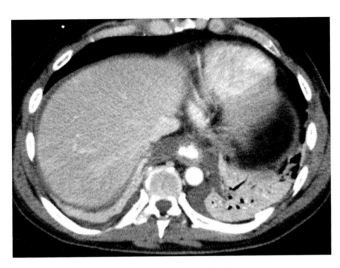

The distal esophagus (*arrows*) is thick walled.

Answers

1. Caustic ingestion is the best diagnosis. It is the best fit for emergent chest and abdominal pain, shaggy esophagus with esophageal, gastric, and duodenal fold and wall thickening and impending gastric perforation (ulcer vs sealed perforation). Upon questioning the ER confessed that there was a history of ingestion of a cocktail of toilet bowl cleaner (contains hydrochloric acid) and Smirnoff vodka.

2. Pancreatitis is not a known complication of acid ingestion. Gastric perforation, intestinal perforation, stricture and gastric obstruction, and UGI hemorrhage are known complications of acid caustic ingestion.

3. The stomach is most commonly and most severely injured in acid ingestion.

4. Acid ingestions cause tissue injury by coagulation necrosis, often resulting in the formation of an eschar. This eschar may protect the underlying tissue from further damage. However, the eschar sloughs in 2 to 4 days and perforation may occur at this time.

5. Gastric outlet obstructions occur 2 to 4 weeks after acid ingestion due to scar tissue contraction. Immediate vomiting may occur after acid ingestion due to pyloric and antral spasm.

Pearl

- Acid ingestions usually have the most adverse effect on the stomach whereas alkalis tend to affect the oropharynx, hypopharynx, and esophagus the most. After acid ingestions, patients are at risk for delayed gastric perforation in about 2 days, which can be fatal. Gastrectomy is sometimes performed to obviate this risk.

Suggested Readings

Doo EY, Shin JH, Kim JH, Song HY. Oesophageal strictures caused by the ingestion of corrosive agents: effectiveness of balloon dilatation in children. *Clin Radiol*. March 2009;64(3):265-271.

Muhletaler CA, Gerlock AJ, de Soto L, Halter SA. Gastroduodenal lesions of ingested acids: radiographic findings. *AJR Am J Roentgenol*. December 1980;135(6):1247-1252.

Nagi B, Kochhar R, Thapa BR, Singh K. Radiological spectrum of late sequelae of corrosive injury to upper gastrointestinal tract. A pictorial review. *Acta Radiol*. February 2004;45(1):7-12.

77-year-old man 2 weeks s/p Dacron grafting and anterior resection of 7 cm aortic aneurysm with heme (+) stool, leukocytosis, and fever

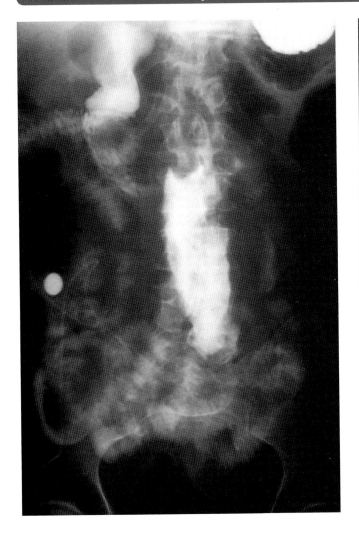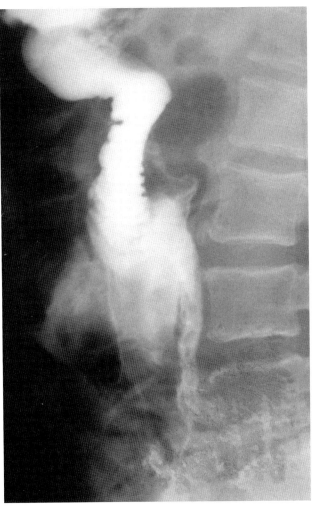

1. What are the findings and what is the best diagnosis?

2. What are the possible signs and symptoms of aortoduodenal fistula?

3. What are the CT findings of aortoduodenal fistula?

4. What are predisposing conditions to primary aortoduodenal fistula?

5. What is the best imaging modality for suspected aortoduodenal fistula?

Case ranking/difficulty:

Category: Duodenum

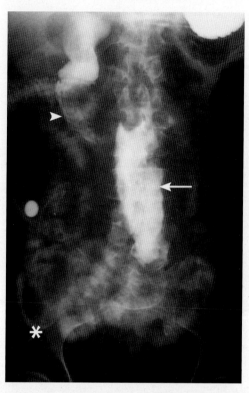

AP (left, A) and lateral (right, B) overheads from water soluble contrast UGI (*arrowhead, arrow* and *asterisk*).

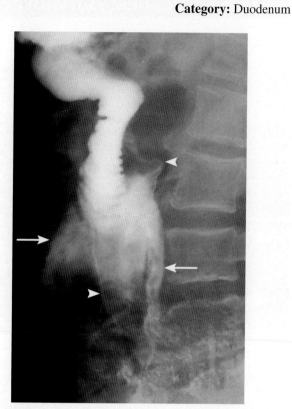

AP (left, A) and lateral (right, B) overheads from water soluble contrast UGI (*arrowheads* and *arrows*).

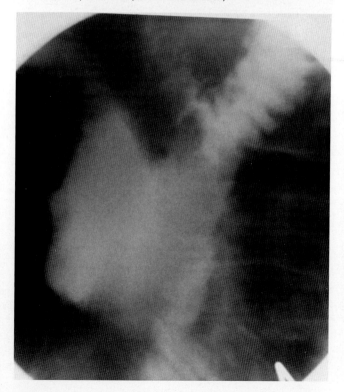

Spot film of duodenum from water soluble contrast UGI showing contrast extravasating out of the third portion of the duodenum.

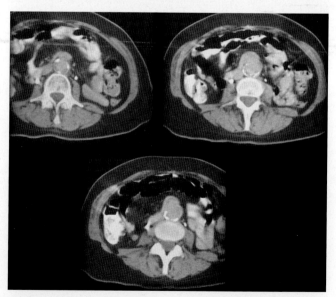

Different case, primary aortoduodenal fistula- elderly man presented with a sentinel bleed. CT shows loss of the fat plane between the transverse duodenum and the aneurysm. Patient exsanguinated five hours later.

Answers

1. The findings are contrast extravasated from the aorta into the paraprosthetic space (large arrows, top left and right) and into the peritoneal cavity outlining the cecum (asterisk top left). The aortic graft is outlines by extravasated contrast (arrowheads, top right). There is mass effect on the duodenum (arrowhead top left). Contrast is shown exiting the duodenum on the spot film (bottom left).

2. The GI bleed is often initially occult, and only later exsanguinating. Weight loss is not a common presenting problem. Unexplained fever, occult GI bleed, abdominal or back pain, and pulsatile abdominal mass may be presenting signs or symptoms.

3. Perigraft soft-tissue edema, fluid, and ectopic gas in a patient postop AAA repair can be normal for 3 to 4 weeks. Extravasation of aortic contrast material into the duodenal lumen; leakage of enteric contrast material into the paraprosthetic space; hematoma after 2 to 3 months postop AAA repair in the retroperitoneum or within the bowel wall or lumen; gas in the native aorta in a patient without surgery or ectopic gas in the graft or paraprosthetic space after 3 to 4 weeks postop AAA repair are all potential CT findings in aortoduodenal fistula.

4. Lymphoma does not predispose patients to aortoduodenal fistula. Atherosclerotic abdominal aortic aneurysm, penetrating ulcer, mycotic aneurysm, and collagen vascular disease do.

5. MRI suffers from long imaging time, poor GI contrast, and insensitivity to gas and calcification. UGI may be normal in patients with aortoduodenal fistula. Sonography is nonspecific. Aortography may fail to show extravasation of contrast.

Pearls

- Patients rarely exsanguinate during first bleeding episode (herald bleed due to focal necrosis and mucosal ulceration not true fistula) with a quiescent periods days to months being common. Classic triad of abdominal pain, pulsatile mass, and GI bleed is infrequent. Presentation with low-grade infection is common.
- CT is the first-line imaging modality for suspected aortoenteric fistula.
- Perigraft soft-tissue edema, fluid, and ectopic gas may be normal CT findings immediately after surgery.
- After 3 to 4 weeks, any ectopic gas is abnormal and should be considered a sign of perigraft infection and possibly fistulization to bowel. Perigraft soft-tissue thickening, fluid, or hematoma should resolve within 2 to 3 months after surgery.
- Hematoma after that in the retroperitoneum or within the bowel wall or lumen is suggestive. Extravasation of aortic contrast material into the enteric lumen or leakage of enteric contrast material into the paraprosthetic space is diagnostic.
- Other CT findings that are suggestive of both perigraft infection and aortoenteric fistula include pseudoaneurysm, loss of the normal fat plane between the aorta and the adjacent bowel, and disruption of the aortic wall.

Suggested Readings

Hughes FM, Kavanagh D, Barry M, Owens A, MacErlaine DP, Malone DE. Aortoenteric fistula: a diagnostic dilemma. *Abdom Imaging*. February 2012;32(3):398-402.

Raman SP, Kamaya A, Federle M, Fishman EK. Aortoenteric fistulas: spectrum of CT findings. *Abdom Imaging*. 2013 Apr;38(2):367-375.

Vu QD, Menias CO, Bhalla S, Peterson C, Wang LL, Balfe DM. Aortoenteric fistulas: CT features and potential mimics. *Radiographics*. February 2012;29(1):197-209.

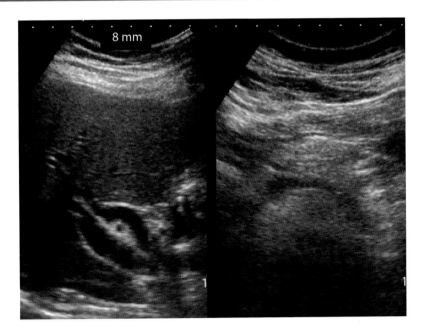

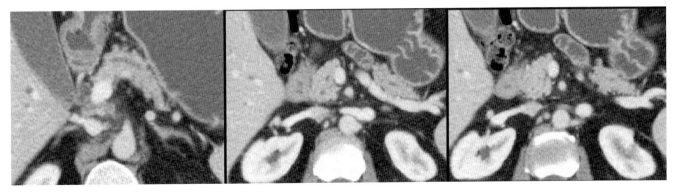

1. Based on the above figures, what is your best diagnosis?

2. What are the signs and symptoms of pancreatic adenocarcinoma?

3. On what imaging modality was the double duct sign originally described?

4. What are the most common causes of the double duct sign?

5. When there is a double duct sign and no demonstrable mass on any modality, what do you suggest as a diagnosis?

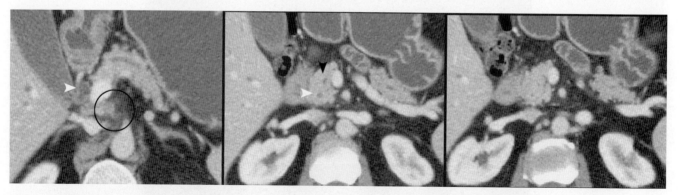

Portal venous phase CT. Left shows mildly dilated pancreatic duct and common bile duct (*arrowhead*). Intrahepatic ducts are mildly dilated. There is subtle infiltration of fat adjacent to the SMA origin (*circle*). Middle image is at the level of caudal ends of the dilated CBD (*white arrowhead*) and dilated pancreatic duct (*black arrowhead*). Right image is next slice down where biductal stenosis is maximum. No mass seen on either. Arterial phase images (*not shown*) were similar.

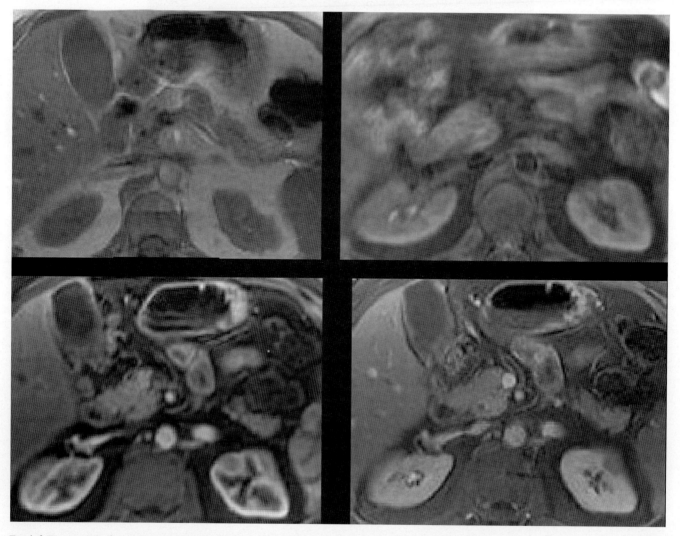

Top left T1, top right fat sat T1, bottom left postgad arterial phase, bottom right postgad delayed all showing no intrapancreatic mass at the level of maximal bile duct stenosis.

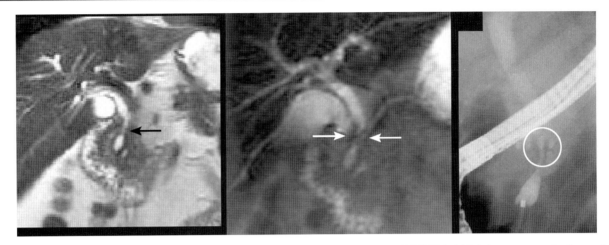

Coronal T2WI left shows a common bile duct stenosis (*arrow*) but no pancreatic mass. MIP MRCP (*middle*) shows anatomically contiguous bile and pancreatic ducts stenoses (*arrows*). Significance of double duct sign not appreciated and erroneous diagnosis of benign bile duct stricture due to stone passage made. Six weeks later after the patient had gotten worse the diagnosis of adenocarcinoma of the pancreas was established by EUS and biopsy. Retrograde cholangiogram at that time on right redemonstrates short segment intrapancreatic bile duct stenosis (*circle*). Pancreatic duct could not be cannulated.

Answers

1. Despite the absence of a demonstrable pancreatic mass, adenocarcinoma of the pancreas is the best diagnosis to explain the double duct sign, especially in view of the infiltration of perivascular fat. Cholangiocarcinoma of the distal CBD is possible but unlikely to cause pancreatic ductal obstruction.

2. Pancreatic cancer symptoms/signs commonly include jaundice, pain (upper or middle abdomen or back), and unexplained weight loss. Other signs/symptoms are anorexia, fatigue, light-colored stools, and dark urine.

3. Originally described on ERCP the double duct sign can also be seen on MRCP, CT, and ultrasonography.

4. The most common causes of the double duct sign are carcinoma of the head of the pancreas and carcinoma of the ampulla of Vater.

   Less common causes: cholangiocarcinoma of the distal CBD, pancreatic lymphoma, metastasis(es) to the pancreas, pancreatitis, and ampullary stenosis.

5. Depending on the site of the double duct sign, ampullary carcinoma and carcinoma of the head of the pancreas are the two best diagnoses. Cholangiocarcinoma and IPMN (biliary obstruction due to mucin coming from pancreatic duct) are possible but less likely.

Pearls

- Double duct sign: Simultaneous dilatation (caused by stenosis/encasement/obstruction) of the common bile and pancreatic ducts.
- Originally described on ERCP now also seen on MRCP, CT, and ultrasonography.
- Most common causes: Carcinoma of the head of the pancreas and carcinoma of the ampulla of Vater.
- When the stenosis/encasement/obstruction of each duct is anatomically contiguous, and each stenosis morphologically consistent with malignancy, the cause is virtually always one of the above two.
- When there is a double duct sign carcinoma of the pancreas (or ampulla) is likely even if no mass lesion can be imaged. If you suspect pancreatic carcinoma and different imaging examinations draw different conclusions, the correct diagnosis is likely to be carcinoma of the pancreas.

Suggested Readings

Ahualli J. The double duct sign. *Radiology*. July 2007;244(1): 314-315.

Kalman RS, Bresnick MA, Huang CS. Now you see it, now you don't: an unusual cause of the "double duct sign." *Gastroenterology*. February 2014;146(2):348-592.

Krishna N, Tummala P, Reddy AV, Mehra M, Agarwal B. Dilation of both pancreatic duct and the common bile duct on computed tomography and magnetic resonance imaging scans in patients with or without obstructive jaundice. *Pancreas*. July 2012;41(5):767-772.

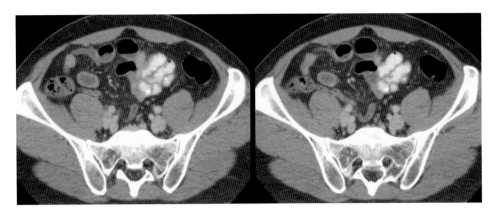

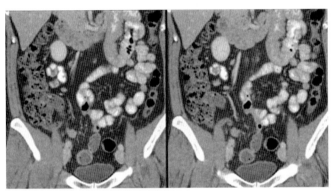 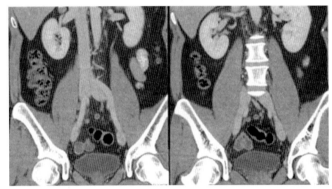

1. What is the most likely diagnosis based on the above figures?

2. What are the CT signs of appendicitis?

3. What do you do when CT for suspected appendicitis does not show a normal appendix, but there are no signs of appendicitis either?

4. What are the potential complications of delayed treatment of appendicitis?

5. When is MRI indicated for suspected appendicitis?

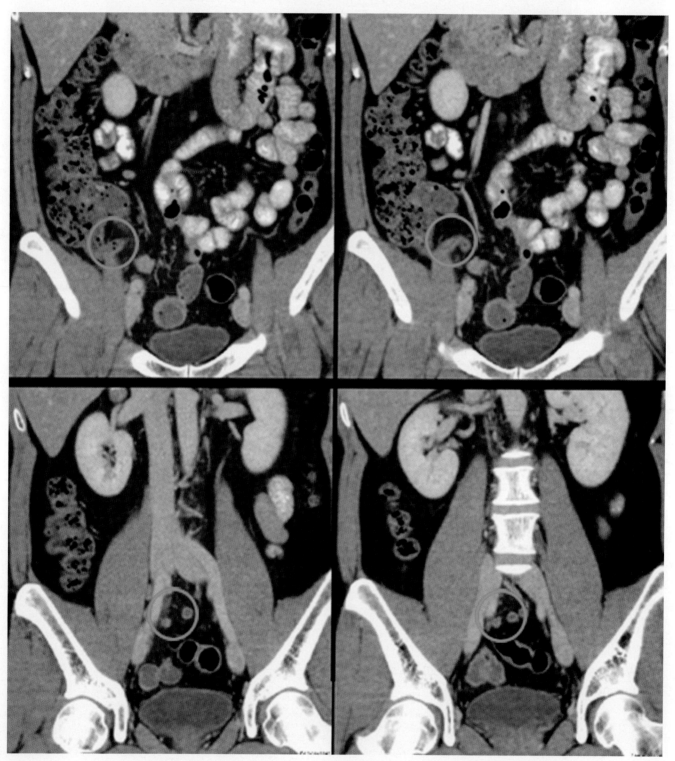

Coronal images show a long appendix (*circles*) with intraluminal fluid, mild enhancement, and mild dilatation distally.

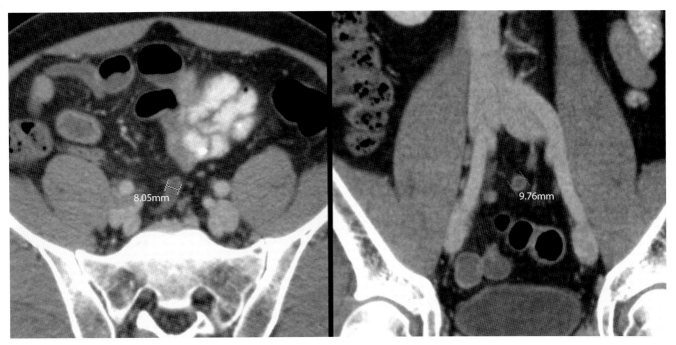

Axial (*left*) and coronal (*right*) images show measurements (8.1 cm axial and 9.8 cm coronal).

Answers

1. Mild enlargement of the fluid-filled distal appendix with mild wall enhancement is consistent with tip appendicitis. Unfortunately the diagnosis was not made and the patient went on to perforate.

2. CT signs of appendicitis are enlargement, increased wall contrast enhancement, and periappendiceal fat stranding. Small amounts of free intraperitoneal fluid may be present. Focal cecal thickening centered on the appendiceal orifice may cause the contrast material in the cecal lumen to assume an arrowhead configuration pointing at the appendix (arrowhead sign). Thickening of the wall of the adjacent terminal ileum may be seen.

3. In CT patients in whom the appendix is not visualized, this finding, in the absence of right lower quadrant inflammation, carries a high negative predictive value for appendicitis. No further imaging is done.

4. The most common complication of acute appendicitis is rupture. Signs of rupture include periappendiceal abscess, extraluminal gas (usually localized), free peritoneal fluid, and focally poor enhancement of the appendiceal wall. Less common complications are diffuse peritonitis (free air is unusual) superior mesenteric and/or portal vein thrombosis, and liver abscess.

5. When pregnant women present with acute abdominal pain, a sonogram is usually done first to exclude ectopic pregnancy and ovarian torsion. In pregnancy the appendix is displaced from its usual RLQ location and is very difficult to visualize on ultrasound. MRI is often then employed.

Pearls

- Optimal CT for appendicitis requires oral and intravenous contrast; coronal reconstructions often are superior to transverse images.
- CT reliably depicts a normal appendix and is better than US for delineating periappendiceal inflammatory changes, abscesses, and other acute diagnoses in the abdomen.
- CT criteria for appendicitis include enlargement, increased contrast enhancement of its wall, and periappendiceal fat stranding. Small amounts of free intraperitoneal fluid may be present. Focal cecal thickening centered on the appendiceal orifice may cause the contrast material in the cecal lumen to assume an arrowhead configuration pointing at the appendix (arrowhead sign). Thickening of the wall of the adjacent terminal ileum may be seen.
- Filling of the appendix by orally or rectally introduced positive contrast material is useful in excluding acute appendicitis. But since isolated involvement of the distal segment of the appendix (tip appendicitis) may occur, the entire appendix must be identified and filled to be called normal by virtue of contrast filling.

Suggested Readings

Kim MS, Park HW, Park JY, et al. Differentiation of early perforated from nonperforated appendicitis: MDCT findings, MDCT diagnostic performance, and clinical outcome. *Abdom Imaging*. June 2014;39(3):459-466.

Orth RC, Guillerman RP, Zhang W, Masand P, Bisset GS 3rd. Prospective comparison of MR imaging and US for the diagnosis of pediatric appendicitis. *Radiology*. July 2014 Mar;272(1):233-240.

Trout AT, Towbin AJ, Zhang B. Journal club: the pediatric appendix: defining normal. *AJR Am J Roentgenol*. May 2014;202(5):936-945.

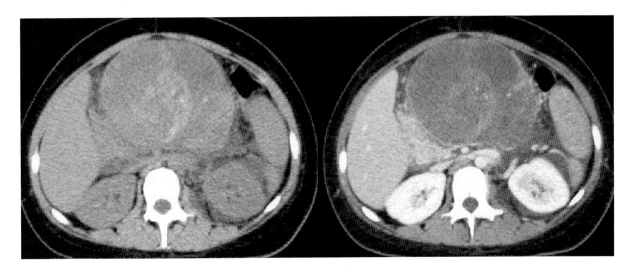

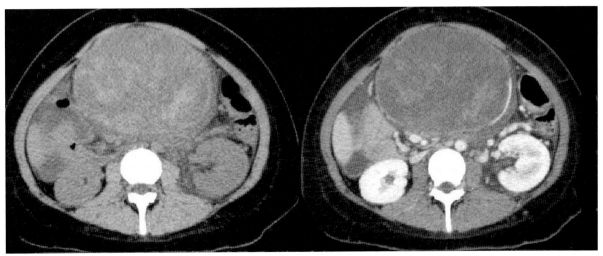

1. What is the most likely diagnosis with this history and CT scan?

2. What are the clinical and demographic features of solid pseudopapillary tumor (SPT) of the pancreas?

3. What are the clinical presenting features?

4. What are the gross pathologic features of SPT?

5. What are the common imaging features of SPT?

Solid pseudopapillary tumor (neoplasm) of pancreas   Case 150 (496)

                              Category: Pancreas

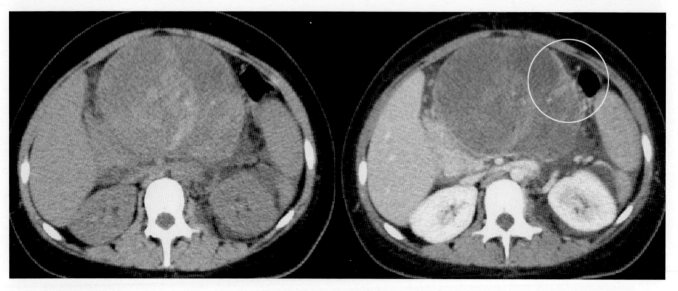

Noncontrast CT (*left*) and enhanced CT (*right*) at the same level shows a large mass in the region of the pancreas with ascites and perirenal edema. There is central punctate calcification. Most of the mass is somewhat less than soft tissue density with no enhancement. There is a central high-density component consistent with blood that does not enhance. There is thin peripheral enhancement and a small wedge-shaped enhancing component at 2:00 (*circle*).

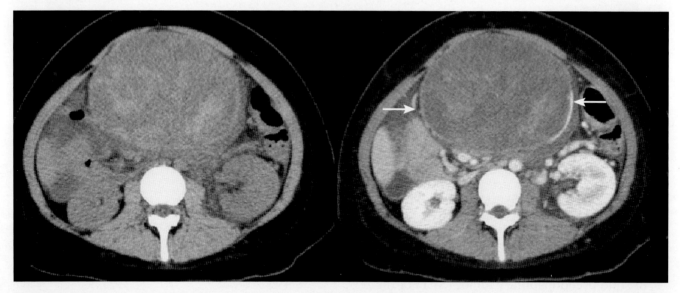

Noncontrast CT (*left*) and enhanced CT (*right*) at the same level shows a large mass in the region of the pancreas with ascites (*arrows*). There are unenhancing somewhat less than soft tissue components and several unenhancing high-density components. The latter are consistent with blood.

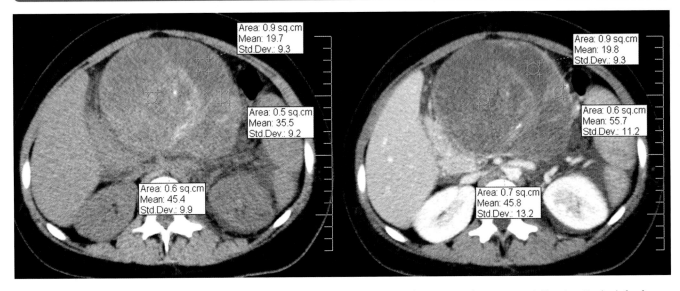

Noncontrast CT (*left*) and enhanced CT (*right*) at almost the same level as Image 1 shows central punctate calcification. To the left of midline is a high-density area (45HU) precontrast that does not enhance, consistent with blood. To the right of midline there is a less than soft tissue component (20HU) precontrast that does not enhance. At 2:00 is a small wedge-shaped area (36HU) precontrast that enhances to 56HU postcontrast consistent with a solid component. In total, the mass is consistent with old and new hematoma with small residual solid tissue.

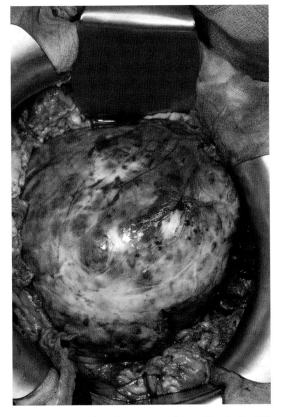

Intraoperative photo of the large mass that at first looked like a huge hematoma to the surgeons.

Answers

1. In an 18-year-old female with a 3-day history of abdominal mass and pain, a large mass with imaging characteristics consistent with central hemorrhagic necrosis is most likely a solid pseudopapillary tumor. Adenocarcinoma does not get this big and rarely calcifies and the patient is too young. Hematoma is unlikely absent coagulopathy or trauma. Nonfunctioning islet cell carcinoma and osteoclast-type giant cell carcinoma are unlikely in an 18-year-old.

2. Mean age of patients is 24, (range 10-50 years), 1/3 are adolescents, F/M = 9.5/1, and patients are usually Asian or African-American. SPT is a low-grade malignancy almost always curable by complete resection (clear margins important), but liver metastases may be present. Lymph node metastasis, peritoneal spread, and multiplicity rare.

3. Patients with SPT are often asymptomatic with the diagnosis made at abdominal examination, US, CT, or MRI performed for other reasons, that is, trauma.

   Patients may present with a gradually enlarging nontender abdominal mass or vague abdominal discomfort. Obstructive symptoms may occur if the mass is large enough to compress adjacent viscera.

   Usually serum amylase levels and cancer markers are normal. Occasional polyarthralgia and/or eosinophilia are present due to intravascular release of lipase.

4. SPTs range from 1.5 to 30 cm, average 10.5 cm. They occur anywhere in the pancreas most frequently in the tail or the head. SPTs are usually well demarcated and externally smooth. Larger SPTs usually have large confluent or geographic areas of hemorrhage, necrosis, cystic degeneration. They may have preserved peripheral solid areas or may look entirely cystic with only a few septa and little peripheral solid neoplasm. Occasionally large SPTs are predominately solid.

5. US: Round well-defined encapsulated tumors, either mixed cystic-solid or solid masses. Occasionally almost completely cystic.

CT: Large, well-encapsulated mass, varying solid and cystic components due to hemorrhagic degeneration. Calcifications and enhancing components seen at the periphery. Central calcification unusual.

MR: Well-defined mass, mix of high and low SI on T1 and T2WI. Blood products often seen: high T1, low T2 SI. Low SI fibrous capsule common on T2WI.

Enhancement pattern (enhanced US, CT or MR): Peripheral rim shows isoenhancement during the early arterial phase, and the interior shows heterogeneous enhancement consisting of regions of isoenhancement, hypoenhancement, and nonenhancement. Progressive washout of the contrast agent during venous phase results in hypoenhancement compared with normal adjacent parenchyma.

- MR: Well-defined mass, mix of high and low SI on T1 and T2WI. Blood products often seen: high T1, low T2 SI. Low SI fibrous capsule common on T2WI.
- Enhancement pattern (enhanced US, CT, or MR): Peripheral rim shows isoenhancement during the early arterial phase, and the interior shows heterogeneous enhancement consisting of regions of isoenhancement, hypoenhancement, and nonenhancement. Progressive washout of the contrast agent during venous phase results in hypoenhancement compared with normal adjacent parenchyma.
- Small SPTs are in middle-aged women and usually (90%) have neither a capsule or intratumoral hemorrhage. They usually exhibit a completely well-defined margin and pure solid consistency. They have low SI on unenhanced T1WI and very high SI on T2WI.
- Early heterogeneous and slowly progressive enhancement has been reported in small SPT's and may turn out to be a characteristic MRI qualitative feature of SPT significantly different from islet cell tumors or adenocarcinoma.

Pearls

- SPT should be primarily considered in a young African-American or Asian female presenting with a large, well-defined partially cystic mass in the pancreas. Complete resection has an excellent prognosis.
- US: Round well-defined encapsulated tumors, either mixed cystic-solid or solid masses. Calcification is sometimes seen, usually peripheral. Occasionally nearly completely cystic. Areas of increased blood flow can be seen in solid areas on color or power Doppler imaging.
- CT: Large, well-encapsulated mass, varying solid and cystic components due to hemorrhagic degeneration. Calcifications and enhancing components seen at the periphery. Central calcification unusual.

Suggested Readings

Choi JY, Kim MJ, Kim JH, et al. Solid pseudopapillary tumor of the pancreas: typical and atypical manifestations. *AJR Am J Roentgenol*. August 2006;187(2):W178-W186.

Cooper JA. Solid pseudopapillary tumor of the pancreas. *Radiographics*. August 2006;26(4):1210.

Yu MH, Lee JY, Kim MA, et al. MR imaging features of small solid pseudopapillary tumors: retrospective differentiation from other small solid pancreatic tumors. *AJR Am J Roentgenol*. December 2010;195(6):1324-1332.

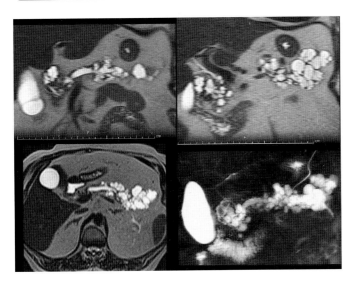

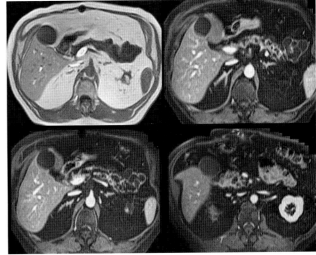

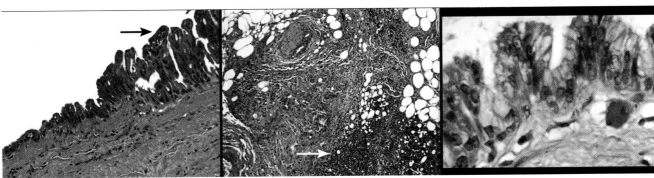

1. What is the diagnosis in this case?

2. What is the distribution predilection of IPMN in the pancreas?

3. What are the pathologic grades of IPMN (benign vs malignant)?

4. What are some of the clinical features of IPMN?

5. What is the key imaging feature differentiating branch duct IPMN from other pancreatic cysts?

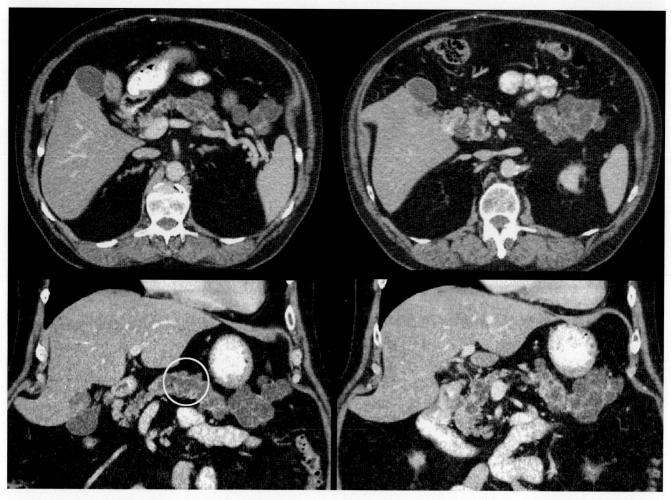

Axial (*top*) and coronal (*bottom*) CECT of the same patient shows innumerable unenhancing low-density small pancreatic masses and a dilated main pancreatic duct (*best seen bottom left, circle*)

Answers

1. On the previous page on the left coronal (top 2) and axial (bottom left) T2WI and MRCP (bottom right) show innumerable small pancreatic cystic masses and a dilated main pancreatic duct. On the previous page on the right axial T1WI without contrast (top left) and post gadolinium T1W1 (top right and bottom 2) show low intensity pancreatic cysts and a dilated low signal main pancreatic duct (seen best bottom left).

2. Originally called ductectatic carcinoma in the radiology literature IPMNs were thought to arise specifically in the uncinate process and were considered unusual. IPMN is now common and diagnosed in all parts of the pancreas. There is a mild preference for branch duct IPMN for the uncinate process.

3. IPMNs are variably aggressive ranging from slow-growing foci to invasive and metastatic neoplasms as are their histologic cousins, mucinous cystic neoplasms. They can be characterized as IPMN adenoma, IPMN borderline lesion (with dysplasia), and intraductal papillary mucinous carcinoma (carcinoma in situ and/or invasive carcinoma). On the previous page histology of IPMN: Left and middle are same patient. Transtition from normal epithelium to IPMN (black arrow, left) with papillary formation. In an adjacent field there is invasive adenocarcinoma (white arrow, middle) infiltrating the pancreas. On right is microscopic field from another patient- papillary formation, atypical nuclei with migration away from the basement membrane. Pathologists could not agree on

moderate dysplasia (borderline) vs. high grade dysplasia (carcinoma in-situ).

4. Branch duct IPMNs are most often incidental findings. IPMNs can present with pain, nausea, diarrhea, steatorrhea, new onset diabetes, jaundice, or pancreatitis. Since patients with IPMN are at risk for both pancreatic and extrapancreatic malignancies, early recognition, treatment, and systemic surveillance are important.

5. Branch duct IPMNs dilate the affected side branch with mucin, resulting in a cystic mass in the pancreas that communicates with the main pancreatic duct. Other neoplastic cystic masses (mucinous cystic neoplasm, serous cystadenoma, and solid pseudopapillary tumor) generally do not communicate with the duct.

Pearls

- Branch duct IPMN—round or oval small lobulated cystic mass(es) on cross-sectional studies often uncinate process but can be anywhere in pancreas. Macrocystic pattern—uni- or multilocular with or without filling defects due to mucin or tumor nodules. Microcystic pattern—multiple thin septa separating small cystic spaces (cluster of grapes). Communication between the cystic mass and the main pancreatic duct sometimes demonstrated by MRI, MRCP, or CT. ERCP may be the only method for showing communication, but sometimes mucin obstructs the flow of contrast. Filling defects on ERCP or MRCP due to tumor nodules (adherent to wall) or mucin.
- Main duct IPMN—segmental (sometimes cystic) or diffuse main pancreatic duct dilatation. Clues versus pancreatitis—smooth dilatation, mural nodules or mucin globs, papilla dilatation with bulging into the duodenum, solid component due to malignancy. Mucin protruding through a bulging, patulous papilla on ERCP is diagnostic. Benign versus malignant: main duct IPMNs with >1 cm diameter are likely malignant, side branch IPMNs <3 cm are likely benign. Mural nodules/thick septa increase likelihood of malignancy. Frankly invasive cancers look like other pancreatic adenocarcinomas and IPMN remnants may coexist.

Suggested Readings

Kang KM, Lee JM, Shin CI, et al. Added value of diffusion-weighted imaging to MR cholangiopancreatography with unenhanced MR imaging for predicting malignancy or invasiveness of intraductal papillary mucinous neoplasm of the pancreas. *J Magn Reson Imaging.* September 2013;38(3):555-563.

Kim JH, Eun HW, Kim KW, et al. Intraductal papillary mucinous neoplasms with associated invasive carcinoma of the pancreas: imaging findings and diagnostic performance of MDCT for prediction of prognostic factors. *AJR Am J Roentgenol.* September 2013;201(3):565-572.

Raman SP, Kawamoto S, Blackford A, et al. Histopathologic findings of multifocal pancreatic intraductal papillary mucinous neoplasms on CT. *AJR Am J Roentgenol.* March 2013;200(3):563-569.

Pancreatic tail mass discovered on ER stone CT for left flank pain in a 47-year-old male. He underwent follow-up CT and MRI

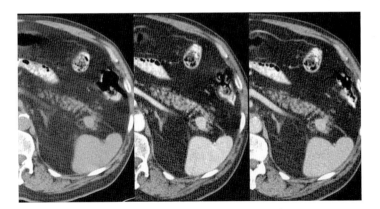

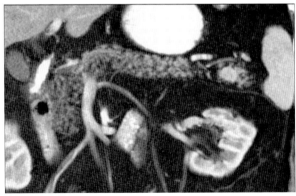

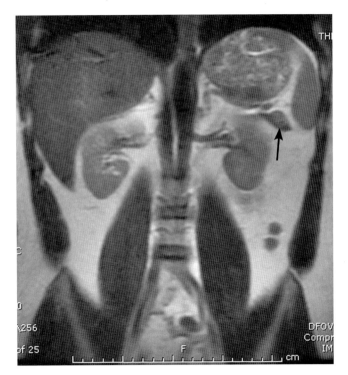

1. What is a reasonable differential diagnosis for this pancreatic tail mass?

2. Which is the best diagnosis?

3. What additional imaging could prove the diagnosis?

4. What is the best modality for proving the diagnosis?

5. What are the clinical characteristics of accessory spleens (AS)?

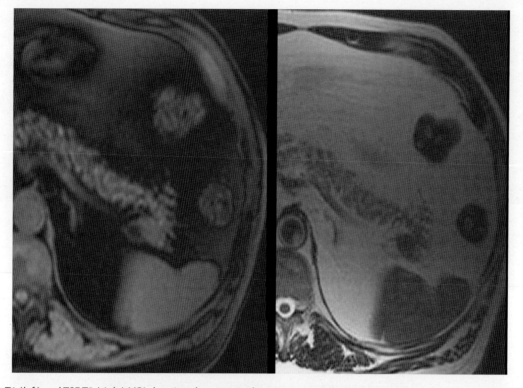

Fat sat T1 (*left*) and TSE T2 (*right*) MRI showing the mass in the pancreatic tail with identical signal intensity to the spleen.

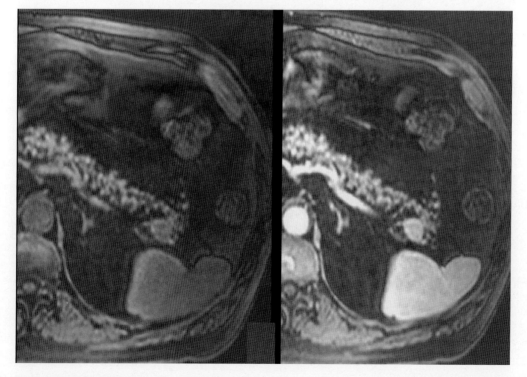

Pre- and postcontrast (*arterial*) T1 VIBE images show that the mass has identical signal intensity to the spleen both before and after contrast. It enhances more than the pancreas.

Answers

1. Garden variety duct cell adenocarcinoma of the pancreas does not enhance with intravenous contrast on arterial phase images and is not a concern in this case. Variant adenocarcinomas of the pancreas can enhance in the arterial phase but are large masses with central necrosis.

2. Nonfunctioning islet cell tumors are usually large and malignant but could be small. They are unlikely to always be identical to normal spleen on multiple modalities/phases. Adenocarcinoma is unlikely see answer 1 above. Absent a known renal cell carcinoma, melanoma, or HCC hypervascular metastasis to the pancreas is unlikely. SPT is usually large with considerable hemorrhagic necrosis and usually seen in teenagers or young adults. A rare variant seen in middle-aged women is small and would be a consideration but the patient is male. Given identical imaging characteristics to normal spleen, the most likely diagnosis is intrapancreatic accessory spleen.

3. Heat damaged red cell scintigraphy, sulfur colloid scintigraphy, superparamagnetic iron oxide MR, contrast-enhanced sonography and image-guided biopsy could all potentially prove the diagnosis.

4. Heat damaged red cell scintigraphy is widely available and has a better target to background ratio and a better spleen to liver ratio than sulfur colloid scintigraphy and is the best choice. Reticuloendothelial (RES) cells show contrast uptake and lower SI in IPAS as well as in normal spleen on T2- or T2*-weighted MR images after SPIO but this agent is no longer widely available. Persistent enhancement for as long as 3 to 5 minutes, due to entrapment of Levovist by RES cells, is a specific finding on contrast-enhanced sonography but this modality is not widely available. Image-guided biopsy will be diagnostic by showing normal spleen but is technically challenging in a small mass, is invasive, and might cause pancreatitis.

5. AS is usually an asymptomatic incidental finding; they are rarely symptomatic because of torsion, spontaneous rupture, or hemorrhage. Masses, most commonly epidermoid cysts, may be seen within accessory spleens. Failure to remove accessory spleens may result in recurrent hematologic disease postsplenectomy. An undamaged accessory spleen may take over splenic function after splenectomy. Accessory spleens are commonly located near the splenic hilum, near the spleen, or adjacent to the pancreatic tail. An accessory spleen may be located along the splenic vessels, in the gastrosplenic or splenorenal ligament, within the pancreatic tail, in the gastric wall, in the greater omentum or the mesentery, or even in the pelvis or scrotum.

Pearls

- Gray-scale US: IPAS oval mass isoechoic to spleen, hypoechoic to pancreas. Color or power Doppler US: Vascular hilum.
- CT: Attenuation of IPAS on all phases is usually the same as that of the spleen. IPAS, if large enough, will demonstrate diagnostic zebra heterogeneous enhancement on early arterial phase CT. IPAS usually brighter than the pancreas on all three dynamic CT phases.
- MRI: SI of IPAS is darker than that of pancreas on T1WI and brighter on T2WI (unhelpful for DDx). SI of IPAS usually identical to that of the spleen on multiple MR pulse sequences. Enhancement of IPAS on MRI is similar to that of the adjacent normal spleen; characteristic zebra enhancement of IPAS may be seen on arterial phase.
- Nuclear medicine: Technetium-99m heat-damaged RBC scintigraphy diagnostic criterion used to detect accessory spleen, including IPAS, is a marked increase in uptake that exceeds that of the cardiac blood pool and the major vessels at the site of suspected accessory spleen.

Suggested Readings

Hu S, Zhu L, Song Q, Chen K. Epidermoid cyst in intrapancreatic accessory spleen: computed tomography findings and clinical manifestation. *Abdom Imaging*. October 2012;37(5):828-833.

Ittrich H, Klutmann S, Adam G. Intrapancreatic accessory spleen—an important differential diagnosis of primary pancreatic tail neoplasia]. *Rofo*. March 2013;185(3):269-272.

Jang KM, Kim SH, Lee SJ, Park MJ, Lee MH, Choi D. Differentiation of an intrapancreatic accessory spleen from a small (<3-cm) solid pancreatic tumor: value of diffusion-weighted MR imaging. *Radiology*. January 2013;266(1):159-167.

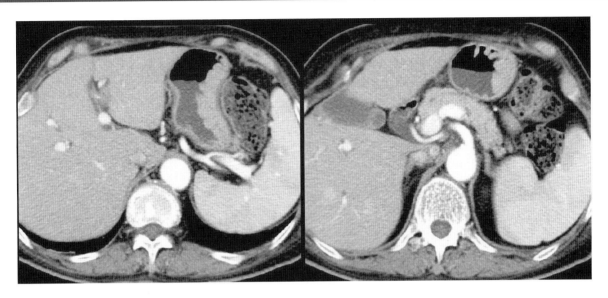

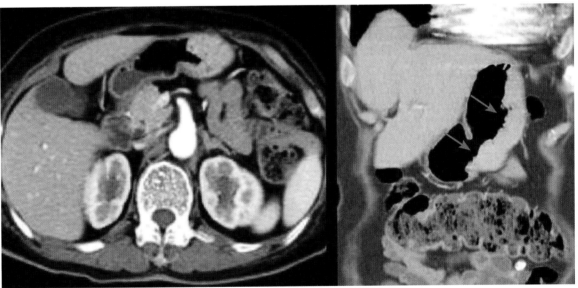

1. What is the best diagnosis?

2. What is the treatment for pediatric Menetrier disease?

3. What is the treatment for adult Menetrier disease?

4. What are the clinical features of Menetrier disease?

5. What are the pathologic features of Menetrier disease?

Case ranking/difficulty:

Category: Stomach

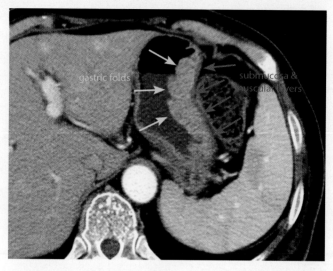

Markedly thickened gastric folds (*green arrows*) and normal thickness of the other layers (*red arrows*).

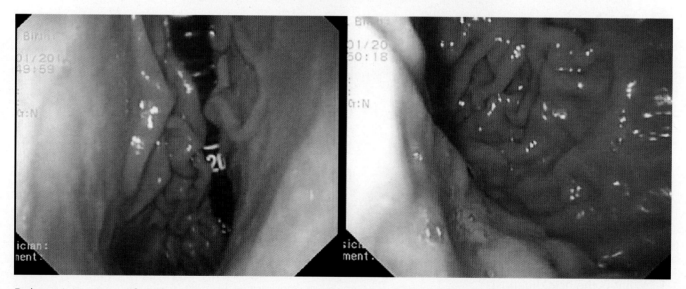

Endoscopic imaging confirmed presence of thickened gastric body folds (*left*). The folds do not compress with additional air insufflation.

Answers

1. Menetrier disease is characterized by massively enlarged, lobulated, irregular rugal folds in the gastric fundus and body with sparing of the antrum, preserved wall stratification, and good contrast enhancement on arterial phase images as seen in this case.

Scirrhous carcinomas have homogeneously enhanced segments with wall thickening and perigastric fat plane infiltration and/or perigastric adenopathy, lack of wall stratification, and gradual transmural enhancement from the arterial phase to the delayed phase.

Because it spreads submucosally, gastric lymphoma lacks wall stratification and causes focal or diffuse gastric fold enlargement. The mucosal layer has normal thin enhancement with a bulky moderately enhancing tumor mass.

Acute gastric mucosal lesions have regular thickening of the gastric folds with preserved stratification.

The thickened folds in pancreatitis are posterior predominant if inflammatory and fundal predominant if due to splenic vein occlusion and varices.

2. Pediatric Menetrier disease cases are usually self-limited and are treated symptomatically for weeks to months.

3. Anticholinergic agents, high protein diet, prostaglandins, proton pump inhibitors, prednisone, and H_2 receptor antagonists are variably effective. Blockers of epidermal growth factor receptors (EGFR) have shown promise. Unresponsive severe disease requires total gastrectomy.

4. Clinical presentation is epigastric pain with variable symptoms of anorexia, vomiting, melena, and hypoproteinemia. Children may present with ascites and edema.

5. The pathologic features of Menetrier disease are:

   • Hyperplasia of surface and glandular mucous cells.

   • Hypoplasia of parietal and chief cells.

   • Inflammation is usually not marked.

   • Menetrier disease is a hypertrophic gastropathy not a gastritis.

Pearls

• UGI: Enlarged and convoluted but pliable rugal folds with intervening linear strands of contrast, which represent contrast material trapped between the enlarged foldings.
• CT: Massive thickening of the gastric folds with masslike protrusions into the lumen. The submucosal layer and serosa are intact.
• Both CT and UGI: There is usually antral sparing.
• When Menetrier disease is suspected on barium studies or CT, full-thickness endoscopic biopsy specimens should be obtained for definitive diagnosis.

Suggested Readings

Chen CY, Jaw TS, Wu DC, et al. MDCT of giant gastric folds: differential diagnosis. *AJR Am J Roentgenol.* November 2010;195(5):1124-1130.

Friedman J, Platnick J, Farruggia S, Khilko N, Mody K, Tyshkov M. Ménétrier disease. *Radiographics.* November 2010;29(1):297-301.

Trout AT, Dillman JR, Neef HC, Rabah R, Gadepalli S, Geiger JD. Case 189: pediatric Ménétrier disease. *Radiology.* January 2013;266(1):357-361.

Chapter Index

Note: Numbers in parentheses refer to Case IDs.

Spleen

Stomach

Subchapter Index

Note: Numbers in parentheses refer to Case IDs.

Alphabetical Subject Index

Note: Numbers in parentheses refer to Case IDs.

Difficulty Level Index

Note: Numbers in parentheses refer to Case IDs.

Author Index

Acknowledgment Index

Note: Numbers in parentheses refer to Case IDs.